The
Human Brain
and
Spinal Cord

The
Human Brain
and
Spinal Cord

*Functional Neuroanatomy
and Dissection Guide*

Lennart Heimer, M.D.

Department of Neurology
University of Virginia

With 213 Illustrations Mostly in Color

Springer-Verlag
New York Berlin Heidelberg Tokyo

Lennart Heimer, M.D.
Professor
Departments of Otolaryngology and Neurosurgery
University of Virginia Medical Center
Charlottesville, Virginia 22908, USA

The figure on the front cover is Fig. 25.
The venous sinuses and the veins of the head, (p. 40).

Library of Congress Cataloging in Publication Data
Heimer, Lennart.
  The human brain and spinal cord.

  Includes index.
  1. Brain—Anatomy. 2. Spinal cord—Anatomy.
3. Human dissection. I. Title. [DNLM: 1. Dissection.
2. Central nervous system. WL 101 H467m]
QM455.H4 1983   611′.8   82–19665
ISBN 0–387–90741–6
ISBN 0–387–90740–8 (pbk.)

Typeset by Kingsport Press, Kingsport, Tennessee
Printed and bound by Kingsport Press, Kingsport, Tennessee
Printed in the United States of America

(Fourth printing, 1988)

ISBN 0–387–90741–6 Springer-Verlag New York Berlin Heidelberg Tokyo (cloth)
ISBN 3–540–90741–6 Springer-Verlag Berlin Heidelberg New York Tokyo (cloth)
ISBN 0–387–90740–8 Springer-Verlag New York Berlin Heidelberg Tokyo (paper)
ISBN 3–540–90740–8 Springer-Verlag Berlin Heidelberg New York Tokyo (paper)

To Hanne-Björg, Hakon, Mikael, Gösta, and Knut

Contents

Preface   ix

Acknowledgments   xi

I. Introduction

1. Basic Design and Terminology   *3*
2. Development of the Nervous System   *9*
3. Meninges and Cerebrospinal Fluid   *37*

II. Dissection of the Brain

Introduction   *51*
First Dissection   *53*
  Meninges and Subarachnoid Cisterns; Superficial Arteries; Vertebral–
  Basilar System; Internal Carotid System; Basal Surface, and Cranial
  Nerves
Second Dissection   *65*
  Midsagittal Section; Lobes, Sulci, and Gyri
Third Dissection   *75*
  White Matter; Blunt Dissection of Major Fiber Systems
Fourth Dissection   *85*
  Ventricular System, Fornix, and Basal Ganglia
Fifth Dissection   *97*
  Fourth Ventricle; Cerebellum; Brain Stem
Sixth Dissection   *111*
  Atlas of the Brain: Frontal, Sagittal, and Horizontal Brain Sections;
  Anatomical Correlation of Computerized Brain Tomography

III. Functional Neuroanatomy

4. Neurohistology and Neuroanatomic Techniques   *127*
5. The Spinal Cord   *151*
6. Ascending Sensory Pathways   *165*
7. The Lower Motor Neuron and the Descending Supraspinal
   Pathways   *183*
8. Basal Ganglia   *199*
9. Cerebellum   *211*
10. Brain Stem, Reticular Formation, and Monoaminergic Pathways   *225*
11. Cranial Nerves   *237*

12. Auditory System *261*
13. Visual System *271*
14. Olfactory System *287*
15. Hypothalamus and the Hypothalamohypophysial System *295*
16. The Autonomic Nervous System *309*
17. Amygdaloid Body, Hippocampal Formation, and "Limbic System" *321*
18. Thalamus *331*
19. Cerebral Cortex *337*
20. Neuronal Transmitters and Modulators *353*
21. Cerebrovascular System *357*

Epilogue *375*

Appendix *377*

Index *391*

Preface

This book was written to serve both as a guide for the dissection of the human brain and as an illustrated compendium of the functional anatomy of the brain and spinal cord. In this sense, the book represents an updated and expanded version of the book *The Human Brain and Spinal Cord* written by the author and published in Swedish by Scandinavian University Books in 1961.

The complicated anatomy of the brain can often be more easily appreciated and understood in relation to its development. Some insight about the coverings of the brain will also make the brain dissections more meaningful. Introductory chapters on these subjects constitute *Part I* of the book.

Part 2 is composed of the dissection guide, in which text and illustrations are juxtaposed as much as possible in order to facilitate the use of the book in the dissection room. The method of dissection is similar to dissection procedures used in many medical schools throughout the world, and variations of the technique have been published by several authors including Ivar Broman in the "Människohjärnan" (The Human Brain) published by Gleerups Förlag, Lund, 1926, and László Komáromy in "Dissection of the Brain," published by Akadémiai Kiadó, Budapest, 1947. The great popularity of the CT scanner justifies an extra laboratory session for the comparison of nearly horizontal brain sections with matching CT scans.

Since there is a tendency to rely heavily on expensive audiovisual aids in medical education, it seems especially important to promote the dissection of the human brain. No brain model or TV movie can match the efficiency of brain dissections in teaching the gross anatomy of the brain, and it is usually possible to secure a certain number of human brains at most medical schools. It seems important to emphasize, however, that a systematic description of the topographic anatomy of the brain is all the more important if brains cannot be obtained for dissection. With this in mind, the dissection guide has been richly illustrated and can be used as an introductory gross anatomy text without dissecting the brain.

Part 3 constitutes an illustrated account of the functional anatomy of the major parts and systems of the brain and spinal cord. Many of the schematic illustrations in part 3 have been modeled after the more elaborate drawings in Part 2, and they can be best appreciated on the basis of a reasonable understanding of the gross anatomy of the brain as outlined in the dissection guide. Considering the clinical importance of cerebrovascular diseases, the blood supply of the brain is discussed separately in the last chapter.

Physiologic, chemical and pharmacologic aspects have been briefly discussed whenever appropriate, but no effort has been made to introduce the basics of these subjects. The clinical relevance of neuroanatomy has been emphasized by including "Clinical Notes" at the end of each chapter, and some commonly seen disorders of the nervous system have been presented in the form of "Clinical Examples" in order to prepare the medical student for the practice of medicine. Many of the "Clinical Examples" have been illustrated with appropriate CT scans or angiograms. The reading lists at the end of the chapters do not pretend to be complete; they are presented as an encouragement for further studies, and they include some of the larger medical school texts, in which the various subjects are more fully discussed. Figures of the distribution of the peripheral nerves, finally, have been included in an appendix.

It is my hope that the book will serve a useful purpose in almost any type of neuroscience education. It should fortify and complement related studies in basic and clinical neuroscience.

Lennart Heimer

Acknowledgements

Many of my friends and colleagues have been kind enough to read one or several of the chapters, and it is with a great deal of gratitude that I acknowledge the help of Drs. Shirley Bayer, Theodore Blackstad, Anders Björklund, Irving Diamond, Björn Folkow, Ann Graybiel, Gunnar Grant, Gary Van Hoesen, Leonard Jarrard, Anders Lundberg, Eugene Millhouse, Enrico Mugnaini, Ulf Norsell, Alan Peters, Jim Petras, Gordon Shepherd, Jan Voogd, and Torsten Wiesel.

Colleagues at the University of Virginia, including Drs. George Alheid, Robert Cantrell, Fritz Dreifuss, John Jane, Ivan Login, Leon Morris, Edwin Rubel, and Richard Winn, have also been very helpful, and I would like to acknowledge specifically Dr. James Bennett, who was kind enough to prepare the "Clinical Examples" and Dr. James Q. Miller, who revised the "Clinical Notes."

The carbon dustings in the dissection guide were prepared by Mrs. Florence Kabir, who spared herself no effort in preparing for the final artwork. Some of the other drawings were prepared by Mrs. Jane Gordon and Mr. János Kálmánfi.

The photographs from various planes of myelin stained sections of the human brain, which appear in the dissection guide, were taken by Mr. Paul Reimann and Dr. Gary Van Hoesen from material in the Yakovlev Collection at the Armed Forces Institute of Pathology in Washington. I would like to thank Dr. Paul Yakovlev for collecting this magnificent material and Mr. Mohamad Haleem for making it easily accessible.

Drs. Victor Haughton and Michael Wolff of the Radiology Department of the Medical College of Wisconsin supplied most of the CT scans, whereas Dr. Leon Morris of the Radiology Department of the University of Virginia furnished the angiograms.

It has been a great pleasure to collaborate with the competent staff of Springer Verlag in New York.

PART 1
Introduction

1
Basic Design and Terminology

THE CENTRAL AND PERIPHERAL NERVOUS SYSTEM

THE NEURON

GRAY AND WHITE MATTER
  Collections of Nerve Cell Bodies
  Collections of Nerve Fibers
  Nervous Pathways

MAJOR SUBDIVISIONS OF THE BRAIN
  Telencephalon
  Diencephalon
  Mesencephalon
  Metencephalon
  Myelencephalon

In freshly cut sections of the brain and spinal cord some regions display a white glistening color, others a grayish color. The white matter represents collections of bundles containing long nerve fibers, which are surrounded by white glistening myelin sheaths. Nerve cell bodies, on the other hand, tend to aggregate in a superficial cortical sheath or in subcortical nuclei, referred to as gray matter.

If the differentiation between gray and white matter is accentuated by appropriate staining methods, it is easily appreciated that the central nervous system is composed of a large number of more or less distinct regions. Although it is important to have an understanding of these various subdivisions and their topography, such knowledge is not very useful by itself. A more meaningful picture will emerge from the knowledge of how the various subdivisions relate to each other and how the individual neurons are interconnected.

THE CENTRAL AND PERIPHERAL NERVOUS SYSTEMS

On the basis of gross anatomic features, the nervous system can be divided into two parts: the *central nervous system* (CNS), which consists of the brain and spinal cord (Fig. 1A), and the *peripheral nervous system* (PNS), which consists of the cranial and spinal nerves and their ganglia. The peripheral nerves connect the CNS with the sense organs and the effector organs (muscles and glands). Although it is useful to subdivide the nervous system in this manner, one should remember that functional–anatomic circuits and systems pay little attention to the boundaries between the central and peripheral nervous systems. For instance, the cranial and spinal nerves are described as part of the PNS, but their cells of origin (motor neurons) or their terminal branches (sensory neurons) are situated within the CNS.

The function of the *autonomic nervous system* is innervation of the internal organs. Although this system was originally conceived of as a peripheral system containing numerous autonomic ganglia and nerve plexuses related to the internal organs, the CNS is intimately involved in the neural control of the visceral organs. The autonomic nervous system, therefore, is composed of both peripheral and central parts. Whereas the peripheral part of the autonomic nervous system can be delineated anatomically from the rest of the PNS, the central components cannot be easily separated from the rest of the CNS.

THE NEURON

The nervous system contains more than 50 billion nerve cells or neurons, and, in addition, an even larger number of neuroglial cells that subserve various supportive, metabolic, and phagocytic functions.

The neurons are specialized to receive, conduct, and transmit nervous impulses, and they have certain characteristics in common, even though they vary widely in shape and size. Two types of processes extend from the cell body (Fig. 2). The receiving processes, the *dendrites,* have a broad base and taper away from the cell body; they branch in the immediate neighborhood of the cell body. There usually are many dendrites per neuron. The *axon,* of which there is only one per cell, conducts

the impulses away from the cell body. Axons vary greatly in length and diameter. The thicker axons, which conduct impulses more rapidly than the thinner ones, are insulated from the environment by a lipoprotein sheath, the *myelin sheath.* Thin axons are either unmyelinated or thinly myelinated. The axon loses its myelin sheath at its destination, and divides into several small branches, which typically end as swellings referred to as *axon terminals* or *boutons.* The boutons establish contacts with other neurons or with an effector organ. The site of interneuronal contact, i.e., where the impulses are transmitted from one cell to another, is called a *synapse* or *synaptic junction.* The neuron and its processes are discussed in more detail in Chapter 4.

GRAY AND WHITE MATTER

The distribution of gray and white matter can be easily appreciated in macroscopic sections through the brain and spinal cord (Figs. 1B and C). The basis for this distinction relates to the structure of the nerve cell. As already indicated, many axons are surrounded by a myelin sheath, which has a white glistening color; consequently, those parts that contain mainly bundles of myelinated axons are white, i.e., *white matter.* The parts that contain aggregations of nerve cell bodies embedded in a network of delicate nerve processes have a gray color, hence the term *gray matter.* There are two major territories of gray substance in the brain, the cerebral cortex on the surface and large subcortical nuclei, e.g., caudate nucleus, thalamus, and lentiform nucleus, in the interior. The gray substance in the spinal cord is located in the center and has a typical H-shaped appearance in transverse sections. It is surrounded by white matter, which contains long ascending and descending pathways.

Collections of Nerve Cell Bodies

Cortex is the superficial coat of gray matter in the cerebral hemispheres and in cerebellum. The nerve cell bodies in the cortex are arranged in more or less well-defined laminae or layers. Groups of nerve cell bodies in other parts of the brain and spinal cord are referred to as *nuclei,* or *columns* if they occur in long rows as they often

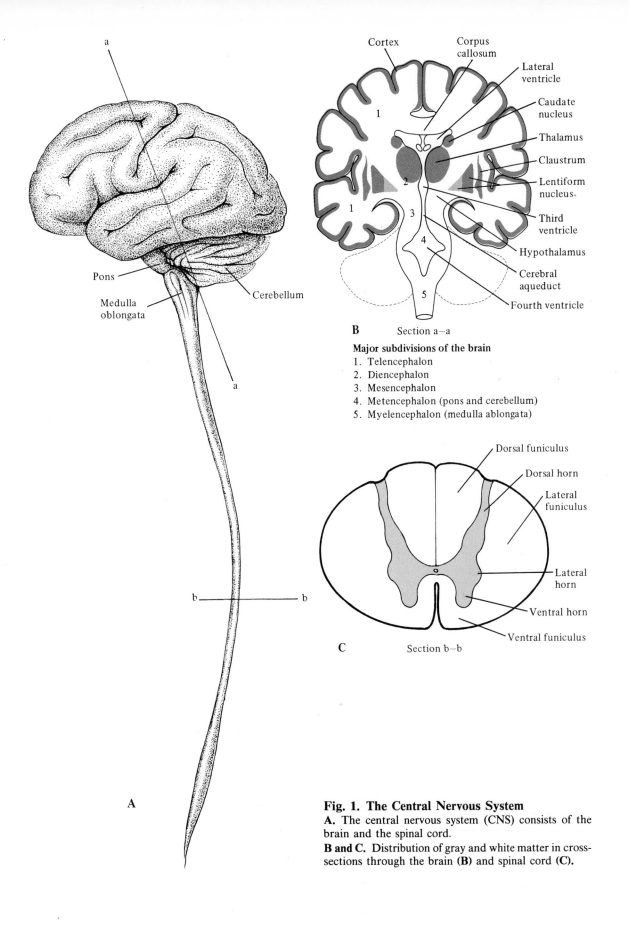

B   Section a–a

Major subdivisions of the brain
1. Telencephalon
2. Diencephalon
3. Mesencephalon
4. Metencephalon (pons and cerebellum)
5. Myelencephalon (medulla ablongata)

C   Section b–b

Fig. 1. The Central Nervous System
A. The central nervous system (CNS) consists of the brain and the spinal cord.
B and C. Distribution of gray and white matter in cross-sections through the brain **(B)** and spinal cord **(C).**

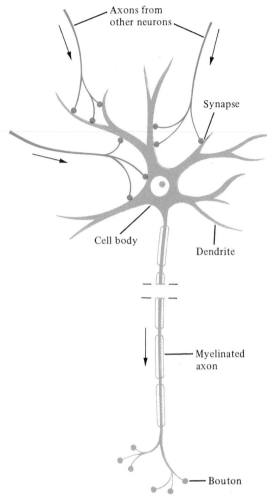

Axons from
other neurons

Synapse

Cell body

Dendrite

Myelinated
axon

Bouton

Fig. 2. The Neuron

Although neurons vary widely in size and shape, they have certain features in common. Most neurons are multipolar, i.e., they have several processes. The dendrites receive impulses from other neurons whereas the axon, of which there is only one to each cell, conducts the impulses away from the cell body.

do in the spinal cord. Note that the term column is also used for the white matter in the dorsal part of the spinal cord (*see below*). Accumulations of nerve cell bodies outside CNS are called *ganglia.*

Collections of Nerve Fibers

A collection of nerve fibers with a common origin and destination constitutes a *tract,* e.g., the corticospinal (or pyramidal) tract. A tract does not necessarily form a well-defined bundle, since the fibers of a tract often intermingle with fibers of neighboring pathways.

A distinct collection of nerve fibers is referred to as a *fasciculus, peduncle,* or *brachium.* Such collections of fibers often contain more than one tract. The term *lemniscus* is specifically used for ascending sensory fiber bundles in the brain stem. The white matter of the spinal cord, which contains the long ascending and descending tracts, is subdivided into *ventral (anterior), lateral,* and *dorsal (posterior) funiculus* (Fig. 1C). The dorsal funiculus, however, is often referred to as the dorsal column, especially in the physiologic literature.

Fibers connecting similar areas on the two sides of the brain form well-defined bundles known as *commissures.* Many fiber bundles cross the midline in their course from one level of the nervous system to another. Such crossing fibers form a *decussation.*

Nerves, *nerve roots, nerve trunks,* and *rami* are examples of bundles of nerve fibers in the PNS.

Nervous Pathways

Efferent pathways project away from the region under consideration. *Afferent pathways* project to the region under consideration. *Extrinsic pathways* project into or out of the region under consideration. *Intrinsic pathways* are confined to the region under consideration.

MAJOR SUBDIVISIONS OF THE BRAIN

The brain is subdivided into five major divisions: telencephalon, diencephalon, mesencephalon, metencephalon, and myelencephalon (Fig. 1B).

Telencephalon

The telencephalon (endbrain) consists of the two *cerebral hemispheres,* which form the largest part of the human brain. The hemispheres are connected by a massive bundle of commissural fibers, the *corpus callosum.* Each hemisphere is covered by a thin layer of gray substance, the *cerebral cortex,* which is heavily folded. The folds are called convolutions, or *gyri,* and the grooves are referred to as *sulci,* or *fissures,* if they are very deep. In the interior of each hemisphere is a centrally placed cavity, the *lateral ventricle,* and a large mass of white substance as well as several large nuclei referred to as the *basal ganglia.* Although

basal ganglia: caudate + lentiform
+(claustrum, thalamus)

thalamus in diencephalon (*see below*) is sometimes included in the basal ganglia, the term is most commonly used for the two telencephalic nuclei, the *caudate* and the *lentiform nuclei,* and some closely related brain stem nuclei, known to be of special importance for control of movements. *Claustrum,* whose functions are unknown, is sometimes included in the term basal ganglia.

Diencephalon

The diencephalon is divided into two halves by a slit-formed median cavity, the *third ventricle,* which is continuous via the small *interventricular foramen* (*of Monro*) with the lateral ventricle in each hemisphere. The *thalamus* and *hypothalamus* are the two major divisions of the diencephalon. Thalamus is a collection of several nuclei with various functions and anatomic relations. Hypothalamus, likewise, contains a variety of different cell groups and pathways. It is well known for its regulation of autonomic and endocrine functions.

Mesencephalon

The mesencephalon (midbrain) is a short segment of the brain between the diencephalon and the metencephalon. Its internal structure is complicated, but its gross anatomic features are simple. It is traversed by a narrow canal, the *cerebral aqueduct,* which connects the third ventricle in the diencephalon with the fourth ventricle in the metencephalon.

Metencephalon

The metencephalon consists of *cerebellum* and *pons* (bridge). Cerebellum, which is concerned with coordination of movements, is located underneath the tentorium cerebelli in the posterior cranial fossa. It consists of the two *cerebellar hemispheres* joined in the midline by a narrow wormlike portion, the *vermis.* Like the cerebral hemispheres, the cerebellum is covered by a layer of gray substance, the *cerebellar cortex,* which is characterized by a large number of parallel folds, *folia,* separated by deep *fissures.*

Although the *pons* is usually said to be located ventral to the cerebellum, it is actually situated in front of cerebellum when the head is in the normal upright position. When viewed from its ventral side, the pons appears as a bridge over a canal (the brain stem).

Myelencephalon

The myelencephalon, or *medulla oblongata,* is continuous with the spinal cord at the level of the foramen magnum. The cavity that is located between cerebellum on one hand and pons and medulla oblongata on the other is referred to as the *fourth ventricle.*

Medulla oblongata, pons, and mesencephalon, which together form the *brain stem,* contain many important nuclear groups including the cranial nerve nuclei. They also contain important pathways connecting the spinal cord and cerebellum with the diencephalon and the telencephalon.

2
Development of the Nervous System

EARLY DEVELOPMENT OF THE CENTRAL
NERVOUS SYSTEM
  Neural Tube
  Neural Crest

SPINAL CORD
  Neuroepithelial, Mantle, and Marginal Layers
  Basal and Alar Plates
  Dorsal Root Ganglia and Spinal Nerves
  Cauda Equina

EARLY DEVELOPMENT OF THE BRAIN
  Primary and Secondary Brain Vesicles
  The Flexures
  Migration and Aggregation of Cells

MAJOR SUBDIVISIONS OF THE BRAIN
  Myelencephalon
  Metencephalon
  Mesencephalon
  Diencephalon
  Telencephalon

CLINICAL NOTES
  Chromosomal Abnormalities and
    Environmental Factors and Their Effect on
    the Brain
  Rachischisis and Spina Bifida
  The Eye
  Craniopharyngioma
  Hydrocephalus

SUGGESTED READING

Knowledge of the important developmental events will facilitate the understanding of the anatomy of the CNS. It will also make it easier to understand malformations of the nervous system that are met in clinical practice.

Although the external shapes of the brain and spinal cord are well developed at birth, the size of the CNS increases dramatically in the neonatal period and during infancy. In addition, pathways mature and neuronal processes develop their complicated branching pattern and synaptic connections both in the pre- and postnatal periods. The factors that influence these various developmental mechanisms are being studied intensively by developmental neurobiologists. In all probability, such knowledge will greatly enhance our efforts to prevent many debilitating nervous system disorders, including malformations, mental retardation, and degenerative diseases.

EARLY DEVELOPMENT OF THE CENTRAL NERVOUS SYSTEM

Neural Tube

The first sign of a nervous system appears in the 3rd week, when the ectoderm on the dorsal side of the embryo thickens to form the *neural plate* (Fig. 3A). The mechanism whereby some of the ectodermal cells are transformed into specialized nervous tissue cells, a process known as induction, is still a puzzling problem. The neural plate soon starts to fold and a groove is formed, which is the *neural groove* (Fig. 3B). The two side walls, the *neural folds,* approach each other in the midline (Fig. 3C) and the groove is gradually transformed into the *neural tube,* which surrounds a fluid-filled central cavity. This tube, in turn, becomes separated from the rest of the ectoderm (Fig. 3D).

The closure of the neural groove begins at the level of C4 and proceeds in both cranial and caudal directions. The last portions of the neural tube to close, located rostrally and caudally, are called the *anterior* and *posterior neuropores.* They are normally closed by the end of the 4th embryonic week.

A defective closure of the neural tube is a common cause of neurologic malformations (see Rachischisis in Clinical Notes). The neuroepithelial cells that form the walls of the neural tube rapidly multiply and eventually give rise to all the neurons and macroglia cells, i.e., astrocytes, oligodendrocytes, and ependymal cells of the brain and the spinal cord. Microglia are believed to be of mesodermal origin, and they apparently invade the CNS at the time the vasculature develops.

Neural Crest

As the neural plate folds to form the neural tube, the most lateral cells are pinched off. These cells, the *neural crest* cells, lie along the dorsolateral part of the tube (Figs. 3C and D). They become segmented into cell groups, which give rise to the sensory ganglion cells of the spinal and cranial nerves, and to postganglionic autonomic neurons. The chromaffin cells of the adrenal medulla and the glial cells in the PNS, i.e., satellite cells and Schwann cells, are also derived from the neural crest. All melanoblasts, likewise, come from the neural crest.

SPINAL CORD

Neuroepithelial, Mantle, and Marginal Layers

When the neural tube has closed, the neuroepithelial cells form a thick pseudostratified epithelium. The cells multiply at a rapid rate in the ventricular zone (Fig. 4A). During the proliferative period the nuclei migrate in a characteristic fashion to and from the lumen at each division (Sauer, 1935; Sidman et al., 1959). In the interphase, when the undifferentiated neuroepithelial cells synthesize DNA, their form is wedge-shaped; the nuclei lie in the outer zone of the primitive ependymal zone and slender cytoplasmic processes extend toward the ventricular surface. During the mitotic cycle the nuclei migrate toward the lumen, where they divide within a few hours following the DNA synthesis. After the division, the nuclei pass away from the lumen and any given cell may continue in a lateral direction and participate in the formation of the *mantle* (intermediate) *layer* (Fig. 4B). These are the neuroblasts, which gradually mature and develop processes. The axons of many of the neurons collect along the periphery of the mantle layer, where they form the *marginal layer.* The neuroepithelial cells also give rise to the *ependymal layer.* The glial cells, which are formed at a somewhat later stage, are located both in the mantle and the marginal layers.

Basal and Alar Plates

A longitudinal groove, *sulcus limitans,* appears on both sides of the central cavity and runs along the length of the neural tube. This sulcus divides the rapidly expanding side walls of the neural tube into a ventral thickening, the *basal plate,* and a dorsal thickening, the *alar plate* (Fig. 4B). The cell bodies in the basal plate form the *ventral* and *lateral gray columns,* which contain somatic and autonomic motor neurons, respectively. The cell bodies in the alar plate form the *dorsal gray column.* These columns are often referred to as the *ventral, lateral,* and *dorsal horns* when viewed in cross-section (Fig. 4C).

The marginal layer, which increases in thickness as more and more neurons send axons into it, forms the white matter of the spinal cord. As a result of continuous enlargement of the walls of the neural tube, the wide central cavity gradually narrows and eventually becomes the *central canal* of the spinal cord.

Dorsal Root Ganglia and Spinal Nerves

The pseudounipolar sensory cells of the dorsal root ganglia (spinal ganglia) develop from the neural crest. The axons of these sensory cells divide in a T-shaped pattern close to the cell bodies. The central processes grow into the spinal cord. These are the *dorsal roots* of the spinal nerve (Fig. 4D). The peripheral processes join the *ventral root* fibers in the region of the intervertebral foramina to form the *spinal nerves.* Most of the axons in the ventral roots arise from somatic and autonomic motor neurons in the ventral and lateral gray columns of the spinal cord.

Cauda Equina

In the embryo, the spinal cord extends the entire length of the vertebral canal, and the spinal nerves pass through the intervertebral foramina at the level of origin in the spinal cord (Fig. 5A). After the 3rd fetal month, however, the vertebral column and dura mater grow more rapidly than the spinal cord, and the various spinal cord segments will eventually lie somewhat higher than the corresponding vertebra. The distance between the spinal cord segment and its corresponding vertebra becomes increasingly greater in the caudal segments. At birth, the spinal cord ends at the level of vertebra L3, but it reaches only vertebra L2 in the adult.

The differential growth of the spinal cord and the vertebral column explains the formation of the *cauda equina* (Fig. 6), which consists of the long lumbar and sacral roots that have been stretched during the development of the cord and the vertebral column. The caudal tip of the tube remains attached to the coccygeal part of the vertebral column and becomes a thin filament, the *filum terminale.* The fact that the spinal cord of the adult reaches only to the second lumbar vertebra is of great clinical relevance (see Lumbar Puncture in Clinical Notes, Chapter 3).

EARLY DEVELOPMENT OF THE BRAIN

Primary and Secondary Brain Vesicles

In the 4th embryonic week, before the closure of the neural tube is completed, the rostral part of the tube forms three primary brain vesicles (Fig. 7A): *prosencephalon* = forebrain; *mesencephalon* = midbrain; and *rhombencephalon* = hindbrain. Subsequently, the prosencephalon is divided into two secondary brain vesicles, the *telencephalon,* which will become the cerebral hemispheres, and a median part, the *diencephalon* (Fig. 7B). At the same time the rhombencephalon divides into the *metencephalon* and the *myelencephalon.*

The Flexures

During early growth, a *midbrain flexure* appears in the region of the midbrain, and a *cervical flexure* at the junction between the hindbrain and spinal cord (Fig. 8A). These flexures appear before the secondary brain vesicles develop. Somewhat later a compensatory flexure, the *pontine flexure,* develops between the other two flexures (Fig. 8B).

Migration and Aggregation of Cells

Many of the neurons in the brain migrate over a considerable distance before they reach a predetermined location where they aggregate with other neurons of a similar type to form a nuclear group or a cortical layer. Although most neurons have reached their ultimate destination before development of processes starts, there are some notable exceptions to this rule (see Development of Cerebellar Cortex). How the axons are able to reach other distant parts of the CNS, or effector organs, is not known. Nor do we know how the neurons and their processes establish specific synaptic relationships.

MAJOR SUBDIVISIONS OF THE BRAIN

Myelencephalon

Myelencephalon develops into the *medulla oblongata,* which is continuous with the spinal cord. The medulla resembles the spinal cord macroscop-

Embryo at 18 days

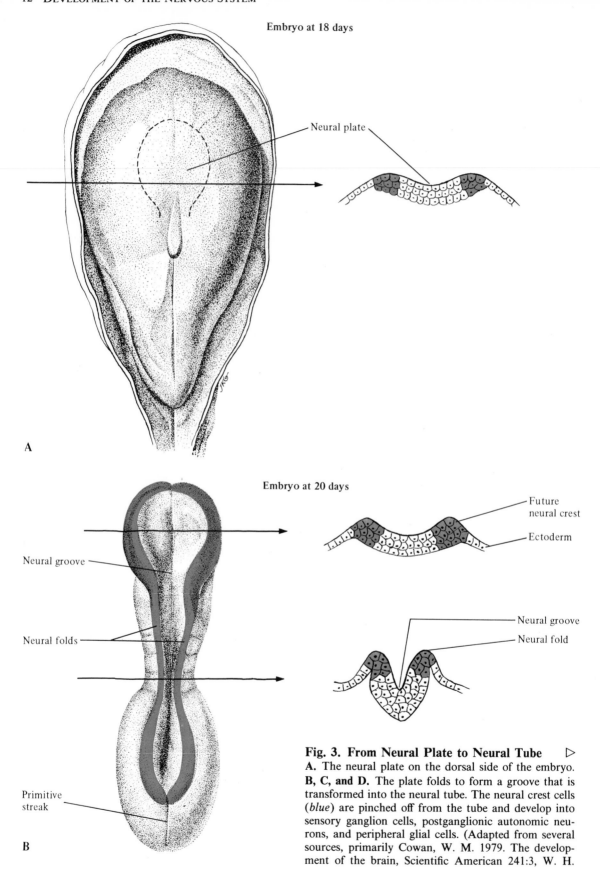

Neural plate

A

Embryo at 20 days

Future
neural crest

Ectoderm

Neural groove

Neural groove

Neural folds

Neural fold

Primitive
streak

B

Fig. 3. From Neural Plate to Neural Tube ▷
A. The neural plate on the dorsal side of the embryo.
B, C, and D. The plate folds to form a groove that is
transformed into the neural tube. The neural crest cells
(*blue*) are pinched off from the tube and develop into
sensory ganglion cells, postganglionic autonomic neurons, and peripheral glial cells. (Adapted from several
sources, primarily Cowan, W. M. 1979. The development of the brain, Scientific American 241:3, W. H.

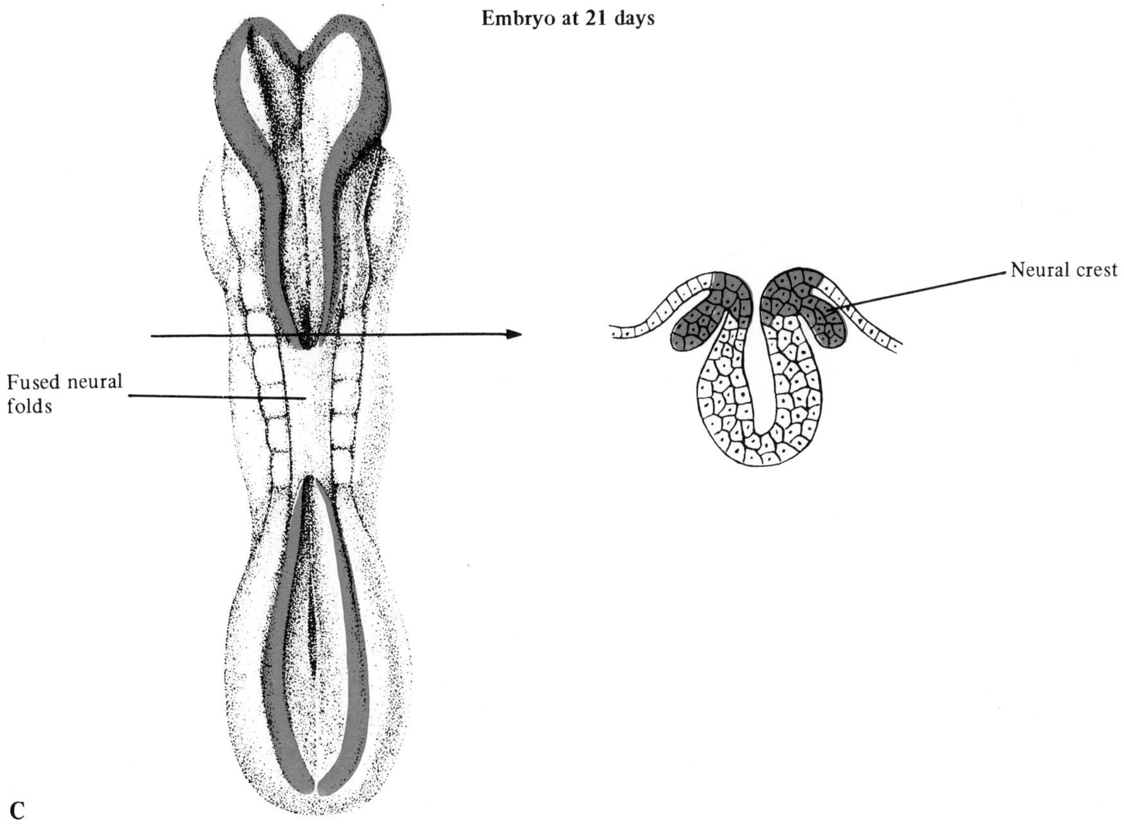

Embryo at 21 days

Neural crest

Fused neural folds

C

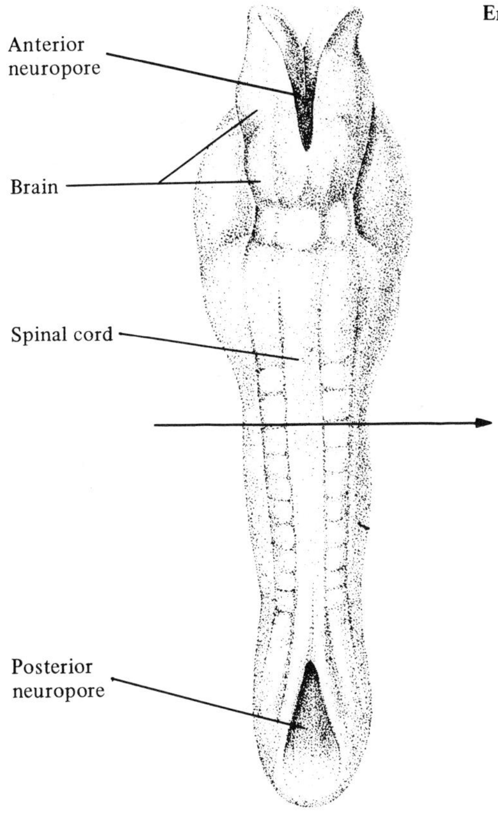

Embryo at 24 days

Anterior neuropore

Brain

Spinal cord

Ectoderm

Neural crest

Neural tube

Posterior neuropore

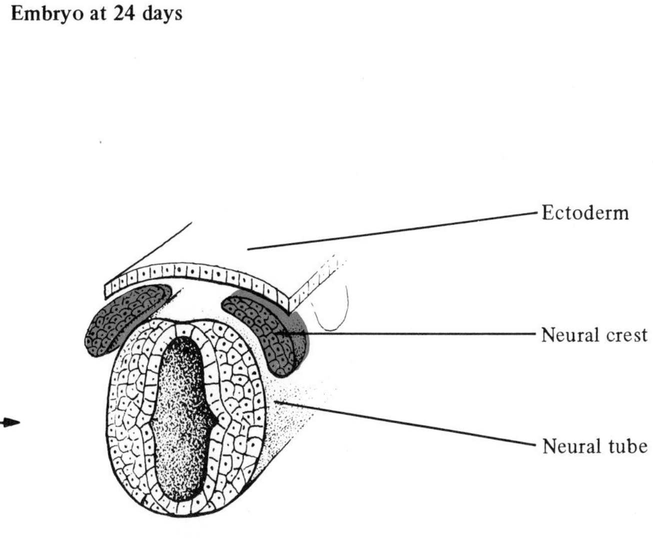

D

Freeman and Company, San Francisco; Crelin, E. S. 1974. Development of the nervous system. A logical approach to neuroanatomy. CIBA Clinical Symposia, 26:2; Hamilton, W. J. and H. W. Mossman, 1972. Hamilton, Boyd and Mossman's Human Embryology: Prenatal development of form and function, 4th ed., 437–525, Heffer, Cambridge; Langman, J. 1981. Medical Embryology, 4th ed., 320–356, Williams and Wilkins, Baltimore.)

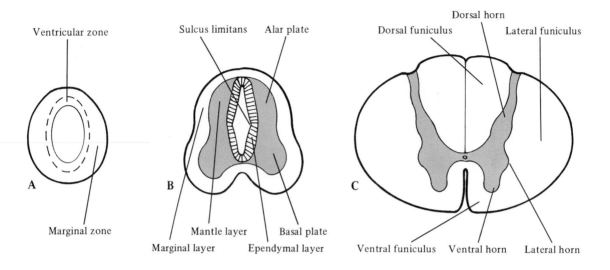

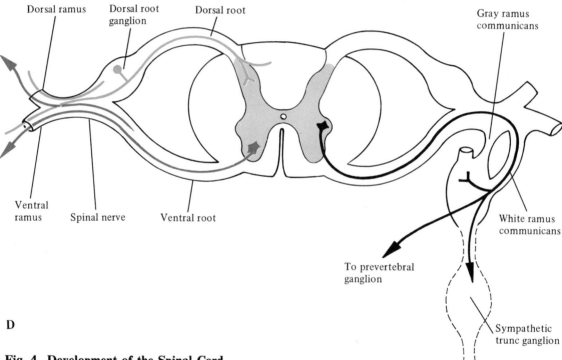

Fig. 4. Development of the Spinal Cord

A. The walls of the neural tube rapidly increase in thickness through cell proliferation.

B. Sulcus limitans indicates the boundary between the basal and alar plates.

C. The basal plates develop into ventral and lateral horns, whereas the alar plates form the dorsal horns.

D. Schematic drawing showing the principal components of the spinal nerves. Somatic motor neuron, *red;* autonomic motor neuron, *black;* sensory neuron, *blue.*

ically, but the typical spinal cord pattern with a centrally placed gray substance surrounded by white substance can not be recognized. Further, the rostral part of the medulla, becomes wider as the alar plates move laterally to give room to the expanding fourth ventricle (Figs. 9A and B). This process results in the development of an extensive but thin roof plate covering the 4th ventricle. It also explains why the cranial sensory neurons as derivatives of the alar plate are located

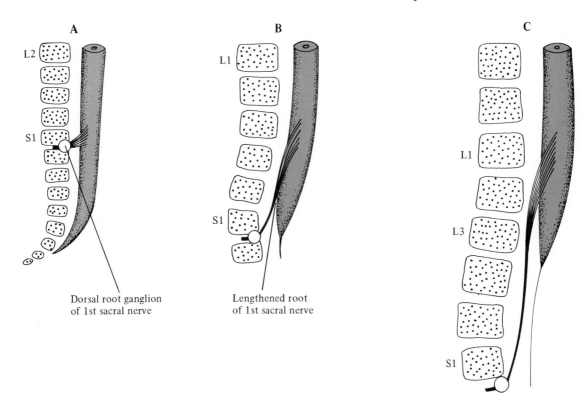

Fig. 5. Cauda Equina
Schematic drawings showing the relationship between the spinal cord and the vertebral column at various stages of development. **A,** approximately at third month; **B,** end of fifth month; **C,** in the newborn (After Streeter, G. L., 1919. Factors involved in the formation of the filum terminale, American Journal of Anatomy 25:1–11 and after Langman, J. 1981. Medical Embryology 4th edition, 320–356, Williams & Wilkins, Baltimore. Langman, 1981. With permission of Williams & Wilkins, Baltimore).

dorsolateral to the columns of cranial motor neurons, which derive from the basal plate (Fig. 9C). The *inferior olivary nucleus,* which is closely related to the cerebellum, derives from the dorsal part of the neural tube and migrates to the ventral part of the medulla, where it forms a prominent landmark. Another prominent structure in the ventral part of medulla is the *pyramid,* which contains corticospinal fibers. The dorsal part of the medulla contains cranial nerve nuclei, long ascending and descending tracts, and reticular nuclei (see Chapter 10).

Metencephalon

Pronounced changes take place in the metencephalon. The *cerebellum* develops from the *rhombic lips,* i.e., symmetric thickenings in the dorsolateral parts of the neural tube (Fig. 10A). Initially the lips bulge into the ventricular cavity, but the extraventricular portions rapidly expand in a dor-

sal direction and fuse in the midline. In the mature cerebellum one can recognize two *hemispheres* and a midline portion, the *vermis.* Both the hemispheres and the vermis contain subcortical nuclear groups, the *intracerebellar nuclei,* and a heavily folded cortex. Cerebellum is of special importance for the coordination of movements.

The ventral part of the metencephalon develops into the *pons,* the basal part of which is characterized by prominent collections of neurons, the *pontine nuclei,* which send their axons to cerebellum. The dorsal, tegmental part of pons is occupied by cranial nerve nuclei, long fiber bundles, and the reticular formation (Fig. 10B). The central cavity of the rhombencephalon becomes the fourth ventricle.

Development of Cerebellar Cortex

The development of the cerebellar cortex has attracted considerable attention. Initially, the cere-

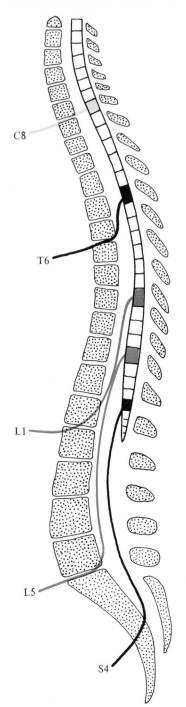

Fig. 6. Relationship between Spinal Cord Segments and Their Corresponding Vertebrae
The distance between the spinal cord segment and its corresponding vertebra becomes increasingly greater in the caudal direction. Cauda equina consists of the long lumbar and sacral roots that have been stretched during the development of the spinal cord and vertebral column.

bellar plate, like the rest of the neural tube, consists of a neuroepithelial, a mantle, and a marginal layer. During further development a number of neuroepithelial cells migrate toward the surface to form the *external granular layer* (Fig. 11A). In contrast with the general rule, this layer retains its capacity to proliferate. Normally, migrating cells in the developing nervous systems are postmitotic; i.e., they have lost their capacity to divide before they start to migrate. This, for instance, is the case with another set of cerebellar neuroblasts that migrate to the superficial part of the mantle layer, where they develop into the large *Purkinje cells.*

The next stage in the development is also exceptional. The external granular cells, which have retained their mitotic activity, give rise to cells that start a second wave of migration in the opposite direction, i.e., inward toward the mantle layer. These cells form the *internal granular layer* (Fig. 11B). Their axons, the parallel fibers (*see below*), and cells that do not take part in the second wave of migration (basket and stellate cells, see Chapter 9) become important constituents of the *molecular layer.*

The various cell types that are released from the external granular layer are closely related to radial glial processes, which seem to guide the migrating cells in their inward radial movement. A close relationship between migrating cells and glial processes is seen in many parts of the developing nervous system.

The majority of the cells in the nervous system generate their processes after they have reached their final destination. However, axonal growth may precede cell migration in some cases. This happens in the cerebellar cortex, where the neuroblasts destined for the internal granular layer develop tangentially oriented axonal processes before they start their inward migration. During the migration, the cell first extrudes a horizontal process and then leaves behind a perpendicular process as it migrates inwardly, giving the axon a characteristic T-shaped appearance (Figs. 11C and D). The tangential part of the axon is referred to as a parallel fiber (see Fig. 120).

Mesencephalon

A gradual thickening of the wall of the mesencephalon reduces the central cavity to a narrow

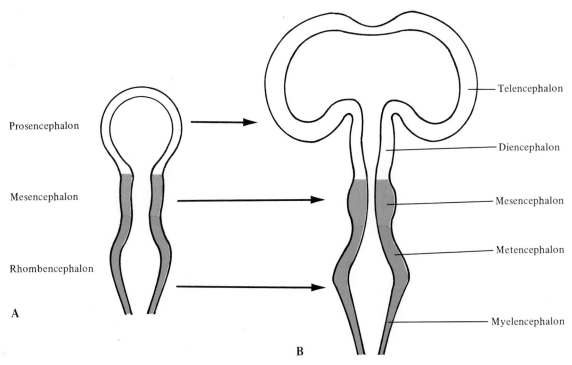

Fig. 7. Primary and Secondary Brain Vesicles

A. The three primary brain vesicles, prosencephalon, mesencephalon and rhombencephalon, develop before the closure of the neural tube is completed.

B. The anterior part of prosencephalon differentiates into the two telencephalic vesicles, which develop into the cerebral hemispheres.

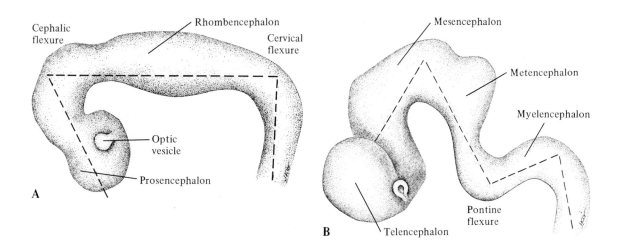

Fig. 8. The Brain Flexures

A. The cervical flexure appears at the junction of the rhombencephalon and the spinal cord, and a cephalic (or midbrain) flexure in the region of mesencephalon.

B. A third flexure, the pontine flexure, develops between the metencephalon and myelencephalon. (Modified after Hochstetter, F., 1919 and 1929. Beiträge zur Entwicklungsgeschichte des menschlichen Gehirns. Deuticke: Vienna and Leipzig.)

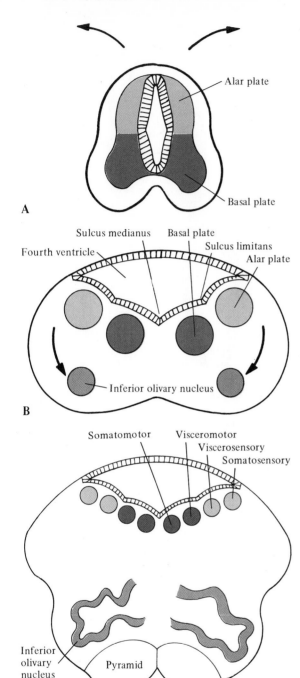

Fig. 9. Development of Medulla Oblongata
A and B. The lateral walls of the neural tube rotate around an imaginary longitudinal axis in a movement resembling the opening of a book. This results in the development of a thin roof plate covering the ventricle. **C.** As a result of this rotation the sensory cranial nerve nuclei will be located in the lateral part of the medulla and the motor nuclei in its medial part.

passage, the *cerebral aqueduct* (Fig. 12). The alar plates develop into the *tectum* with the two paired *superior* and *inferior colliculi*. The superior colliculi are important centers for visual reflexes and the inferior colliculi serve as relay centers for auditory impulses. The *central gray* around the cerebral aqueduct is also believed to come from the alar plate. Neuroblasts in the basal plate give rise to the oculomotor and trochlear nerve nuclei (3rd and 4th cranial nerve nuclei), which are located ventral to the central gray. The *substantia nigra* and *red nucleus* are two prominent nuclei in the ventral part of mesencephalon. As more and more fibers connect the rapidly expanding forebrain with regions in the brain stem and spinal cord, the ventral part of mesencephalon develops into the two prominent *cerebral peduncles*. Most of the descending projection fibers from forebrain regions accumulate in the base of the cerebral peduncle, whereas its dorsal part, the *tegmentum,* contains both ascending and descending pathways as well as reticular and cranial nerve nuclei.

Diencephalon

Major Subdivisions

Three swellings in the lateral wall of the third ventricle give rise to the main divisions of the diencephalon: the *epithalamus, thalamus,* and *hypothalamus* (Fig. 13).

Epithalamus, which is the smallest division, develops into the *habenular nuclei* and *pineal gland* (epiphysis). The pineal gland seems to play a role in gonadal function until puberty. After this time the gland has a tendency to calcify, and since it is normally located in the median plane it serves as an important landmark on an X-ray film of the skull. An expansive lesion on one side of the brain tends to push the pineal gland away from the midline toward the opposite side.

The *sulcus hypothalamicus,* which appears as a longitudinal groove in the lateral wall of the third ventricle, separates the thalamus from the hypothalamus. The development of the thalamus, which is the largest part of the diencephalon, is closely related to the development of the cerebral cortex, and the two structures are closely interrelated in the mature brain. Many of the cell groups in the hypothalamus are closely associated with autonomic and endocrine functions.

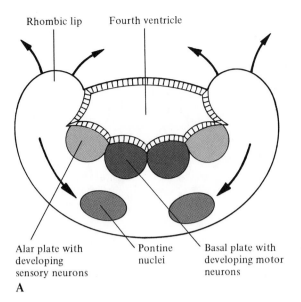

Rhombic lip   Fourth ventricle

Alar plate with developing sensory neurons

Pontine nuclei

Basal plate with developing motor neurons

A

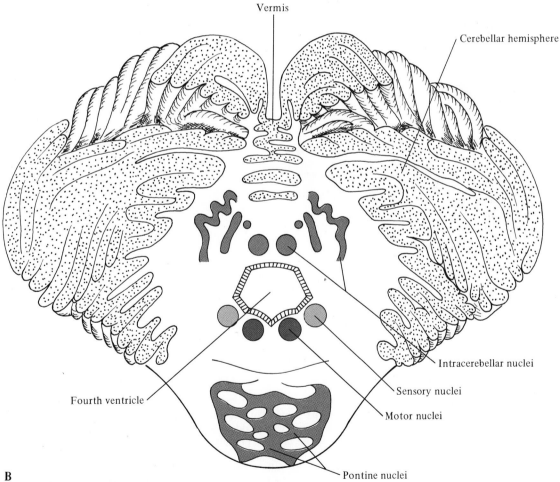

Vermis

Cerebellar hemisphere

Intracerebellar nuclei

Sensory nuclei

Motor nuclei

Fourth ventricle

Pontine nuclei

B

Fig. 10. Development of Metencephalon
A. The rhombic lips expand rapidly in a dorsal direction and give rise to cerebellum.
B. The ventral part of metencephalon, the pons, can be subdivided into a small dorsal part and a large basal part, which contains the pontine nuclei.

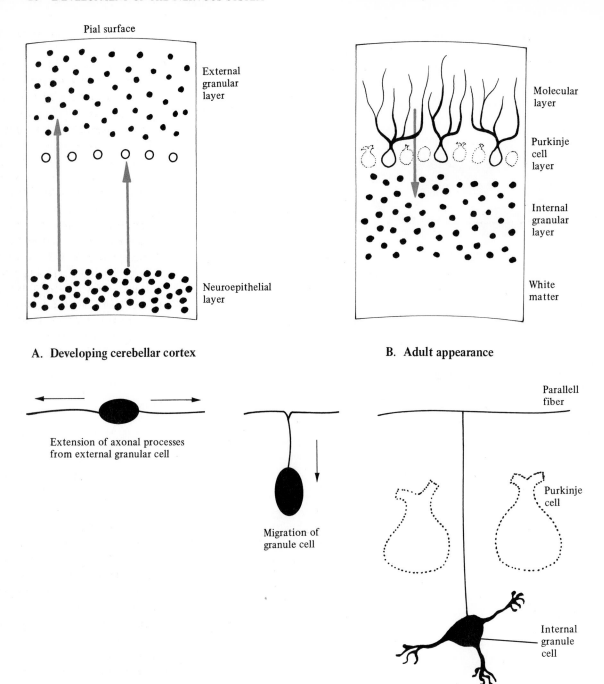

A. Developing cerebellar cortex

B. Adult appearance

C. Development of the granule cell axon

D. Adult appearance

Fig. 11. Development of Cerebellar Cortex

A and B. Neuroepithelial cells first migrate to the surface of the cerebellum, where they form the external granular layer. The cells in this layer retain the capacity to divide and many of the daughter cells migrate in the opposite direction and develop into neurons of the internal granular layer.

C and D. The cells in the external granular layer develop tangentially oriented axonal processes before they start the inward migration. During the migration, the cells leave behind a perpendicular process, giving the axon a typical T-shaped appearance. (Modified after Lund, R. D., 1978. Development and Plasticity of the Brain: An Introduction, Oxford University Press, New York.)

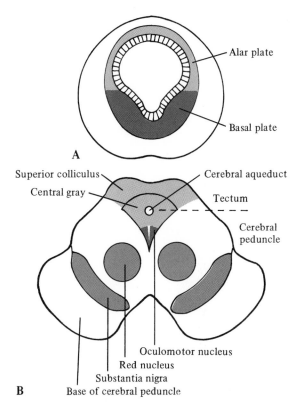

Fig. 12. Development of Mesencephalon
A. A gradual thickening of the wall of the neural tube reduces the central cavity to a narrow passage, the cerebral aqueduct.
B. An imaginary horizontal line through the aqueduct divides the mesencephalon into a dorsal part, the tectum, and a massive ventral part consisting of the two cerebral peduncles.

As the thalamus and hypothalamus develop in the lateral walls of the diencephalon, the central cavity is gradually transformed into the slitlike *third ventricle*. Its roof is formed by a single layer of ependymal cells covered by a highly vascular mesenchyme. The invagination of these two structures into the third ventricle forms the choroid plexus (see below). *Lamina terminalis,* a derivative of the telencephalon, forms the rostral wall of the third ventricle. This is believed to be the area where the final closure of the anterior neuropore occurred. At an early stage, three swellings can be recognized in the floor of the third ventricle. These are, from rostral to caudal, the *optic chiasm, infundibulum,* and *mammillary body*.

Development of the Eye

Ventrally, on both sides of the forebrain, an *optic vesicle* appears in the 3rd embryonic week (Fig. 14A). This vesicle, which remains attached to the brain by the *optic stalk* (Fig. 14B), apposes the ectoderm, in which a thickening is formed. This is the *lens placode,* which develops into the *lens* of the eye. The optic vesicle invaginates to form the *retina* with associated pigment layer, and as the nervous retina apposes the pigment layer, the cavity of the optic vesicle is obliterated. The optic stalk, whose lumen gradually becomes occluded by ingrowing axons from the retina, develops into the *optic nerve*. The nerves from each eye converge at the base of the brain to form the *optic chiasm,* in which the fibers from the medial halves of the two retinae cross the midline.

As the mouth of the optic cup closes around the lens to become the *iris,* a groove, the *choroid fissure,* remains on the ventral side of the optic cup (Fig. 14D). The hyaloid vessels, which reach the interior of the cup through this fetal cleft, develop into the *central artery and vein* of the retina (Fig. 14E). If the edges of the choroid fissure do not fuse properly, a malformation known as coloboma will result (see Clinical Notes).

Development of the Hypophysis (Pituitary)

Each lobe of the hypophysis has a different origin. The *adenohypophysis* (anterior lobe) develops from *Rathke's pouch,* an ectodermal diverticulum in the mouth cavity, whereas the neurohypophysis (the infundibular stem and neural lobe) develops from a downward evagination of the diencephalon, the *infundibulum* (Fig. 15). Cells from the adenohypophysis extend along and around the pituitary stalk, forming the *pars tuberalis* (Fig. 15D). The gross anatomic developmental events seem simple enough; Rathke's pouch apparently elongates and comes in contact with the funnel-shaped infundibulum and the two fuse. Remnants of the pouch sometimes give rise to a tumor called craniopharyngioma (see Clinical Notes).

Telencephalon

Cerebral Hemispheres

The most dramatic developmental changes are seen in the forebrain where the two telencephalic vesicles (Fig. 7B) develop into the cerebral hemispheres, which rapidly expand to cover more and more of the rest of the brain (Fig. 16). The expan-

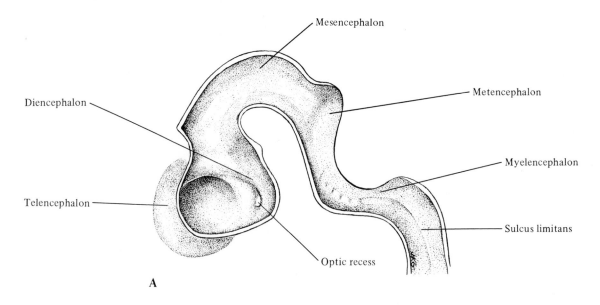

A

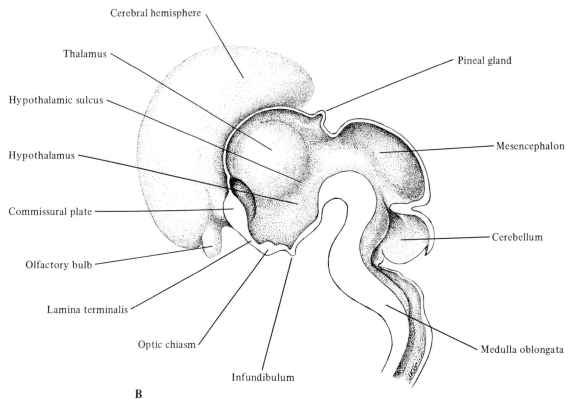

B

Fig. 13. Development of Diencephalon

A. Medial surface of the right half of the cranial part of the CNS in a 11-mm embryo showing the five brain vesicles.

B. The medial surface of the brain in a 43-mm human embryo. Sulcus hypothalamicus separates the thalamus from the hypothalamus. (Modified after Hines, M., 1922. Studies in the growth and differentiation of the telencepahlon in man: The fissura hippocampi: Journal of Comp. Neurol. 34:73–171.)

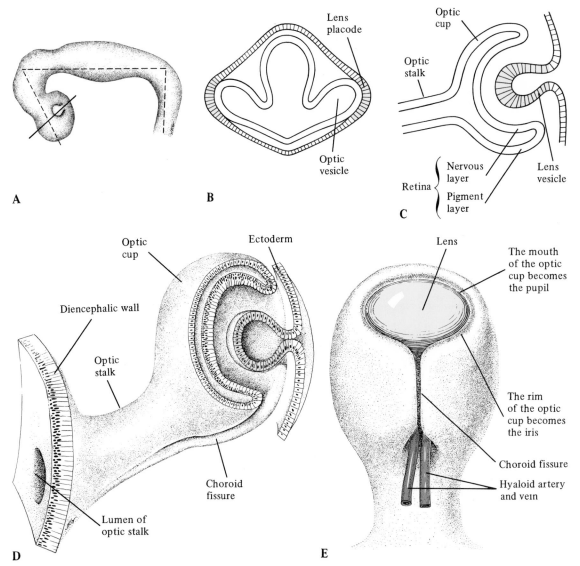

A

B

C

Lens
placode

Optic
vesicle

Optic
cup

Optic
stalk

Retina { Nervous
layer / Pigment
layer

Lens
vesicle

Optic
cup

Diencephalic wall

Optic
stalk

Lumen of
optic stalk

Ectoderm

Choroid
fissure

Lens

The mouth
of the optic
cup becomes
the pupil

The rim
of the optic
cup becomes
the iris

Choroid fissure

Hyaloid artery
and vein

D

E

Fig. 14. Development of the Eye
A–C. The optic vesicles invaginate to form the retina, whereas the lens placod develops into the lens.
D and E. Three-dimensional drawings showing the optic cup and the choroid fissure with the hyaloid vessels, which develop into the central artery and vein of the retina. (Modified after Mann, J. C., 1950. The development of the human eye. Cambridge Univ. Press, London.)

sion is not symmetric in all directions. The postero-ventral part of the telencephalic vesicle, for instance, curves down and forward to form the temporal lobe. The lateral part of the telencephalic vesicle, on the other hand, is characterized by a more modest expansion, and this area, the future *insula,* is gradually covered by the dorsomedial and posterior parts of the expanding hemisphere. These overlying parts are referred to as the *frontal, frontoparietal,* and *temporal opercula* (Fig. 16C). A small swelling, which appears on the anteroven-tral surface of the hemisphere at an early stage, enlarges and can soon be recognized as the olfactory bulb (Figs. 13B and 16B).

To allow for additional expansion within the skull cavity, the cortex of the hemisphere becomes folded, which results in the formation of grooves, *sulci,* that demarcate the different brain convolutions, *gyri.* Some of the more pronounced grooves, i.e., the *lateral fissure, parieto-occipital sulcus,* and *preoccipital notch,* divide the hemisphere into four lobes: the *frontal, parietal, occipital,* and *temporal*

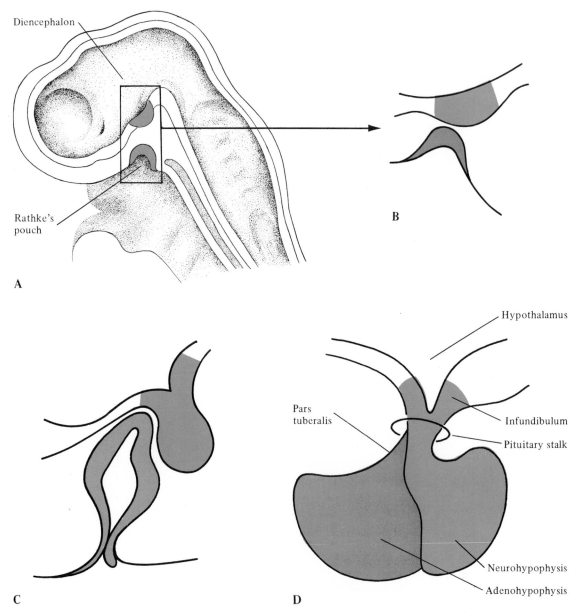

Fig. 15. Development of the Hypophysis
A–D. Successive stages in the development of the pituitary gland, which has two different origins. The neurohypophysis develops from the infundibulum in the floor of the diencephalon, whereas the adenohypophysis comes from the Rathke's pouch in the primitive mouth cavity. (From Moore, K. L., 1977. The developing human: clinically oriented embryology. 2nd ed., W. G. Saunders and Co., Philadelphia. With permission of the publisher.)

lobes (Fig. 16C). The fifth lobe, the *insula,* is hidden in the depth of the lateral sulcus.

The histogenesis of the cerebral cortex follows a characteristic pattern. Most of the cortical cells originate from the primitive ependyma of the lateral ventricle and they are generated in an "inside-

out" sequence, in the sense that cells that form at successively later stages in embryonic life migrate outward past their predecessors (Angevine and Sidman, 1961). In other words, older neurons are located in the basal layers of the cortex while younger neurons are located more superficially.

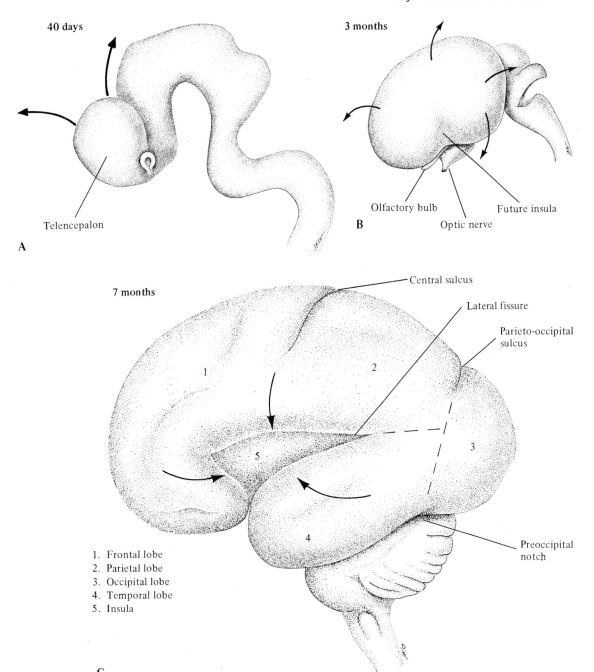

40 days

Telencepalon

A

3 months

Olfactory bulb
Optic nerve
Future insula

B

7 months

Central sulcus

Lateral fissure

Parieto-occipital
sulcus

Preoccipital
notch

1. Frontal lobe
2. Parietal lobe
3. Occipital lobe
4. Temporal lobe
5. Insula

C

Fig. 16. Development of the Cerebral Hemisphere

A and B. The telencephalic vesicle expands rapidly to cover the rest of the brain, and the posteroventral part of the vesicle curves down and forward to form the temporal lobe.

C. The lateral surface of the human brain at approximately 7 months pregnancy. The insular region is bounded by the frontal, frontoparietal, and temporal opercula. Some of the more pronounced grooves have appeared and the hemisphere can be divided into five lobes: the frontal, parietal, occipital, and temporal lobes, and the insula.

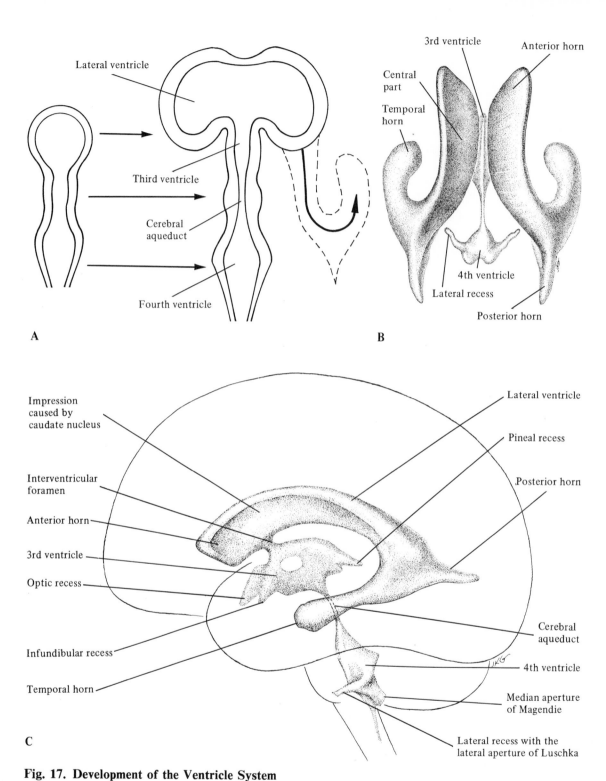

Fig. 17. Development of the Ventricle System

A. With the appearance of the temporal lobe, the lateral ventricle develops into a long curved cavity.

B and C. Superior and lateral views of the ventricle system. (Modified after Bailey, P., 1948. Intracranial tumors. Charles C. Thomas, Publisher, Springfield, IL.)

The Ventricle System

The cavity in the rostral part of the neural tube develops into the ventricle system of the brain. The greatest morphologic changes take place in the cerebral hemisphere, in which develops a long curved cavity, the *lateral ventricle* (Fig. 17). Its shape can best be understood if one conceives of the development of the temporal lobe as a semicircular expansion of the ventral part of the hemisphere (Fig. 16). The different parts of the lateral ventricle are referred to as the *anterior horn, central part, posterior horn,* and *temporal horn.* The lateral ventricle is continuous with the *third ventricle* in the diencephalon through the *interventricular foramen* (of Monro). The third ventricle, in turn, is continuous with the *fourth ventricle* in the rhombencephalon through a narrow canal in the mesencephalon, the *cerebral aqueduct.* The brain ventricles are filled with a clear, colorless fluid, the *cerebrospinal fluid* (CSF), which is produced by the choroid plexus (see below). The fluid leaves the ventricular system through three openings in the 4th ventricle, the *median aperture of Magendie* in the midline and the two *lateral apertures of Luschka* in the lateral recesses.

It is important to be familiar with the normal configuration of the ventricular system, especially for the analysis of X-ray films based on its visualization. Some of the more prominent recesses, such as the *optic, infundibular,* and *pineal recesses* in the third ventricle and the *lateral recess* in the fourth ventricle (Fig. 17C) are valuable landmarks. Enlargement of the ventricle system occurs in hydrocephalus (see Clinical Notes).

Choroid Plexus

In certain regions of the developing brain, i.e., the medial surface of the telencephalic vesicles and the roof of the diencephalon and rhombencephalon, the wall remains very thin, consisting only of an ependymal layer. This layer invaginates into the ventricular cavity together with a highly vascularized mesenchyme to form the choroid plexus (Fig. 18), which produces the CSF. Where the telencephalic vesicle attaches to the diencephalon, i.e., the *hemisphere stalk* (Fig. 18B), the invagination in the medial wall of the telencephalon is continuous with the invagination in the roof of the diencephalon. The choroid plexus of the lateral ventricle, therefore, is directly continuous with the choroid plexus of the third ventricle at the level of the interventricular foramen. In the subsequent development, more and more fibers connect the rapidly developing hemispheres with the diencephalon and brain stem. These projection fibers gather primarily in the ventral and caudal walls of the hemisphere stalk, which increase rapidly in thickness thereby producing a broad attachment between the telencephalon and diencephalon, as if the two parts had fused (Fig. 18B and C). Some fusion, however, does apparently take place at the region where the thin telencephalic (ependymal) wall of the lateral ventricle is attached to the dorsal surface of the thalamus, hence the name *lamina affixa thalami* (Fig. 18C).

After further expansion the two hemispheres finally meet in the midline over the diencephalon. The mesenchyme, which thus becomes trapped between the hemispheres and the diencephalon, forms a highly vascularized connective tissue sheath, the *tela choroidea* or velum interpositum (Fig. 18D). Tela choroidea is located in the *transverse fissure* underneath the corpus callosum and the fornix in the fully developed brain (see below). The choroid plexus of the lateral ventricle appears as an invagination from the lateral edge of tela choroidea, whereas the choroid plexus of the third ventricle represents invaginations from the inferior surface of the tela (Fig. 18D). As already indicated, however, the plexus in the lateral ventricle is continuous with the plexus in the third ventricle at the level of the interventricular foramen (Fig. 18E). Further, the choroid plexus is continuous with the pia mater through the *choroid fissure,* which indicates the site of invagination (black line in Fig. 18E). Since the choroid plexus in the central part of the lateral ventricle continues into the temporal horn, the choroid fissure forms a semicircular curve similar to that described by the developing temporal horn of the lateral ventricle.

Corpus Callosum and Fornix

Fibers projecting from one developing hemisphere to the other, i.e., commissural fibers, cross the midline in the upper part of lamina terminalis, which increases rapidly in thickness to form the *commissural plate* (Fig. 19A). With the expansion of the hemispheres, the plate increases in size, overgrows the tela choroidea and the roof of the third ventricle, and emerges as the dorsally convex *corpus callosum* (Fig. 19B). Its curvature indicates the

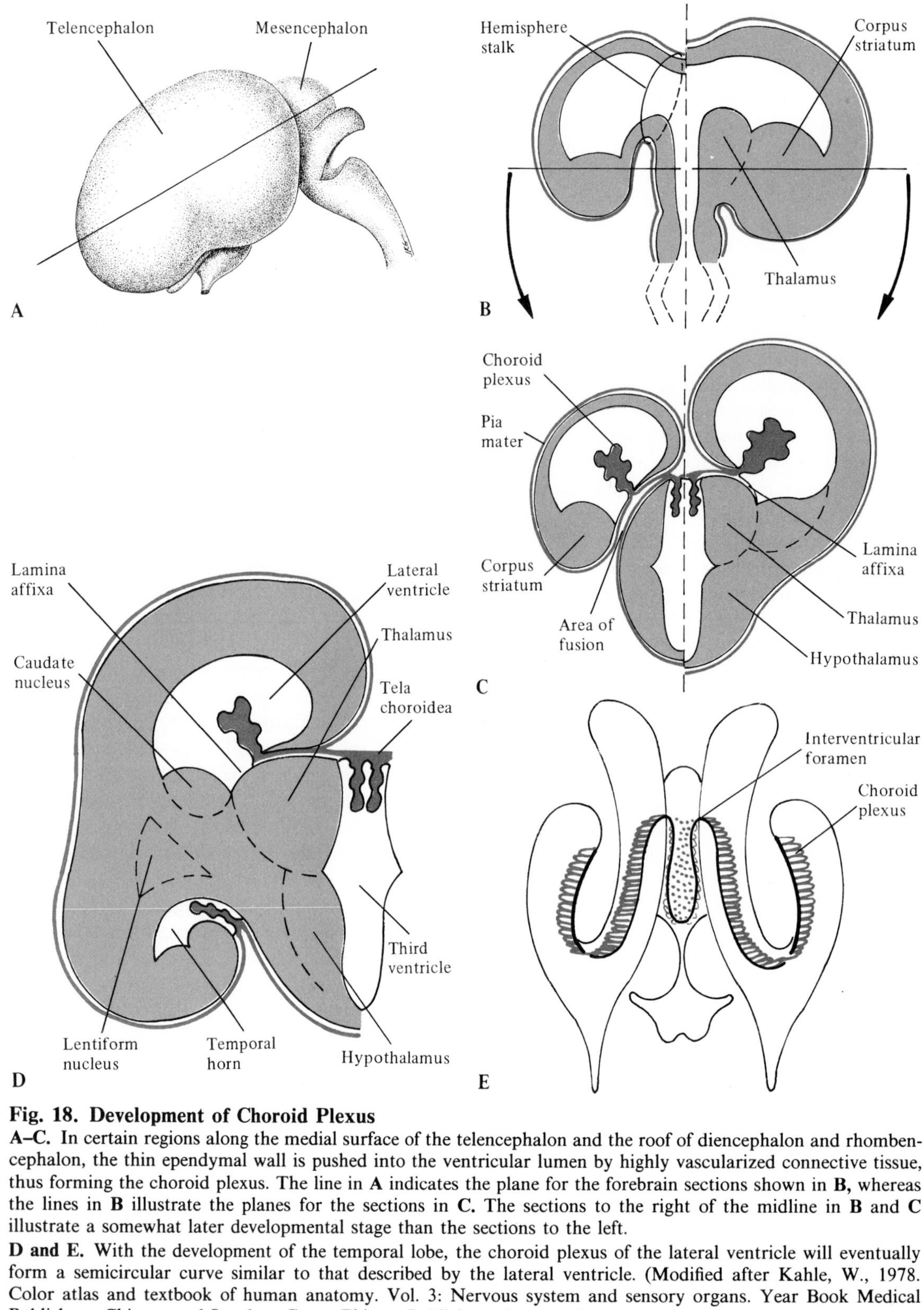

Fig. 18. Development of Choroid Plexus

A–C. In certain regions along the medial surface of the telencephalon and the roof of diencephalon and rhomben-cephalon, the thin ependymal wall is pushed into the ventricular lumen by highly vascularized connective tissue, thus forming the choroid plexus. The line in **A** indicates the plane for the forebrain sections shown in **B**, whereas the lines in **B** illustrate the planes for the sections in **C**. The sections to the right of the midline in **B** and **C** illustrate a somewhat later developmental stage than the sections to the left.

D and E. With the development of the temporal lobe, the choroid plexus of the lateral ventricle will eventually form a semicircular curve similar to that described by the lateral ventricle. (Modified after Kahle, W., 1978. Color atlas and textbook of human anatomy. Vol. 3: Nervous system and sensory organs. Year Book Medical Publishers, Chicago and London. Georg Thieme Publishers. Stuttgart.)

direction in which the hemispheres expanded. The different parts of the corpus callosum are referred to as the *rostrum, genu, body,* and *splenium.* The *anterior commissure* is another important bundle of commissural fibers, which interconnect parts of the temporal lobes with each other. It crosses the midline just behind the upper part of lamina terminalis (Fig. 19B).

The *septum pellucidum* is a thin wall that separates the anterior horns of the lateral ventricles behind the genu of corpus callosum. In the ventral free edge of the septum, a bundle of nerve fibers appears on each side of the midline. This is the *fornix,* which forms an arch over the thalamus. The two fornices diverge markedly as they sweep down as the *crura fornicis* behind the two thalamic nuclei into the temporal lobes. The last flattened part of the fornix, the *fimbria,* reaches the hippocampus in the medial wall of the temporal horn (Fig. 19C). The two crura fornices meet to form the *body of fornix* underneath the corpus callosum. However, they separate again and proceed forward and downward as the *columns of fornix* in the ventral free edge of the septum to reach the *mammillary bodies* in the hypothalamus.

Commissural fibers connecting the hippocampal formations on the two sides cross over between the two crura fornices to form the *hippocampal commissure.* It is situated underneath the splenium of the corpus callosum to which it is intimately attached (Fig. 19C).

Corpus Striatum

Soon after the telencephalic vesicles have appeared, their basal portion thickens rapidly through the proliferation of cells. The fibers connecting the telencephalic vesicle with the diencephalon and the brain stem pass through this cell mass, which therefore acquires a striated appearance, hence the name *corpus striatum* (Fig. 20B). The dorsal part of the hemisphere, the pallium, which covers the striate body like a mantle, develops into the *cerebral cortex.*

With the rapid growth of the cerebral hemispheres, there is a concomitant increase in the number of fibers that connect the expanding hemispheres with the thalamus and the rest of the brain. The hemisphere stalk, which connects the hemisphere with the diencephalon (Fig. 18B), increases in thickness as more and more fibers accumulate,

especially in the basal and posterior walls of the interventricular foramen. As a result, the interventricular foramen becomes smaller and the hemisphere gradually acquires a broad attachment to the diencephalon (Figs. 20C and E).

In the further development, two events deserve special notice. One is the fact that the fibers projecting through the striate body tend to concentrate in the *internal capsule.* This is a massive sheet of white substance that divides the corpus striatum into the *caudate nucleus* and *lentiform nucleus* (Figs. 20C and E). The dorsomedially located caudate nucleus bulges into the lateral ventricle (Fig. 17C), whereas the lentiform nucleus is located close to the lateral surface of the hemisphere.

The other important event concerns the development of the caudate nucleus, which is closely related to the lateral ventricle throughout its extent. The caudal part of the caudate, the tail, describes a semicircular curve similar to that displayed by the temporal horn of the lateral ventricle as it reaches into the temporal lobe. Since the caudate nucleus is situated in the floor of the central part of the lateral ventricle, it is easily appreciated that the tail of the caudate forms part of the roof of the temporal horn (Fig. 21A). The lentiform nucleus, which is situated close to the lateral surface underneath the future insula, is not affected to the same extent by the development of the temporal lobe.

Corpus striatum also contains the primordial tissue for the *amygdaloid body* in the temporal lobe. This large collection of cell groups, which is located in front of the temporal horn of the lateral ventricle (Fig. 21A), is an important part of the limbic system (see Chapter 17).

Topography of Corpus Striatum, Thalamus, and Internal Capsule

The development of the corpus striatum in the telencephalon is matched by the growth of another nuclear mass, the *thalamus,* in the wall of the diencephalon (Figs. 13B and 20B). Whereas thalamus is in direct contact with the caudate nucleus it is separated from the lentiform nucleus by the *internal capsule.* These relationships can be appreciated in Figs. 20–22.

The internal capsule, which is V-shaped in horizontal sections, is located on the medial side of the lentiform nucleus (Fig. 21B). The anterior limb

Fig. 19. Development of Corpus Callosum and Fornix ▷
A. Median section in a 10-week embryo showing the commissural plate and its development into the corpus callosum.
B. Median section through the corpus callosum and diencephalon.
C. Three-dimensional drawing illustrating the relationships between corpus callosum, fornix, and hippocampus.

of the capsule is located between the head of the caudate and the lentiform nucleus, whereas the posterior limb separates the thalamus from the lentiform nucleus. The angle between the two limbs is referred to as the *genu*. The extent of the internal capsule becomes more evident in a three-dimensional drawing (Fig. 22). The posterior part of the internal capsule literally wraps around the posterior half of the lentiform nucleus, forming the *retrolenticular* and *sublenticular* parts of the internal capsule.

The fibers on the outside of the lentiform nucleus form the *external capsule* (Fig. 21B), whereas the *extreme capsule* separates another nucleus, the *claustrum,* from the cortex of the insula.

The shape of the lentiform nucleus resembles a somewhat compressed ice cream cone with the tip directed medially. It is not a homogenous structure like the caudate nucleus, but can be easily separated, even on macroscopic inspection, into *putamen* and *globus pallidus* (Fig. 21B). The putamen and caudate nucleus are characterized by a large number of densely packed small neurons, and their common origin from the striate body is further revealed by the fact that the two structures are in continuity with each other through cell bridges located between the fiber bundles of the internal capsule. This is especially evident in the anterior limb of the internal capsule (Fig. 21B). Globus pallidus is characterized by large spindle-shaped cells that lie rather far apart. It also contains a large number of myelinated fibers, which explains its pale color. Considering these morphologic and developmental aspects, it seems reasonable to underscore the distinction between *pallidum* (globus pallidus) and the *striatum* (caudate nucleus and putamen). *Corpus striatum* is used as a collective term for the caudate nucleus, putamen, and globus pallidus. These three nuclei represent the main components of the basal ganglia (Chapter 8).

The topographic anatomy of the basal ganglia and the internal capsule is complicated and does not lend itself easily to verbal descriptions and illustrations. The relationships, however, are beautifully revealed in brain dissections.

CLINICAL NOTES

Chromosomal Abnormalities and Environmental Factors and Their Effect on the Brain

Many genetic disorders may damage the developing nervous system, and its protracted maturation makes it especially vulnerable to a variety of harmful environmental factors. It is not always possible to identify the specific factor, or *teratogen,* that causes congenital neurologic malformations. Development of the nervous system starts by the third embryonic week. Although cell multiplication and migration usually are completed before birth, some of the cells in the brain, e.g., granular cells in hippocampus and cerebellum, arise postnatally. Further, development of neuronal processes and establishment of synaptic connections continue into early childhood and probably even beyond. Most of the glial cells also seem to arise postnatally, and some of the fiber systems are not fully myelinated until the 2nd or 3rd year after birth.

Chromosomal and Genetic Factors

Chromosomal anomalies and abnormal genes are responsible for many forms of *mental retardation.* One example is *mongolism* (Down's syndrome or trisomy 21). The child has 47 chromosomes instead of 46, with an extra chromosome 21 from meiotic nondisjunction. It is recognizable at birth because of characteristic body features, including medial epicanthal folds with concomitant slanting of the eyes. The chromosomal abnormality can be diagnosed in utero by cytogenetic examination of the amniotic fluid, a procedure now frequently recommended for older mothers, who have increased risk of chromosomal abnormalities. Cytogenetic study would provide an opportunity for abortion to prevent the birth of a child with mongolism if the parents so desire.

A variety of *metabolic disorders,* including phenylketonuria, are also characterized by mental retardation. Phenylketonuria is one of the most com-

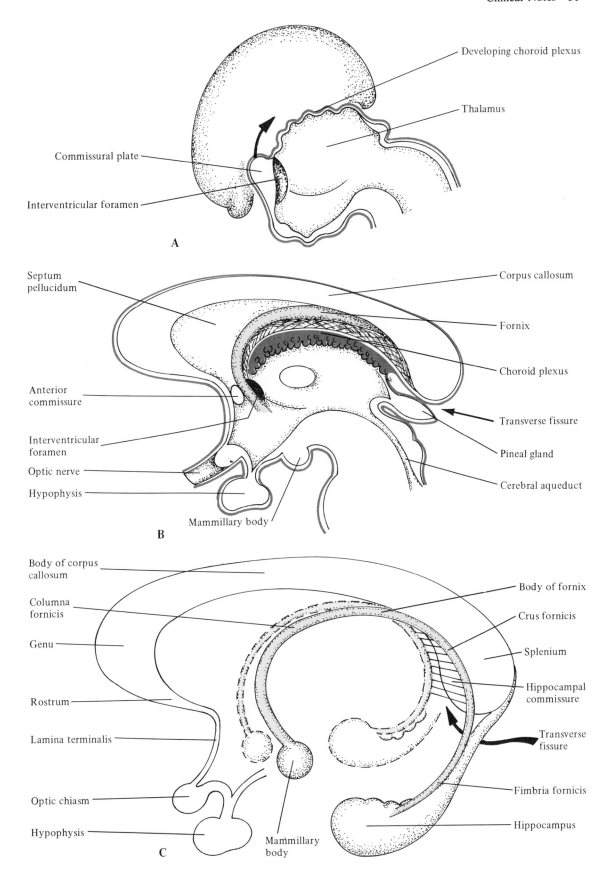

A

B

C

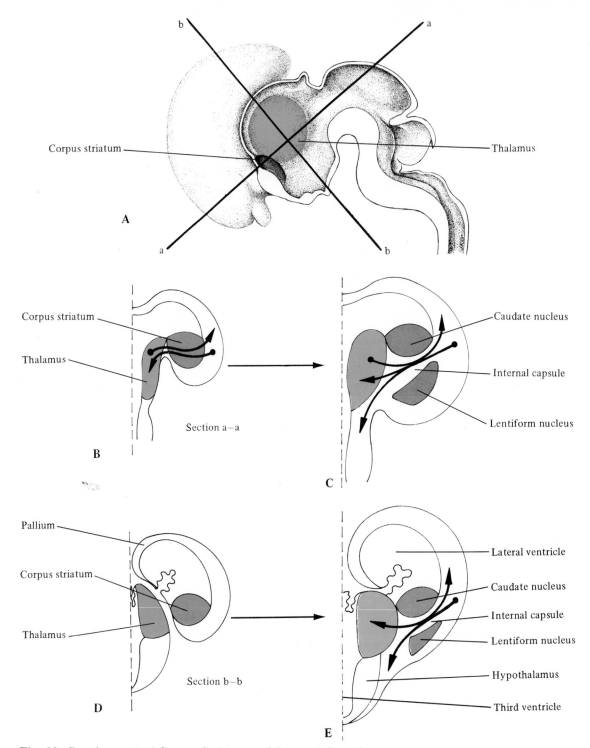

Fig. 20. Development of Corpus Striatum and Internal Capsule

A. The medial surface of the brain in a 43-mm embryo. Thalamus (*blue*) is developing in the diencephalon, and corpus striatum in the basal part of telencephalon. Part of corpus striatum (*red*) can be seen through the interventricular foramen.

B and C. Horizontal sections (a-a in A) through the developing brain showing the concentration of projection fibers in the internal capsule, which divides the corpus striatum into caudate and lentiform nuclei.

D and E. Transverse sections (b-b in A) through the developing brain.

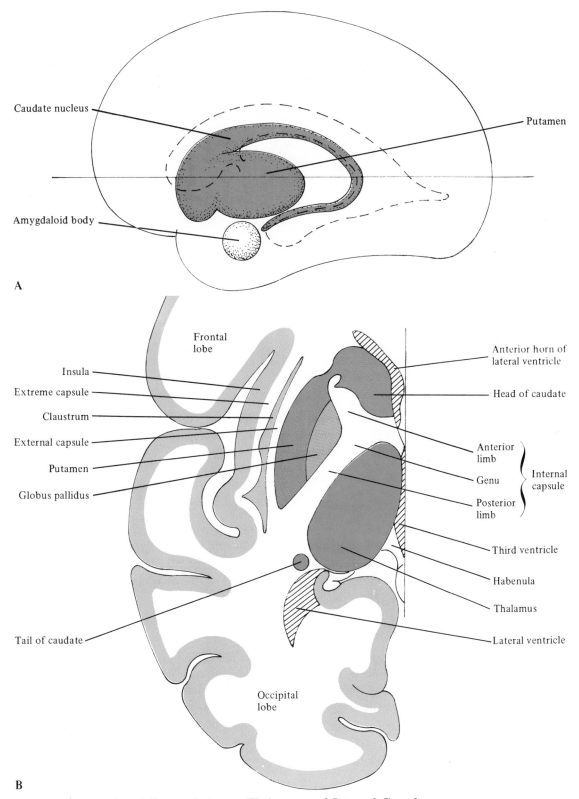

Fig. 21. Topography of Corpus Striatum, Thalamus, and Internal Capsule
A. A schematic drawing showing the location of the striatum and amygdaloid body and their relationship to the ventricle system in the cerebral hemisphere (side view).
B. Horizontal section (as indicated in **A**) through the corpus striatum, thalamus, and internal capsule.

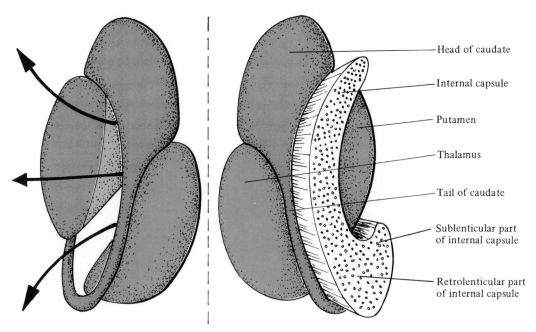

Head of caudate

Internal capsule

Putamen

Thalamus

Tail of caudate

Sublenticular part
of internal capsule

Retrolenticular part
of internal capsule

Fig. 22. Internal Capsule
Three-dimensional drawing showing the topography of the internal capsule, corpus striatum, and thalamus (Modified after Benninghoff, A., 1954. Lehrbuch der Anatomie des Menschen. Dritter Band: Nervensystem, Haut und Sinnes-organe. Urban & Schwarzenberg, München-Berlin.)

mon forms of aminoaciduria. It is characterized by deficiency of the hepatic enzyme phenylalanine hydroxylase, which is necessary for the conversion of phenylalanine to tyrosine.

Maternal Infections

A congenital *rubella* (measles) infection, especially in the first or second trimester, may cause mental retardation and malformations of the eyes, the ears, and the heart. Every female who has not had a rubella infection should therefore be vaccinated against the disease before reaching childbearing age.

Toxoplasmosis, which can cause mental retardation and severe malformations of the brain, is usually not recognized in the pregnant woman. It is therefore difficult to estimate the frequency with which the intracellular parasite *Toxoplasma gondii* affects the neonatal brain.

Radiation, Chemical Substances, and Drugs

Among the many toxic substances known to be harmful to the developing brain are *radiation, steroid hormones,* and various *chemical substances*

including some drugs taken by the pregnant woman. *Thalidomide* is a well-known example, but there may be other potentially harmful drugs, including some *antiepileptic, antipsychotic,* and *antianxiety* drugs (tranquilizers).

Although we know too little about the teratogenicity of "street drugs" such as marijuana, lysergic acid diethylamide (LSD), and phencyclidine ("angel dust"), they are certainly not without potential danger and should therefore be avoided, especially by pregnant women.

Alcohol

Excessive alcohol consumption is generally recognized as a formidable health problem, but it is worth remembering that alcohol is also recognized as a fetal pathogen by most experts, and it should therefore be avoided, especially by the pregnant woman.

Malnutrition

Malnutrition and protein deficiencies adversely affect neurologic and mental maturation, and since malnutrition is rampant in many parts of the

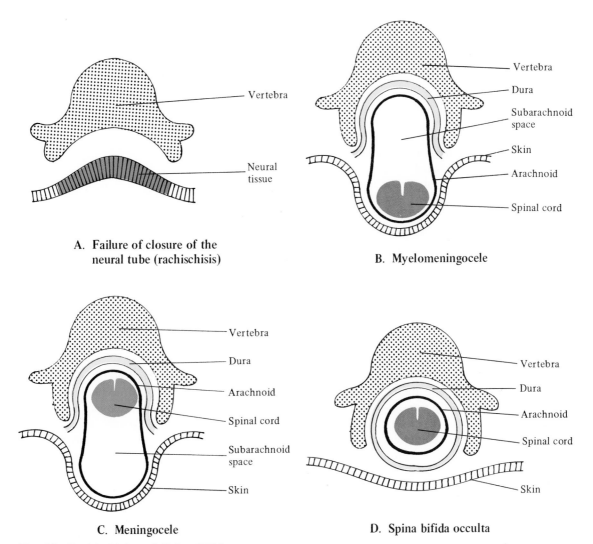

A. Failure of closure of the neural tube (rachischisis)

B. Myelomeningocele

C. Meningocele

D. Spina bifida occulta

Fig. 23. Rachischisis and Spina Bifida
Diagrammatie features of various types of spina bifida. (From Escourolle, R. and J. Poirier, 1978. Manual of basic neuropathology. Translated to english by L. J. Rubinstein. 2nd. ed. W. B. Saunders Co. Philadelphia. With permission of Masson S. A. Paris.)

world, it is a health problem of gigantic proportions. The remedy for this grave condition seems obvious, but the cures are far from simple, primarily because the crucial factors and decisions involved are political rather than medical.

Rachischisis and Spina Bifida

The development of the neural tube is a critical process. If the neural groove fails to close, neural tissue remains exposed to the surface. The many variations of this serious condition are usually included in the term *rachischisis* (Fig. 23A). A defective closure of the neural tube at the cranial end may prevent development of the brain and lead

to a malformation known as *anencephaly*. The hemispheres or the whole forebrain are usually absent, and the little brain tissue that is present is exposed to the surface. Anencephaly is almost always accompanied by severe *myeloschisis* (cleft spinal cord), and the infants are usually born dead.

Spina bifida refers to a defect of the vertebral column. It often is accompanied by posterior midline protrusion of the spinal cord (Fig. 23). There are many variations ranging from *spina bifida occulta* (Fig. 23D), in which the abnormality is confined to the vertebrae only (unclosed posterior arch), to defects that involve the spinal cord and the meninges. If only the meninges protrude through the defect, the condition is referred to as a *meningocele* (Fig. 23C). A more severe form is *myelomeningocele* (Fig. 23B), in which elements of the CNS protrude as well. This condition is often associated with neural deficits and hydrocephalus (see below).

The Eye

The development of the eye presents many aspects of great importance in clinical medicine. Of special significance is the fact that the retina is an outgrowth of the prosencephalon and that the optic nerve is a central brain tract. When clinicians look at the retina through the ophthalmoscope, they are actually looking at a part of the CNS.

Papilledema

The optic nerve is surrounded by the same membranes that cover the brain, and the subarachnoid space that surrounds the brain is in direct communication with a similar potential space around the optic nerve. An increase in the intracranial pressure, therefore, is directly transmitted to the subarachnoid space surrounding the optic nerve, with subsequent swelling of the optic disc, i.e., papilledema, which is one of the cardinal signs of increased intracranial pressure (see Fig. 155, Chapter 13).

Coloboma

This malformation results from an incomplete fusion of the choroid fissure. It may be restricted to a cleft in the iris or may extend into the retina and the optic nerve.

Retinal Detachment

Retinal detachment is a pathologic separation of the retina from the pigment layer. It is in effect a reformation of the space originally present in the optic vesicle, and it can be caused by many conditions, including tumors and infections. It can also occur in response to trauma, especially in myopic eyes.

Craniopharyngioma

Epithelial rests of Rathke's pouch in the region of the hypophysis sometimes give rise to a tumor that usually expands in a dorsal direction into the third ventricle. Although the tumor can occur at all ages, it is especially common in children.

Hydrocephalus

This is a condition characterized by an accumulation of CSF. Congenital hydrocephalus often results from an obstruction occurring somewhere along the CSF pathway, especially where the passage is narrow, as in the cerebral aqueduct or in the region of the foramina of the fourth ventricle. Hydrocephalus causes enlargement of the cerebral ventricles and thinning of the cerebral substance. Congenital hydrocephalus is often apparent at birth or soon thereafter because of enlargement of the head, widening of the sutures, and bulging fontanelles (see also Clinical Notes, Chapter 3).

SUGGESTED READING

1. Cowan, W. M., 1979. The Development of the Brain. Scientific American, 241 (3): 107–117.
2. Hamilton, W. J. and H. W. Mossman, 1972. Hamilton, Boyd and Mossman's Human Embryology; Prenatal Development of Form and Function, 4th ed. Heffer: Cambridge, England, pp. 437–535.
3. Jacobson, M., 1978. Developmental Neurobiology, 2nd ed. Plenum Press: New York.
4. Lou, H. C., 1982. Developmental Neurology. Raven Press: New York.
5. Lund, R. D., 1978. Development and Plasticity of the Brain: An Introduction. Oxford University Press: New York.
6. Sidman, R. L. and P. Rakic, 1982. Development of the Human Central Nervous System. In W. Haymaker and R. D. Adams (eds.): Histology and Histopathology of the Nervous System. Charles C Thomas: Springfield, Illinois, pp. 3–145.
7. Volpe, J. J., 1981. Neurology of the Newborn. W. B. Saunders: Philadelphia, pp. 3–59.

3

Meninges and Cerebrospinal Fluid

DURA MATER
  Dural Folds
  Dural Venous Sinuses

PIA–ARACHNOID

CEREBROSPINAL FLUID

MENINGES OF THE SPINAL CORD
  Dura Mater Spinalis
  Pia Mater and Arachnoidea Spinalis

CLINICAL NOTES
  Head Injuries
  Subdural and Extradural Hemorrhage
  Transtentorial Herniation
  Meningitis
  Hydrocephalus
  Lumbar Puncture

SUGGESTED READING

The brain and the spinal cord are surrounded by three mesodermal coverings or meninges: the dura mater, the arachnoid, and the pia mater. The space between the pia mater and the arachnoid, i.e., the subarachnoid space, is filled with CSF, which serves as a cushion between the delicate CNS and the rigid skull.

The meninges and their various specializations have important protective and supportive functions. In addition special meningeal features are related to the production, circulation, and absorption of CSF, and endothelial-lined sinuses of the dura mater convey the venous blood to the internal jugular veins.

The meninges and their relationships to the brain and the CSF system are of great relevance in a number of clinical conditions including head injuries, intracranial hemorrhages, infections, and hydrocephalus.

DURA MATER

The tough and fibrous dura mater, or pachymeninx, is partly attached to the inner surface of the cranial cavity. Two large sheets of dura, the falx cerebri and tentorium cerebelli, divide the cranial cavity into three communicating compartments i.e., two supratentorial compartments, and one infratentorial compartment (Fig. 24).

Dural Folds

1. The *falx cerebri* is suspended vertically in the longitudinal cerebral fissure between the two cerebral hemispheres, thereby dividing the supratentorial compartment into a right and a left half (Fig. 24B). The falx cerebri is attached to the crista galli of the ethmoid bone in the front and to the horizontally suspended tentorium cerebelli in the back (Fig. 24C).
2. The *tentorium cerebelli* is a tent-like partial partition between the middle and posterior cranial fossae. It divides the cranial cavity into supratentorial and infratentorial compartments (Fig. 24B), and separates the cerebellum from the occipital lobes. Its free anterior edge forms the major part of a large oval opening, the *tentorial notch* or *incisure* (Fig. 24C), which surrounds the midbrain.
3. The *falx cerebelli* is a small midline dural fold in the posterior fossa. It is attached to the posterior inferior surface of the tentorium cerebelli and projects forward into the posterior cerebellar notch, which partly separates the two cerebellar hemispheres.
4. The *diaphragma sellae* is a small circular dural fold that bridges over the sella turcica and covers the pituitary gland. The stalk of the pituitary, which is attached to the base of the brain, passes through an opening in the center of the diaphragma sellae (Fig. 24C).

Dural Venous Sinuses

The cerebral veins are divided into external and internal veins, all of which eventually drain into venous sinuses. The sinuses are endothelium-lined spaces between two layers of dura. They occur along the attachments of the dural folds (Figs. 24B and 28).

Many of the external veins that drain the cerebral cortex on the convexity of hemisphere empty into the superior saggital sinus (Fig. 28). The external veins on the ventral surface of the brain connect with sinuses located in more basal parts of the skull cavity. The blood finally reaches the internal jugular vein through the sinuses.

1. The *superior sagittal sinus* runs along the attachment of the falx cerebri (Fig. 25). It widens as it approaches the internal occipital tuberance to form the *confluence of sinuses,* and next continues as one of the transverse sinuses, usually the right transverse sinus. The superior sagittal sinus receives tributaries from the superior cerebral veins on the convexity of the cerebral hemisphere (Fig. 28).
2. The *inferior sagittal sinus* is situated along the inferior free margin of the falx cerebri (Fig. 25). It receives blood from the medial aspects of the hemisphere and from the falx cerebri.
3. The *straight sinus,* which represents the continuation of the inferior sagittal sinus, is situated along the attachment of the falx cerebri to the tentorium cerebelli (Fig. 25). The straignt sinus receives the *great cerebral vein of Galen* (v. cerebri magna), which collects the venous blood from the left and right *internal cerebral veins* (Fig. 25) as well as from the two basal veins. The two internal cerebral veins drain the central parts of the brain. The left and right basal veins, which pass dorsally around the cerebral peduncles to enter the great cerebral vein of Galen, drain the basal parts of the brain. The straight sinus is usually continuous with the left transverse sinus at the confluence of the sinuses.
4. The *transverse sinus* (lateral sinus) runs horizontally along the bony attachment of the tentorium cerebelli, which extends from the internal occipital tuberance to the base of the petrous portion of the temporal bone (Fig. 26).
5. The *sigmoid sinus,* which is a continuation of the transverse sinus, drains into the internal jugular vein passing through the jugular foramen (Fig. 26).
6. The *cavernous sinus* is located on the lateral surface of the body of the sphenoid bone and is in close relation to the internal carotid artery (Fig. 26). It is connected with its counterpart on the opposite side through intercavernous sinuses. The cavernous sinus, which receives blood from the pituitary, from the orbita through the ophthalmic veins, and from the middle cerebral veins, is drained by the superior and inferior petrosal sinuses.
7. The *superior and inferior petrosal sinuses* lie

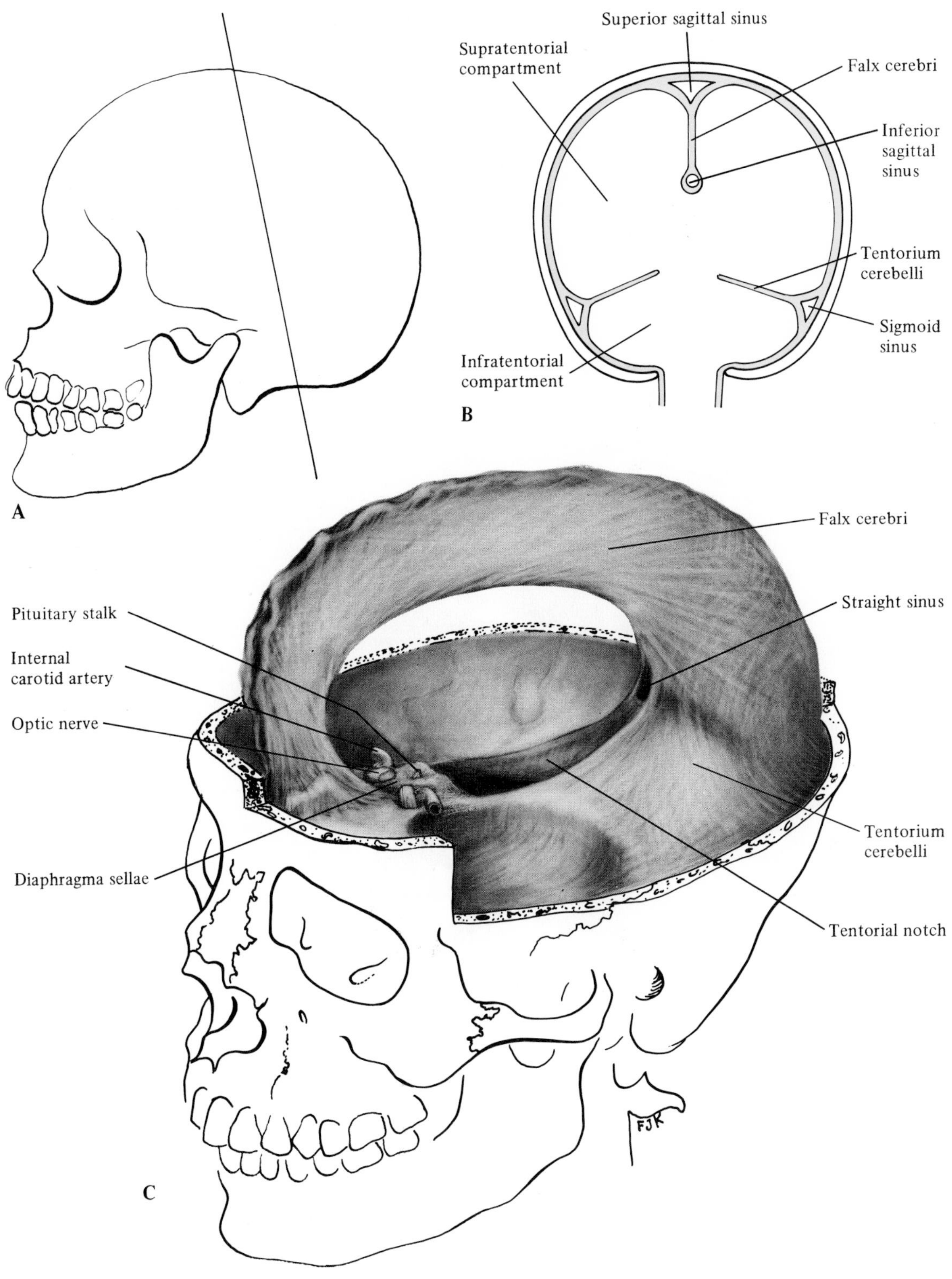

Fig. 24. Falx Cerebri and Tentorium Cerebelli

A illustrates the plane for the cross-section in **B,** which shows how the falx cerebri and tentorium cerebelli divide the skull cavity into supratentorial and infratentorial compartments. The thickness of the dura is exaggerated. **C** shows the attachment of falx cerebri to the crista galli and the tentorium.

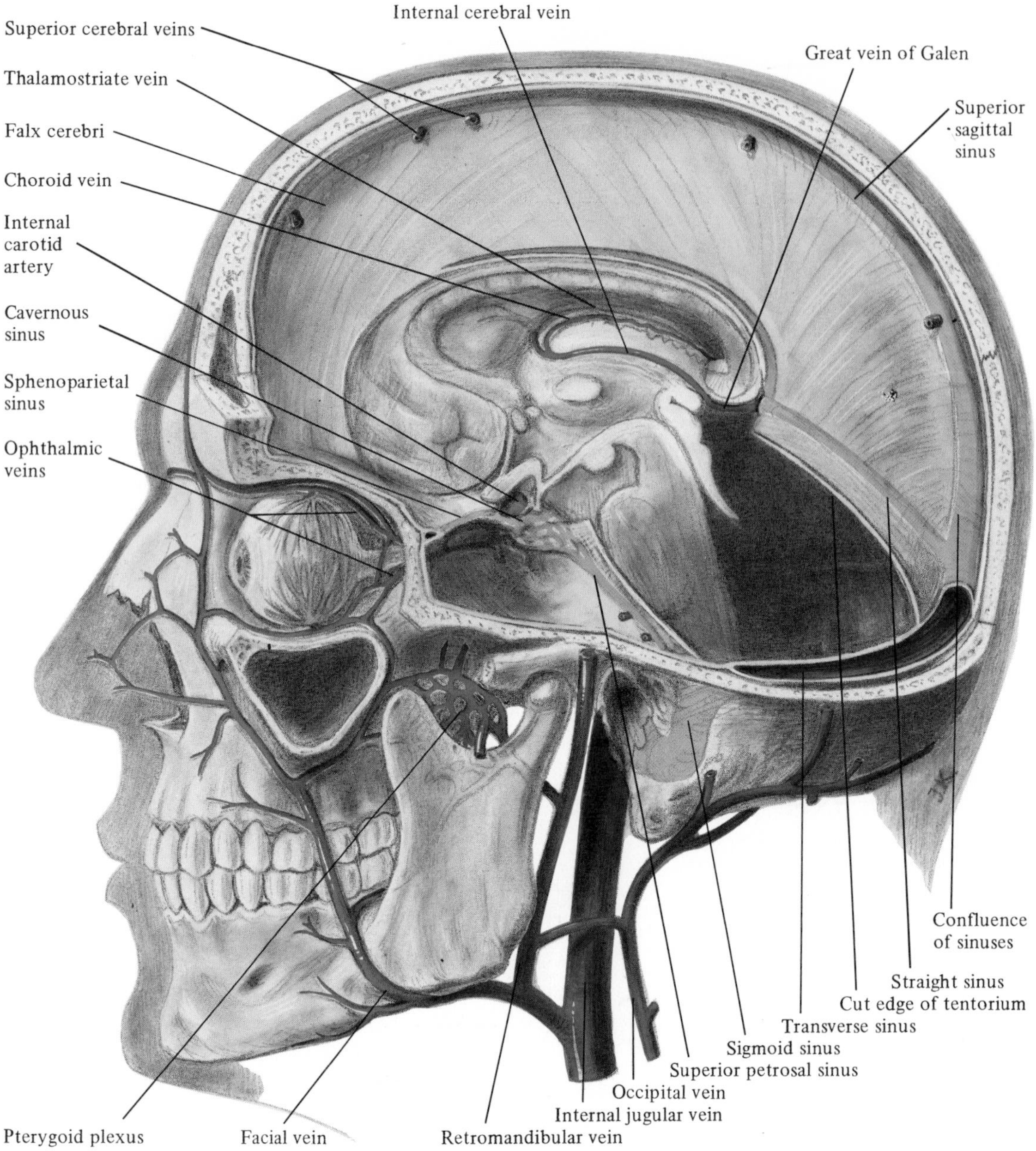

Superior cerebral veins

Thalamostriate vein

Falx cerebri

Choroid vein

Internal carotid artery

Cavernous sinus

Sphenoparietal sinus

Ophthalmic veins

Internal cerebral vein

Great vein of Galen

Superior sagittal sinus

Confluence of sinuses

Straight sinus

Cut edge of tentorium

Transverse sinus

Sigmoid sinus

Superior petrosal sinus

Occipital vein

Internal jugular vein

Retromandibular vein

Facial vein

Pterygoid plexus

Fig. 25. The Venous Sinuses and the Veins of the Head
Dissection of the dural venous sinuses and the deep veins of the brain. The left half of the brain and the entire cerebellum have been removed. The deep veins in the floor of the right lateral ventricle have been exposed by removing septum, fornix, and part of corpus callosum.

upon the superior and posterior margins of the petrous temporal bone (Fig. 26). The superior petrosal sinus connects the cavernous sinus with the junction of the transverse and sigmoid sinuses. The inferior petrosal sinus is continuous with the internal jugular vein.

PIA–ARACHNOID

The very thin pia mater is intimately associated with the surface of the brain, dipping into its fissures and sulci. The arachnoid, however, bridges over the various irregularities of the brain. The

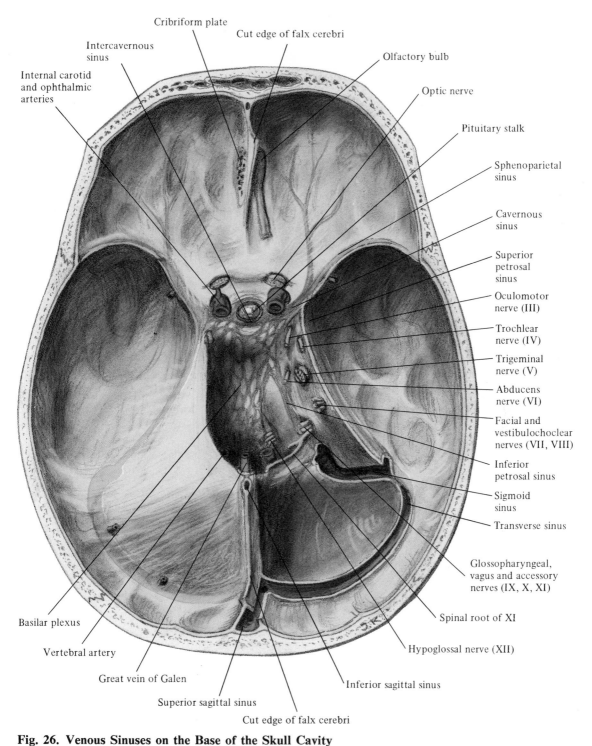

Cribriform plate

Cut edge of falx cerebri

Intercavernous sinus

Olfactory bulb

Internal carotid and ophthalmic arteries

Optic nerve

Pituitary stalk

Sphenoparietal sinus

Cavernous sinus

Superior petrosal sinus

Oculomotor nerve (III)

Trochlear nerve (IV)

Trigeminal nerve (V)

Abducens nerve (VI)

Facial and vestibulochoclear nerves (VII, VIII)

Inferior petrosal sinus

Sigmoid sinus

Transverse sinus

Glossopharyngeal, vagus and accessory nerves (IX, X, XI)

Spinal root of XI

Hypoglossal nerve (XII)

Basilar plexus

Vertebral artery

Great vein of Galen

Superior sagittal sinus

Inferior sagittal sinus

Cut edge of falx cerebri

Fig. 26. Venous Sinuses on the Base of the Skull Cavity

Tentorium cerebelli has been removed on the right side to expose the sigmoid and inferior petrosal sinuses as well as the exits of the cranial nerves.

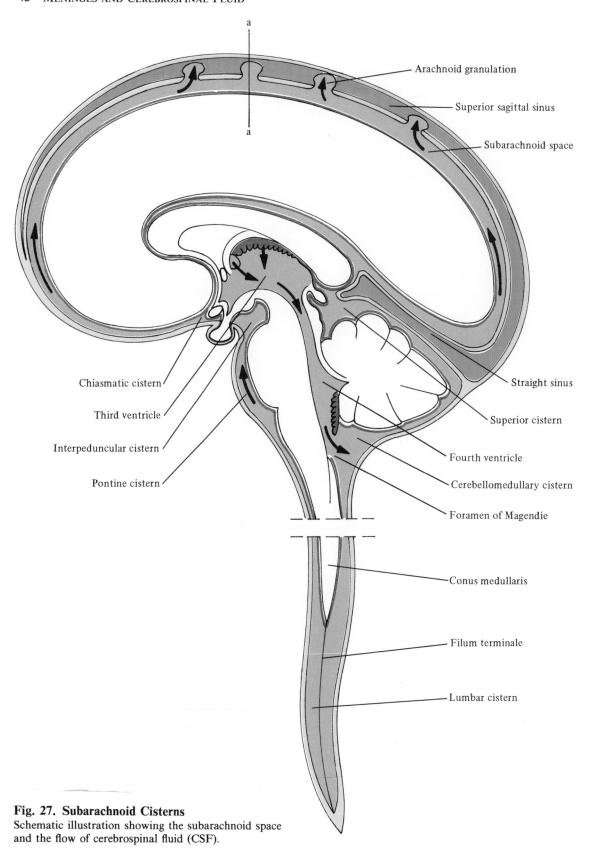

a

a

Arachnoid granulation

Superior sagittal sinus

Subarachnoid space

Chiasmatic cistern

Third ventricle

Interpeduncular cistern

Pontine cistern

Straight sinus

Superior cistern

Fourth ventricle

Cerebellomedullary cistern

Foramen of Magendie

Conus medullaris

Filum terminale

Lumbar cistern

Fig. 27. Subarachnoid Cisterns
Schematic illustration showing the subarachnoid space
and the flow of cerebrospinal fluid (CSF).

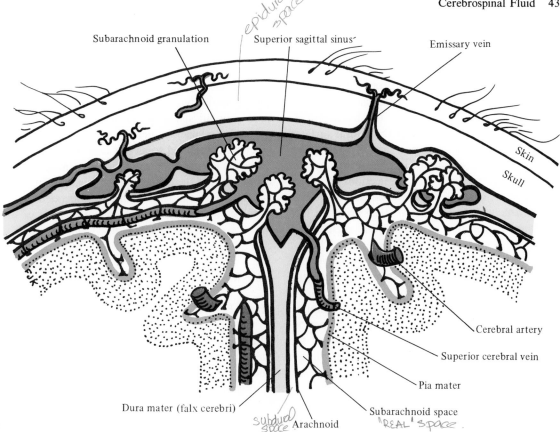

Subarachnoid granulation

Superior sagittal sinus

epidural space.

Emissary vein

Skin

Skull

Cerebral artery

Superior cerebral vein

Pia mater

Dura mater (falx cerebri)

subdural space   Arachnoid

Subarachnoid space
"REAL" space.

Fig. 28. Superior Sagittal Sinus and Arachnoid Granulations
Transverse section (indicated in Fig. 27) through the superior sagittal sinus showing the arachnoid granulations and the relationships between the different meninges.

space between the pia and arachnoid, the *subarachnoid space,* contains CSF, which serves as a protective "water cushion" for the brain and spinal cord. The pia and the arachnoid, together known as the leptomeninges, are connected by fine connective tissue strands or trabeculae. The relationships between the two membranes are in many areas so intimate that they can be regarded as one entity, the *pia–arachnoid.* In certain regions, however, the subarachnoid space widens to form cavities, the subarachnoid cisterns (Fig. 27):

1. *Cerebellomedullary cistern* (cisterna magna), between the cerebellum and the medulla oblongata

2. *Pontine cistern,* surrounding the pons

3. *Interpeduncular cistern,* between the two cerebral peduncles

4. *Superior cistern* between the splenium and the superior surfaces of the midbrain and the cerebellum. The superior cistern and the interpeduncular cistern are continuous with the

5. *Cisterna ambiens* on the sides of the midbrain

6. *Cistern of the lateral fossa* on the lateral side of the hemisphere where the arachnoid bridges over the lateral fissure

7. *Chiasmatic cistern* below and anterior to the optic chiasm.

CEREBROSPINAL FLUID

The CSF fills the ventricular system and the subarachnoid space. It is a clear and colorless waterlike fluid that is formed primarily by the choroid plexus in the lateral ventricles and, to a lesser degree, by the choroid plexus of the third and fourth ventricles. The formation of CSF is complex and includes both passive filtration and active secretory mechanisms.

CSF produced in the lateral ventricles enters the third ventricle through the interventricular foramen and flows through the cerebral aqueduct into the fourth ventricle (Fig. 27). It then reaches the subarachnoid space through three openings, the *median aperture* (foramen of Magendie) in the posterior medullary velum and the two *lateral apertures* (foramina of Luschka) in the lateral recesses of the fourth ventricle. From the cerebello-medullary cistern and the pontine cistern, the CSF flows through the cisterns on the basal surface of the brain and upward over the lateral surfaces to the region of the superior sagittal sinus. Here most of the fluid is absorbed into the venous system through the *arachnoid villi.* Collections of microscopic arachnoid villi form macroscopic elevations, *arachnoid granulations,* that protrude into the lateral expansions of the superior saggital sinus through openings in the dura mater (Fig. 28).

The flow of CSF is fairly rapid. The total volume of CSF in the ventricle system and the subarachnoid space is only about 125 ml, but it is estimated that more than 4 times that amount, or about 500 ml, is formed during a 24-h period. A small amount of CSF seeps down around the spinal cord, but little is known about its circulation and absorption in the spinal subarachnoid space.

MENINGES OF THE SPINAL CORD

Dura Mater Spinalis

The spinal cord is enveloped by membranes that are directly continuous with those covering the brain. Unlike the situation in the skull cavity, in which the dura mater is attached to the periosteum of the skull, the *spinal dura mater* forms a tubular sac that is firmly attached to the bone only at the margin of the foramen magnum. The dural sac ends at the level of the second sacral vertebra. A filamentous extension of the spinal cord, the *filum terminale* stretches from the caudal tip of the spinal cord to the bottom of the dural sac, where it is closely united with the dural sheath to form a cord, which stretches further caudally to become continuous with periosteum of the coccygeal bone (Fig. 31). Between the spinal dura mater and the periosteum of the vertebral canal is the *extradural space,* which it filled with a venous plexus and adipose tissue. The anterior and posterior spinal nerve roots are surrounded by a common dural sleeve that is continuous with the epineurium of the spinal nerve at the level of the intervertebral foramen.

Pia Mater and Arachnoidea Spinalis

Whereas the *pia mater* is intimately attached to the surface of the spinal cord, the *arachnoid* is closely associated with the spinal dura mater. The subarachnoid space, which is filled with CSF, is particularly spacious below the conus medullaris, where it is referred to as the *lumbar cistern.* This cistern is occupied by the filum terminale and the nerve roots of the cauda equina (Fig. 6). Throughout its length the spinal cord is suspended in the dural sac by 21 pairs of lateral extensions of the pia, the *denticulate ligaments.*

CLINICAL NOTES

Head Injuries

The brain is well protected by the skull and the dura mater. Nevertheless, brain damage is a frequent complication in head injuries, which are common in motorized and industrial societies. The brain injury may take the form of a "knock-out" or *concussion,* with transient loss of consciousness but no obvious injury to the brain, or there may be ecchymosis in the brain tissue, referred to as *contusion.* Finally, hemorrhage or laceration may occur and cause severe and permanent symptoms.

The most important consideration in the case of a skull fracture is the extent and nature of damage to the brain. Fractures of the base of the skull, which are difficult to detect in X-ray films, are more apt to cause severe damage to the brain or cranial nerves than are simple linear fractures of the vault. Leakage of CSF from the nose or bleeding from the auditory canal indicates the presence of a basal fracture. Although the brain can be severely damaged without any evidence of skull fracture, fractures of the cranial cavity always increase the risk of meningeal infections and bleeding.

Subdural and Extradural Hemorrhage

These are serious and not infrequent complications of head injuries. A *subdural hematoma* is a common complication that may result from even trivial head trauma. The subdural bleeding, which is most often located over the convexity of the frontal or parietal lobes, is usually attributable to the tearing of veins that bridge the space between the brain and the superior sagittal sinus (Fig. 28). The condition may develop slowly, and recovery following prompt evacuation is usually good. Rapidly developing subdural hematoma is usually associated with cerebral contusion and venous and arterial bleeding. Such an acute subdural hematoma is often fatal.

A skull fracture may be associated with rupture of one of the meningeal arteries or dural sinuses. The middle meningeal artery (Fig. 29), the largest of the meningeal arteries, is often damaged as a result of a linear fracture in the parietotemporal region. The subsequent bleeding between the dura and the skull results in a rapidly expanding mass, an *epidural haematoma,* that can cause irreversible damage to the brain if it is not removed.

Transtentorial Herniation ✻ PROBLEM II

Intracranial pathologic processes, such as hemorrhages, tumors, or infections, tend to cause a displacement and deformation of brain tissue with subsequent rise in intracranial pressure. Herniations usually develop along lines of decreased resistance to expansion. Herniation of part of the temporal lobe through the tentorial notch, for instance, is a very serious complication of an expanding supratentorial lesion, e.g., an extradural or subdural hematoma. The herniating parts of the temporal lobe, the uncus and parahippocampal gyrus, compress the midbrain as well as other structures within the tentorial incisure (Fig. 30A).

Although the uncal herniation syndrome can be fully appreciated only on the basis of a more comprehensive understanding of the functional anatomy of the brain (see clinical case in Chapter 11), the main pathologic events will nevertheless be summarized at this point. The syndrome is characterized by an alarming *deterioration of consciousness* to a state of deep coma (unconsciousness) within minutes or hours. The 3rd cranial nerve, the oculomotor nerve, is likely to be affected at an early stage, as it is caught between the posterior cerebral artery and the superior cerebellar artery. This usually causes initial constriction followed by *dilation of the pupil* on the side of the herniation (Fig. 30B). The cerebral peduncle contralateral to the herniation is compressed against the free edge of the tentorium. This is likely to

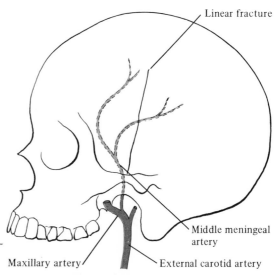

Fig. 29. Middle Meningeal Artery and Epidural Hematoma
Diagram showing the location of the middle meningeal artery on the inside of the skull. Epidural hematoma is often caused by a linear fracture in the parietotemporal region associated with rupture of the middle meningeal artery.

affect the descending corticofugal fiber bundles including the corticospinal (pyramidal) tract, which is of crucial importance for motor functions. Since the corticospinal tract crosses over to the opposite side in the pyramidal decussation in the lower part of the medulla oblongata, there will be a loss of motor functions on the same side as the uncal herniation, i.e., *ipsilateral hemiparesis* ("false localizing sign"). Compression of the posterior cerebral artery may cause obstruction of blood circulation with subsequent necrosis of the tissue (infarction) in the distribution area of the posterior cerebral artery. With further herniation hemorrhages in the brain stem decrease the chance of survival.

Herniations of brain tissue can also occur underneath the falx cerebri, i.e., *cingulate herniation,* or down through the foramen magnum, *tonsillar herniation* (Fig. 30C).

Meningitis

Infections of the meninges are relatively common. It is especially important to recognize those bacterial, protozoal, or fungal infections that can be successfully treated with antibiotics. The inflammatory reaction is usually related to the pia–

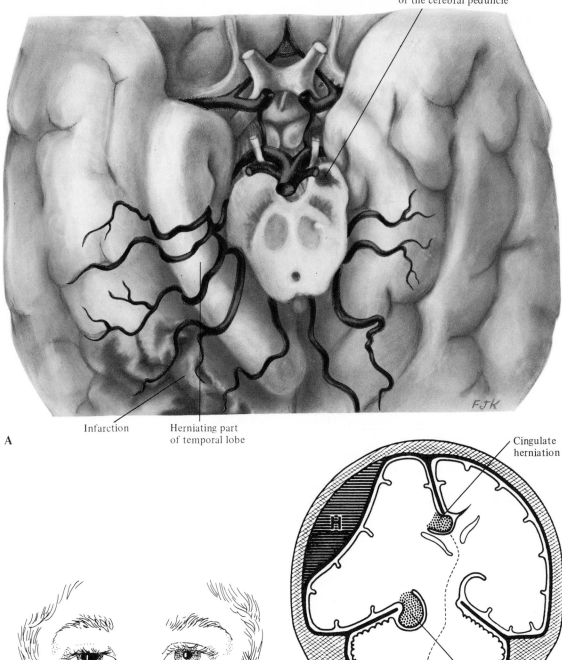

Hemorrhage in the base
of the cerebral peduncle

Infarction   Herniating part
of temporal lobe

A

Cingulate
herniation

Transtentorial
herniation

Tonsillar
herniation

B   **C**

Fig. 30. Transtentorial Herniation

A. Expanding supratentorial lesions may cause downward transtentorial herniation of the uncus and parahippocampal gyrus (*left side of figure*) with compression of the brain stem and injury to third nerve. (Based on a photograph provided by L. Rubinstein.)

B. Third nerve damage may lead to dilation of the ipsilateral pupil and ptosis of the upper lid.

C. Summary diagram of the major types of cerebral herniations. (From Escourolle and Poirier, 1978. Manual of basic neuropathy. Translated to english by L. J. Rubinstein. 2nd ed., W. B. Saunders Co., Philadelphia. With permission of Masson et Cie, Paris.)

arachnoid and to the subarachnoid space. Since the subarachnoid space is continuous, not only around the brain and the spinal cord, but also with the ventricular system, the infection rapidly reaches most parts of the CNS. The risk of complications increases if therapy is delayed. One example of a serious complication is the formation of fibrous adhesions between the pia and arachnoid, which may interfere with the circulation of CSF and cause hydrocephalus. Fever, headache, and stiff neck are common symptoms in a patient with meningitis, and the diagnosis is made by examining the CSF, which contains an increased number of white blood cells.

Hydrocephalus

This condition is characterized by an excessive amount of CSF in the ventricular system. Clinically important hydrocephalus are those cases in which the fluid is under increased pressure. This can happen because of increased production of the fluid, or because of disturbances in its circulation or absorption into the dural venous sinuses. Most cases of hydrocephalus with increased intracranial pressure are due to an obstruction in the circulation of CSF. The ventricular system contains several narrow passages, such as the interventricular foramen and the cerebral aqueduct, where a pathologic process can easily block the flow of CSF. If hydrocephalus occurs in childhood before the sutures have closed, the head may reach an enormous size unless the condition is treated. In older children and adults, in whom the sutures are closed, there is a gradual ventricular dilation with compression and thinning of brain tissue.

Lumbar Puncture

The composition of CSF, as well as its pressure, varies in different pathologic conditions. The analysis of the CSF can be of great help in establishing a diagnosis. The simplest and safest method of obtaining CSF is to insert a lumbar puncture needle into the lumbar cistern, which can be reached by placing the needle in the sagittal plane between the third and fourth, or the fourth and fifth lumbar spinal processes (Fig. 31). The spinal cord ends above L2; thus, there is no risk that the spinal cord will be damaged.

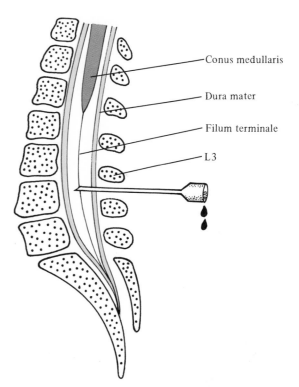

Fig. 31. Lumbar Puncture
CSF is obtained by inserting a needle into the lumbar cistern between the 3rd and 4th or 4th and 5th lumbar spinal processes.

Normal CSF contains very little protein (15–45 mg/ml) and only a few lymphocytes per cubic millimeter. Its sugar content is somewhat lower than that of the blood, although the concentration of NaCl is somewhat higher. The amount of the different components, however, may change drastically when inflammation or bleeding involve part of the ventricular system or the meninges. An increase of red blood cells, for instance, may indicate subarachnoid bleeding. The pressure of the CSF, which is a good indicator of the intracranial pressure, can be estimated by attaching a manometer to the lumbar puncture needle. The normal pressure is between 6 and 14 cm water. Lumbar puncture is occasionally performed for the purpose of introducing therapeutic substances or local anesthetics into the subarachnoid space, and radiologists use lumbar puncture for introducing air or an opaque medium into the subarachnoid space.

There are certain instances in which removal of CSF by lumbar puncture is dangerous. If, for instance, the intracranial pressure is greatly increased as a result of a brain tumor or bleeding, a sudden withdrawal of CSF from the spinal canal may cause downward herniation of the cerebellar tonsils through the foramen magnum (Fig. 30C).

A *tonsillar herniation* ("cerebellar pressure cone") will cause compression of the medulla oblongata, which may compromise vital respiratory and circulatory functions.

SUGGESTED READING

1. Browder, J. and H. A. Kaplan, 1976. Cerebral Dural Sinuses and Their Tributaries. Charles C Thomas: Springfield, Illinois.
2. DeJong, R. N., 1979. The Neurologic Examination, 4th ed. Harper & Row: Hagerstown, Maryland, pp. 743–795.
3. Fishman, R. A., 1980. Cerebrospinal Fluid in Diseases of the Nervous System. W. B. Saunders: Philadelphia.
4. Greenlee, J. E., 1979. Anatomic Considerations in Central Nervous System Infection. In G. L. Mandell, R. G. Douglas, and J. E. Bennett (eds.): Principles and Practice of Infectious Diseases. John Wiley: New York, pp. 725–738.
5. Jennett, B. and G. Teasdale, 1981. Management of Head Injuries. F. A. Davis: Philadelphia.
6. Wood, J. H., 1980. Neurobiology of Cerebrospinal Fluid. Plenum Press: New York.

PART 2
Dissection of the Brain

Introduction

First Dissection: Meninges and Subarachnoid Cisterns; Superficial Arteries; Vertebral–Basilar System; Internal Carotid System; Basal Surface and Cranial Nerves

Second Dissection: Midsagittal Section; Lobes, Sulci, and Gyri

Third Dissection: White Matter; Blunt Dissection of Major Fiber Systems

Fourth Dissection: Ventricular System, Fornix, and Basal Ganglia

Fifth Dissection: Fourth Ventricle; Cerebellum; Brain Stem

Sixth Dissection: Atlas of the Brain: Frontal, Sagittal, and Horizontal Brain Sections; Anatomical Correlation of Computerized Brain Tomography

Introduction

The dissection of the human brain is a rewarding experience for both teachers and students if it proceeds in a systematic fashion. How to arrange the dissection course in the most practical manner depends to a certain extent on time and number of brains available. Although a general goal should be to have the students participate actively in the dissections, an insufficient number of brains may restrict the laboratory activities to a series of prosections. The following dissection guide is suitable for a 15–20 hours dissection course. Although it would be ideal to have two brains available, the dissections can be completed with one whole brain in addition to one half brain obtained by subdividing a brain in the midsagittal plane.

The dissection course will be considerably more rewarding if a group of 10–15 students can be assigned a teaching assistant. If arrangements are made ahead of time, neurology, psychiatry, or neurosurgery residents may be willing to assist in the dissections. This makes it especially enjoyable for the students because the residents tend to relate the anatomy of the central nervous system to clinically relevant problems. In return, the residents get a welcome review of the brain anatomy.

To make it easier for the students to proceed with the dissections in a systematic fashion, it is advisable to have the assistants perform prosections of the different portions. This can, for instance, be arranged in the form of a preview of next day's session. As there is considerable variation in background and experience among the different teaching assistants, it may even be advisable to prepare the assistants by arranging a few practice sessions before the course starts. This ensures a certain uniformity in the teaching.

Following the autopsy, the brains are usually stored in strong formalin. To avoid the formalin fumes and reduce the risk of ecxema and conjunctivitis, the brains should be soaked in water for a few days before use. It is recommended that a pair of surgical gloves or thin plastic gloves be used. To prevent the brain specimens from drying between sessions, it is recommended that they be stored in alcohol or wrapped in a wet cloth in a plastic bag. The following instruments are needed for the brain dissection: brain knife, scalpel, scissors, forceps with fine terminals, anatomic forceps, and a probe.

The dissection described in this guide requires the use of at least one and a half brain. The whole brain will be used for the study of the surface anatomy and of inspection of the meninges and the superficial arteries. It will also be used for the exploration of the ventricular system and for the study of the basal ganglia and the internal capsule. The half brain will be used for the blunt dissection of major fiber tracts and the dissection can be facilitated by placing the brain in a freezer for several days. While the brain is in the freezer, it is advisable to store it in a plastic container filled with 10% formalin. Before the dissection, the brain is thawed in running cold water overnight. This deep freezing procedure, which was developed by Klingler, can with advantage be repeated several times.

First Dissection

Meninges and Subarachnoid Cisterns, Superficial Arteries, Vertebral-Basilar System, Internal Carotid System, Basal Surface, and Cranial Nerves

MENINGES AND SUBARACHNOID CISTERNS

The brain and the spinal cord are surrounded by three membranes, or meninges, which have protective and supportive functions.

Dura Mater (Pachymeninx)

Dura mater, which is partly attached to the inner surface of the cranial cavity, usually remains in the skull when the brain is removed at autopsy, and is therefore best studied in relation to the dissection of the head.

Arachnoidea and Pia Mater (Leptomeninx)

These two membranes are in many places so closely attached to each other by delicate fibrous strands, trabeculae, that they cannot be separated, and it is common practice to refer to them as an entity, the *pia–arachnoid*. However, there is a significant difference between the pia mater and the arachnoid in the sense that the pia closely follows the contour of the brain and dips into all irregularities of its surface, whereas the arachnoid follows the dura mater and therefore bridges over the irregularities. In places where the irregularities are pronounced, especially on the base of the brain, large cisterns are formed in the subarachnoid space between the pia and the arachnoid.

Subarachnoid Space and Subarachnoid Cisterns

The space between the pia and the arachnoid, the subarachnoid space, is filled with *cerebrospinal fluid* (CSF), which serves as a cushion for the delicate brain. This fluid comes from the ventricles of the brain and enters the subarachnoid space through three apertures in the fourth ventricle (see below). When the brain is removed from the skull, the fluid escapes and the subarachnoid space collapses. However, it should still be possible to identify some of the major cisterns on one of the brains before the meninges and the blood vessels are removed. Review the location of the following important subarachnoid cisterns (Fig. 27):

(large sub-arach. spaces)

1. *Cisterna magna* (cerebellomedullary cistern) in the angle between the cerebellum and the medulla oblongata. It receives CSF through the median aperture (Magendie) and the two lateral apertures (Luschkae) of the fourth ventricle.

2. *Superior cistern* (cistern of the great cerebral vein of Galen) is situated between the splenium of corpus callosum and the superior surface of mesencephalon. It is continuous with cisterna ambiens on the sides of the midbrain.

3. *Interpeduncular cistern* is located in the interpeduncular fossa in front of pons. *front of midbrain*

4. *Pontine cistern* surrounds the pons. *front of pons*

5. *Chiasmatic cistern* is situated below and anterior to the optic chiasm.

6. *Cistern of the lateral fossa* is an elongated expansion of the subarachnoid space at the place where the arachnoid bridges over the cleft formed by the lateral fissure.

7. *Lumbar cistern* of the spinal subarachnoid space is a large cavity, which extends from the second lumbar vertebra to the sacrum. It contains the cauda equina, and it can easily be reached by the aid of a lumbar puncture needle, if one needs to obtain CSF for diagnostic purposes (see Clinical Notes, Chapter 3).

Pneumoencephalography and CAT Scan

By injecting air or oxygen into the subarachnoid space, the subarachnoid cisterns as well as the ventricular system can be visualized on X-ray films. The procedure is called pneumoencephalography. The air is usually injected into the lumbar cistern with the patient sitting upright. By holding the head in different positions, it is possible to direct the air to the various cisterns as well as to different parts of the ventricular system. The use of pneumoencephalography makes it possible to detect intracranial lesions, which distort the normal anatomy of the subarachnoid and ventricular spaces. To be able to use the procedure effectively, however, it is necessary to have a good understanding of the normal anatomy of the subarachnoid cisterns and the ventricular system.

The newly developed technique of *computerized axial tomography* (CAT), which does not depend on the introduction of air into the subarachnoid space, has partly replaced pneumoencephalography for the visualization of many intracranial structures. The method is based on the use of a fine X-ray beam and a ring of sensitive detectors that rotate around the head. The information is fed into a computer, which builds up a cross-sectional picture of the head including the brain (Figs. 75–79). However, pneumoencephalography is still valuable, especially for studying the structures at the base of the cranial cavity, where thick bone formations tend to distort the CAT scan.

SUPERFICIAL ARTERIES

The brain holds a unique position in the human body in regard to blood supply. Although it is responsible for only 2% of the body weight in the adult, about one-fifth of the oxygenated blood that comes from the heart is carried to the brain. The blood reaches the brain through two pairs of arterial trunks, the *internal carotid arteries* and the *vertebral arteries* (see Fig. 180). Each internal carotid artery, which is a terminal branch of the common carotid artery, enters the skull through the carotid canal. The two major branches of the internal carotid artery, the *middle* and *anterior cerebral arteries*, supply the rostral parts of the brain including most of the basal ganglia and the internal capsule. The caudal parts of the brain, including the cerebellum and most of the brain stem, receive blood from the two vertebral arteries. The vertebral artery arises from the subclavian artery and ascends through the transverse processes of cervical vertebrae 1–6, whereupon it enters the skull through the foramen magnum. The vertebral arteries of the two sides unite at the caudal border of the pons to form the *basilar artery,* which in turn divides to form the two *posterior cerebral arteries* at the rostral border of the pons. Study the following arteries and arterial formations related to the vertebral–basilar system and the internal carotid system.

VERTEBRAL–BASILAR SYSTEM

Vertebral Artery (Fig. 32)

1. *Posterior inferior cerebellar artery* (PICA) is the largest branch of the vertebral artery. It pursues a tortuous course between the medulla oblongata and cerebellum, and supplies the dorsolateral part of the medulla oblongata, the choroid plexus of the fourth ventricle, and the posterior and inferior parts of the cerebellum.
2. *Anterior spinal artery* is a single artery formed by a contribution from each vertebral artery. It supplies the median and paramedian parts of the medulla oblongata before it descends into the vertebral canal, where it is reinforced by radicular branches as it continues along the length of the spinal cord.

Basilar Artery

The unpaired basilar artery is formed at the inferior border of the pons by the combination of the two vertebral arteries (Fig. 32). It lies in the midline on the ventral surface of pons and divides into the two posterior cerebral arteries at the upper margin of the pons. The basilar artery gives off the following branches:

1. *Anterior inferior cerebellar artery* (AICA) arises from the caudal end of the basilar artery. It supplies the upper medulla and lower pons before it reaches the inferior surface of the cerebellum.
2. *Internal auditory artery* (*labyrinthine artery*) is a branch of the basilar artery or the anterior inferior cerebellar artery. It reaches the membranous labyrinth of the inner ear through the internal auditory canal.
3. *Pontine arteries.* Numerous median and paramedian branches enter directly into pons.

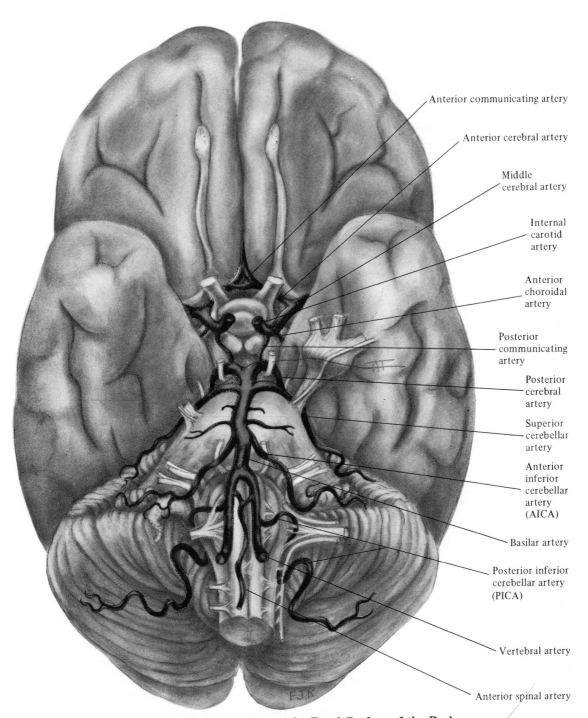

Anterior communicating artery

Anterior cerebral artery

Middle cerebral artery

Internal carotid artery

Anterior choroidal artery

Posterior communicating artery

Posterior cerebral artery

Superior cerebellar artery

Anterior inferior cerebellar artery (AICA)

Basilar artery

Posterior inferior cerebellar artery (PICA)

Vertebral artery

Anterior spinal artery

Fig. 32. Major Arteries on the Basal Surface of the Brain

4. *Superior cerebellar artery* arises from the rostral end of the basilar artery and passes posteriorly along the upper border of pons to reach the superior surface of the cerebellum. Note that the IIIrd cranial nerve, the oculomotor nerve, passes between the superior cerebellar artery and the posterior cerebral artery.

Posterior Cerebral Artery

Each of the two posterior cerebral arteries, which are terminal branches of the basilar artery, curves around the lateral aspect of the midbrain to reach the medial and inferior surfaces of the temporal +occipital lobes.

and occipital lobes of the cerebral hemisphere (Fig. 33). Branches from the proximal segment of the posterior cerebral artery penetrate the posterior perforating space to reach structures in the interior of the brain. Cortical branches from the posterior cerebral artery supply the visual cortex in the occipital lobe. The posterior cerebral artery is connected to the internal carotid artery on the same side through the *posterior communicating artery* (Fig. 32).

INTERNAL CAROTID SYSTEM

Internal Carotid Artery

The internal carotid artery is a terminal branch of the common carotid artery, and it enters the skull through the carotid canal and gives off several collateral branches before it divides into the two terminal branches, the *middle cerebral artery* and the *anterior cerebral artery*. The *hypophysial arteries* and the *ophthalmic artery* come off the internal carotid artery as soon as the artery has entered the skull and they are usually not present on the part that is attached to the brain specimen. Identify the following two branches of the internal carotid artery (Fig. 34):

1. *Posterior communicating artery* varies considerably in length and caliber. It runs in a caudal direction to join the posterior cerebral artery.

2. *Anterior choroidal artery,* which sometimes comes off the middle cerebral artery, passes in a caudolateral direction beside the optic tract before it enters the choroid fissure to reach the choroid plexus in the inferior horn of the lateral ventricle. The choroid plexus also receives one or several posterior choroidal arteries from the posterior cerebral artery (Fig. 34).

Middle Cerebral Artery (Figs. 35 and 36)

This is the largest branch of the internal carotid artery and it runs in a lateral direction between the temporal lobe and the frontal lobe toward the lateral fissure. Many perforating branches, *striate arteries,* emerge from the initial segment of the middle cerebral artery, and penetrate the anterior perforated space to supply important structures in the interior of the brain (Fig. 35). On reaching the lateral fissure, the middle cerebral artery divides into several large branches on the surface of the insula. These branches continue laterally and emerge on the lateral surface of the hemisphere between the lips of the lateral fissure. Practically the whole lateral surface of the hemisphere, including important motor and sensory areas of the cortex, is supplied by branches of the middle cerebral artery (Fig. 36).

Anterior Cerebral Artery

This terminal branch of the internal carotid artery runs in a medial and rostral direction between the optic nerve and the anterior perforated space to the region of the longitudinal fissure, where it is connected with the corresponding artery on the opposite side by the short *anterior communicating artery* (Fig. 35). Perforating arteries to the hypothalamus and to other important structures in the basal part of the brain arise from the proximal part of the anterior cerebral artery.

Distal to the anterior communicating artery, the two anterior cerebral arteries ascend in the longitudinal fissure, where they curve upward and backward above the corpus callosum. Although the two arteries lie close together during their course in the longitudinal fissure, they are separated by falx cerebri. The terminal ramifications of the anterior cerebral artery on the medial surface of the frontal and parietal lobes cannot be seen until the medial aspect of the hemisphere is exposed (Fig. 33).

Circle of Willis

The anterior and posterior communicating arteries help form an arterial circle, circulus arteriosus cerebri or Circle of Willis, which is of great clinical importance (see below). The very short anterior communicating artery connects the two anterior cerebral arteries in front of the optic chiasm, and the two posterior communicating arteries complete the posterior part of the circle by connecting the internal carotid artery with the posterior cerebral artery on each side. Small perforating arteries, which emanate from the different components of the Circle of Willis, supply the basal parts of diencephalon and mesencephalon. The initial segment of the anterior cerebral artery also gives rise to the *recurrent artery of Heubner,* which supplies the rostral limb of the internal capsule and adjacent parts of the basal ganglia (Fig. 35).

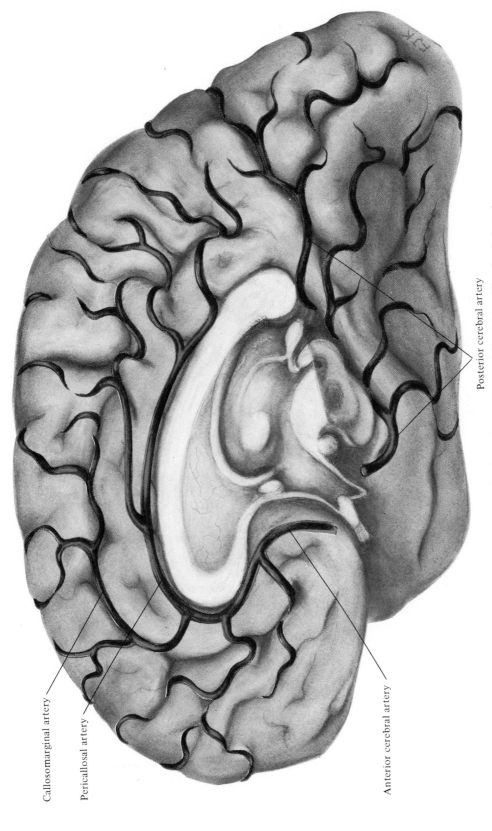

Posterior cerebral artery

Callosomarginal artery

Pericallosal artery

Anterior cerebral artery

Fig. 33. Cortical Distribution of Anterior and Posterior Cerebral Arteries

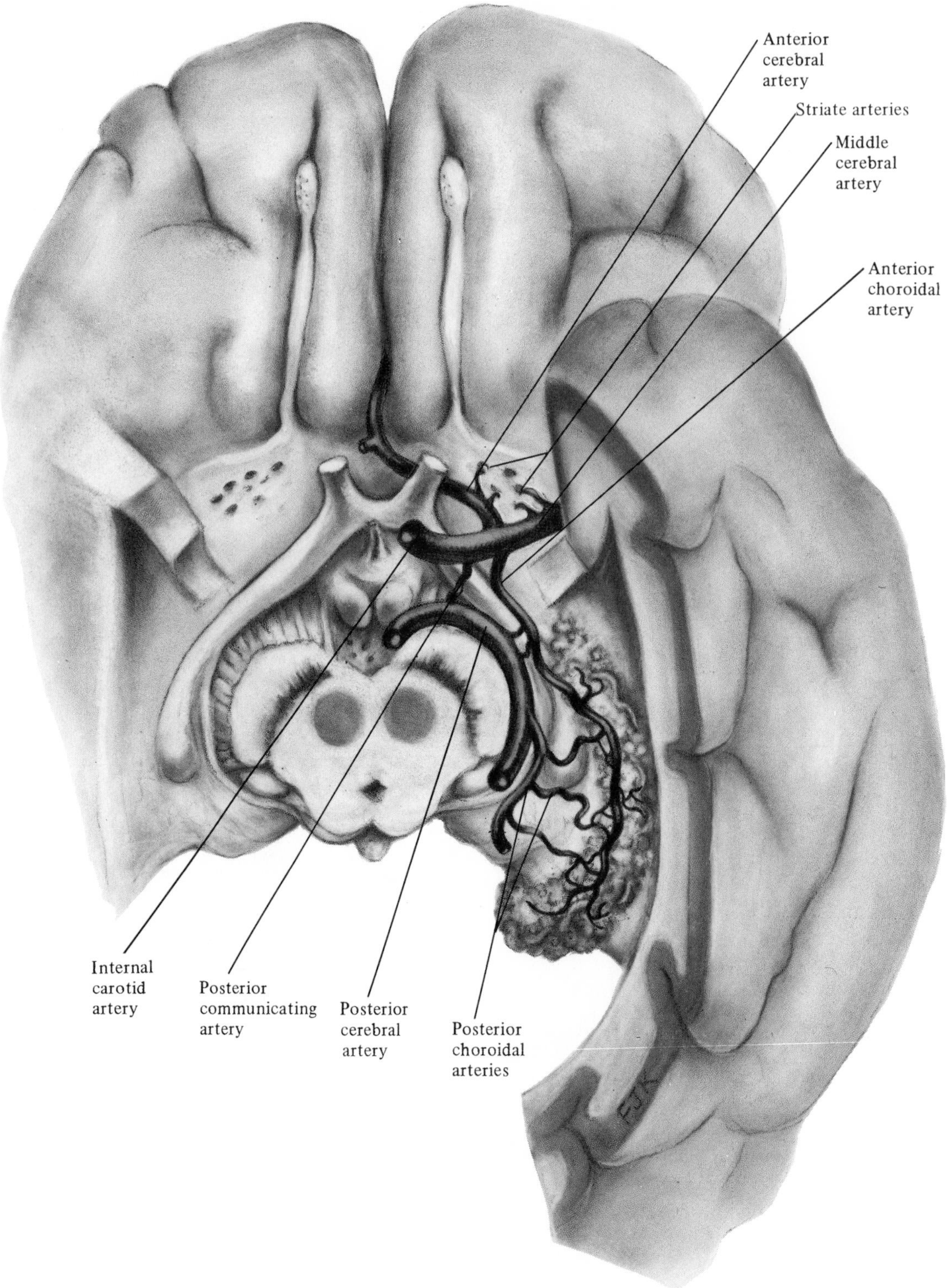

Fig. 34. Choroidal Arteries
The medial parts of the temporal lobes have been removed to illustrate the blood supply of the choroid plexus in the lateral ventricle.

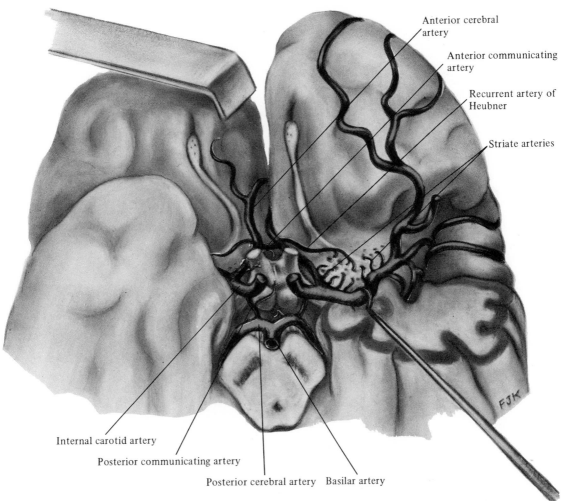

Anterior cerebral artery

Anterior communicating artery

Recurrent artery of Heubner

Striate arteries

Internal carotid artery

Posterior communicating artery

Posterior cerebral artery   Basilar artery

Fig. 35. Circle of Willis, Striate Arteries, and Anterior Perforated Space
The middle cerebral artery is retracted to show the striate arteries.

Clinical Notes

Disorders related to the blood vessels of the brain are very common. The functional anatomy of the cerebrovascular system will therefore be treated more fully in a separate chapter following the presentations of the different functional–anatomic systems of the brain.

Circle of Willis

The Circle of Willis is of great clinical importance because it provides for the possibility of collateral circulation in the event of occlusion in one of the major arteries proximal to the circle. A thrombosis in the internal carotid artery on one side, for in-

stance, may go unnoticed if sufficient collateral circulation can be established, either from the opposite internal carotid artery via the anterior communicating artery, or through the basilar artery via the posterior communicating artery. There are, however, great variations in the configuration of the circle, and an effective collateral circulation may not always be possible.

Cerebral Angiography

The vessels of the brain can be visualized by injecting a contrast medium into one of the large arterial trunks carrying blood to the brain. This is usually done by puncturing the femoral artery and passing a catheter to the top of the aortic arch, from where

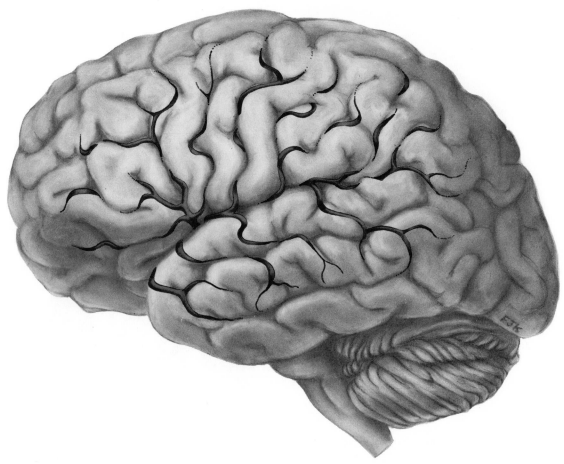

Fig. 36. Cortical Distribution of the Middle Cerebral Artery

the big arterial trunks leading to the brain can be reached by the tip of the catheter (Fig. 187, Chapter 21).

Subarachnoid Hemorrhage (SAH)

Bleeding in relation to the meninges is a serious and often fatal disorder. Whereas clinically significant hemorrhage related to the dura mater, i.e., subdural and extradural hematomas, are usually caused by head injuries (see Clinical Notes, Chapter 3), subarachnoid hemorrhage of clinical significance is usually of nontraumatic origin. A subarachnoid bleed often results from a ruptured arterial aneurysm in the Circle of Willis or one of its major branches. Because most aneurysms lie in one of the large subarachnoid cisterns on the base of the brain, the extravasated blood tends to spread widely in the subarachnoid space. A subarachnoid bleed is a medical emergency, and

if the patient survives, the condition calls for angiographic investigation, possibly followed by surgical isolation of the aneurysm from the rest of the circulation.

BASAL SURFACE AND CRANIAL NERVES

After having studied the arrangement of the major arteries on the base of the brain, cut through the superior cerebellar arteries as well as the posterior and middle cerebral arteries at their origin, and the anterior cerebral arteries where they disappear into the longitudinal fissure. Remove the Circle of Willis together with the basilar and the vertebral arteries with their branches. By leaving the anterior, the middle, and the posterior cerebral arteries intact, it will be possible to study the distribution of these arteries on the medial and lateral side of the hemisphere in more detail later. Remove the remaining parts of the pia–arachnoid on the basal surface. The pia, which is attached to the cranial nerves, should be cut with scissors around the exit of the nerves. Identify the following structures (Fig. 37):

Medulla Oblongata

1. *Pyramis* is a cone-shaped eminence formed by the corticospinal (pyramidal) tract. The corticospinal tract contains fibers passing from the cerebral cortex to the spinal cord.
2. *Pyramidal decussation* is situated at the lower end of the bulb. Here, most of the fibers in the corticospinal tract cross the median plane. The pyramidal decussation explains why the cortical motor areas for voluntary control of motor functions primarily affect the contralateral side of the body.
3. *Olive* derives its name from the *inferior olivary nucleus*, which appears as a large wrinkled bag-shaped mass just beneath its surface. The inferior olivary nucleus is closely related to the cerebellum.

Cerebellum

Cerebellum, which is an important structure for control of motor functions, is divided into a medial part, (medial)
1. *Vermis,* and two lateral lobes or
2. *Cerebellar hemispheres* (lateral lobes)
3. *Choroid plexus* of the fourth ventricle protrudes through the lateral *apertures of Luschkae* into the subarachnoid space in the angle between the medulla oblongata and the cerebellum.

Pons

The *middle cerebellar peduncles* connect the pons with the cerebellum. The transverse striations on the ventral surface of the pons represent pontocerebellar fibers connecting the base of the pons with the cerebellum. The other two pairs of cerebellar peduncles, the *inferior* and the *superior cerebellar peduncles,* cannot be seen from the basal side. They will therefore be studied later in relation to the dissection of cerebellum.

Mesencephalon

1. *Cerebral peduncles,* one on each side, form the ventral surface of the mesencephalon. The basal part of the cerebral peduncle, the basis pedunculi, contains the majority of the fibers that descend from the cerebral cortex to the brain stem and the spinal cord.
2. *Interpeduncular fossa* is a deep depression between the two peduncles. Many small blood vessels perforate the floor of the fossa to reach the interior of the brain. When the vessels are stripped away during the dissection, the area exhibits a perforated appearance, the *posterior perforated space.*

Hypothalamus

1. *Mammillary bodies* (so named because of their resemblance to a woman's breasts) represent characteristic landmarks in the posterior part of the hypothalamus.
2. *Tuber cinereum,* which is hidden behind the hypophysis in Fig. 37, is a small slightly elevated area of gray matter in front of the mammillary bodies.
3. *Optic chiasm* is formed by the junction of the two *optic nerves.* Fibers from the nasal half of each retina cross the median plane in the optic chiasm and enter the contralateral *optic tract,* which swings around the lateral side of the cerebral peduncle to reach the *lateral geniculate body* in the thalamus. The partial decussation of the optic nerve fibers in the optic chiasm, and the fact that many units in the lateral geniculate body and the visual cortex receive input from the same part of the visual field of both eyes, provides for a high degree of stereoscopic vision in primates.
4. *Hypophysis* (pituitary gland) is lodged in the cella turcica and covered from above by diaphragma sellae. The hypophysis is usually ripped off from the base of the hypothalamus when the brain is removed from the cranium during autopsy. The *hypophysial stalk,* which still attaches to the brain, contains an opening representing the infundibular recess of the third ventricle.

Telencephalon

The major part of the basal surface of the brain is represented by the *frontal* and *temporal lobes.*

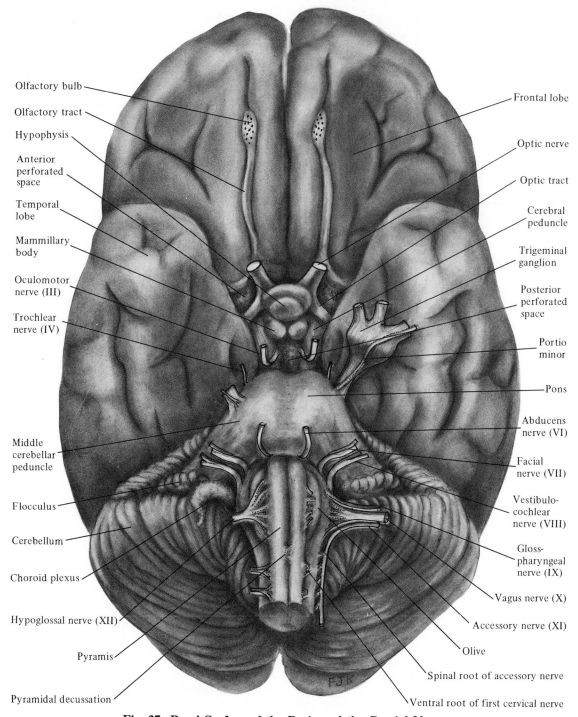

Olfactory bulb

Olfactory tract

Hypophysis

Anterior perforated space

Temporal lobe

Mammillary body

Oculomotor nerve (III)

Trochlear nerve (IV)

Middle cerebellar peduncle

Flocculus

Cerebellum

Choroid plexus

Hypoglossal nerve (XII)

Pyramis

Pyramidal decussation

Frontal lobe

Optic nerve

Optic tract

Cerebral peduncle

Trigeminal ganglion

Posterior perforated space

Portio minor

Pons

Abducens nerve (VI)

Facial nerve (VII)

Vestibulo-cochlear nerve (VIII)

Gloss-pharyngeal nerve (IX)

Vagus nerve (X)

Accessory nerve (XI)

Olive

Spinal root of accessory nerve

Ventral root of first cervical nerve

Fig. 37. Basal Surface of the Brain and the Cranial Nerves

A conspicuous structure on the ventral surface of the frontal lobe is the:

1. *Olfactory bulb,* which is situated in a groove, the *olfactory sulcus,* on the ventral surface of the frontal lobe.

2. *Olfactory tract* is the caudal continuation of the olfactory bulb. It attaches to the base of the brain in front of the

3. *Anterior perforated space,* whose perforations represent points of entrance for numerous arterial branches, that have been ripped off from the ante-

Table 1. Exits of Cranial Nerves from the Brain and the Cranial Cavity.

Name	Its Ganglion	Exit from Brain	Exit from Skull
I. Olfactory nerve	Corresponds to the olfactory receptor cells in the olfactory mucosa	Olfactory bulb	Cribriform plate
II. Optic nerve	Corresponds to the ganglion cells in retina	Optic chiasm	Optic canal
III. Oculomotor nerve	Ciliary ganglion (parasympathetic)	In front of pons in the interpeduncular fossa	Superior orbital fissure
IV. Trochlear nerve	—	Dorsally, behind the inferior colliculus	Superior orbital fissure

V. Trigeminal nerve
  1. Ophthalmic nerve
  2. Maxillary nerve
  3. Mandibular nerve
	Trigeminal ganglion (som.) pterygopalatine ganglion, otic ganglion and submandibular ganglion (all parasympathetic) are topographically related to the Vth nerve	Anterolateral part of pons	1. Superior orbital fissure
			
			2. Foramen rotundum
			
			3. Foramen ovale

VI. Abducens nerve	—	Between pons and the pyramid of the medulla oblongata	Superior orbital fissure
VII. Facial nerve	Geniculate ganglion (somatic)	Between pons and olive in the cerebellopontine angle	Internal acoustic meatus, facial canal and stylomastoid foramen

VIII. Vestibulocochlear nerve
  1. Cochlear nerve
  2. Vestibular nerve
	
	Spiral ganglion
	Vestibular ganglion
		Lateral to VII in the cerebellopontine angle	Internal acoustic meatus

IX. Glossopharyngeal nerve	Superior ganglion Inferior ganglion	On the lateral side of the olive	Jugular foramen
X. Vagus nerve	Superior ganglion	On the lateral side of the olive, behind IX	Jugular foramen
XI. Accessory nerve	—	1. On the lateral side of the olive, behind X. 2. From the 5 or 6 first segments of the cervical part of the spinal cord	Jugular foramen
XII. Hypoglossal nerve	—	Between the pyramid and the olive	Hypoglossal canal

Cranial Nerves

rior part of the circle of Willis and the middle cerebral artery during the removal of the blood vessels and the pia–arachnoid (Fig. 35).

Identify the cranial nerves and study the place of their exits from the brain and the skull (Fig. 37, Table 1).

Clinical Notes

Visual Pathways

Lesions of the visual pathways cause characteristic defects in the visual fields. A visual field is that area seen by one eye. The right and left eyes' respective fields overlap. The visual pathways run from rostral to caudal as they course from eyeball to visual receptive cortex in the occipital lobes. The optic chiasm sends fibers from the left half of each retina into the left optic tract and vice versa. Thus, visual pathway lesions in or behind the chiasm cause bilateral visual field defects, whereas prechiasmal lesions are associated with monocular abnormalities. Visual field defects can thus be specific localizing neurologic signs (see Clinical Notes, Chapter 13).

Cerebellopontine Angle Tumor

Tumors in the cerebellopontine (CP) angle, where the Vth, VIIth, and VIIIth cranial nerves are located, usually arise from the Schwann cells of the VIIIth cranial nerve (acoustic neurinoma) within the internal auditory canal and expand centrally to occupy the cerebellopontine angle. The first symptom is often tinnitus (noise in the ear) followed by loss of hearing. The triad of deafness (VIIIth nerve), loss of corneal reflex (Vth nerve), and cerebellar signs on one side almost certainly indicates an angle tumor on the same side. If facial weakness (VIIth nerve) is present, the tumor is usually very large. The CP tumor is usually benign and the patient can be treated successfully, especially if the diagnosis is made when the tumor is still confined to the internal auditory canal (see also Clinical Notes, Chapter 12).

Second Dissection

Midsagittal Section; Lobes, Sulci, and Gyri

MIDSAGITTAL SECTION

If two whole brains are available, place the brain knife on the corpus callosum of one of them and bisect it by gently pulling the moistened knife through the brain. Do not press the knife into the tissue. Save one half for the preparation of frontal brain sections at the end of the course.

Study the distribution of the anterior cerebral artery on the medial surface of the hemisphere (Fig. 33). The artery ascends toward the genu of the corpus callosum and describes a wide curve backward on the dorsal side of this massive commissural plate, where it is sometimes referred to as the *pericallosal artery.* Another branch is called the *callosomarginal artery.* Study the distribution of the posterior cerebral artery on the medial side of the temporal and occipital lobes. Remove the pia–arachnoid on the medial surface of the hemisphere, and identify the following structures (Figs. 38 and 39):

Myelencephalon (Medulla Oblongata)

Medulla oblongata continues caudally without sharp boundary into the spinal cord. The *central canal* of the spinal cord contines up into the lower part of the medulla oblongata but gradually moves dorsally and opens into the fourth ventricle when it reaches the upper half of the medulla.

Metencephalon

1. *Pons* consists of a large ventral or basal part and a smaller dorsal part. The ventral part is characterized by many fiber bundles and scattered gray matter, the *pontine nuclei.*

2. *Cerebellum* is characterized by deep fissures separating narrow folds, folia. The tree-like outline of the white matter is referred to as arbor vitae. Cerebellum is an important center for coordination of movements. It is separated from pons and medulla oblongata by the fourth ventricle.

3. The *fourth ventricle* is continuous caudally with the central canal and rostrally with the cerebral aqueduct. The rostral part of the roof of the fourth ventricle is formed by the *superior medullary velum,* which fills the angular space between the superior cerebellar peduncles. The caudal portion of the roof, the *inferior medullary velum,* is very thin and it has a large hole, the *median aperture, of Magendie* in its caudomedial part. Through the median aperture and the two *lateral apertures of Luschkae* in the lateral recess, the CSF escapes from the ventricular system into the subarachnoid space. The *choroid plexus* of the fourth ventricle is attached to the ventricular surface of the inferior medullary velum.

Mesencephalon (Midbrain)

1. *Cerebral aqueduct* connects the third and the fourth ventricles.

2. *Tectum* contains the *superior* and *inferior colliculi.* Superior colliculus contains visual reflex centers, whereas the inferior colliculus is an important relay center in the auditory pathways.

3. Ventral to the aqueduct is the *cerebral peduncle,* one on each side. Mesencephalon, pons, and medulla oblongata are usually referred to as the *brain stem.* Occasionally, thalamus or even the whole of diencephalon is included. Cerebellum, however, is not included in the term.

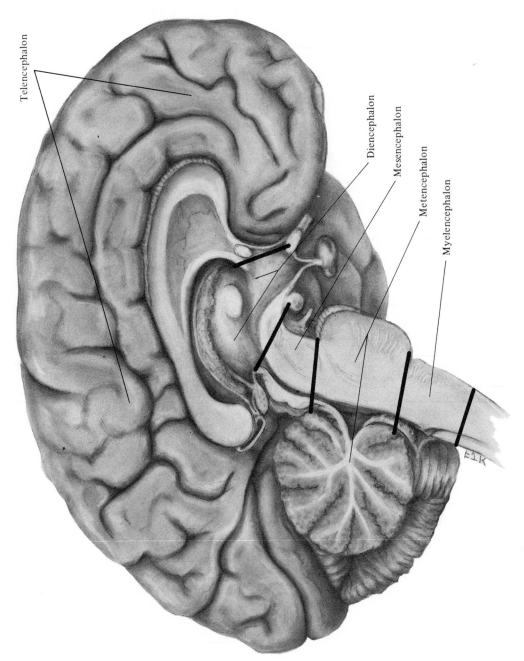

Fig. 38. Major Subdivisions of the Brain

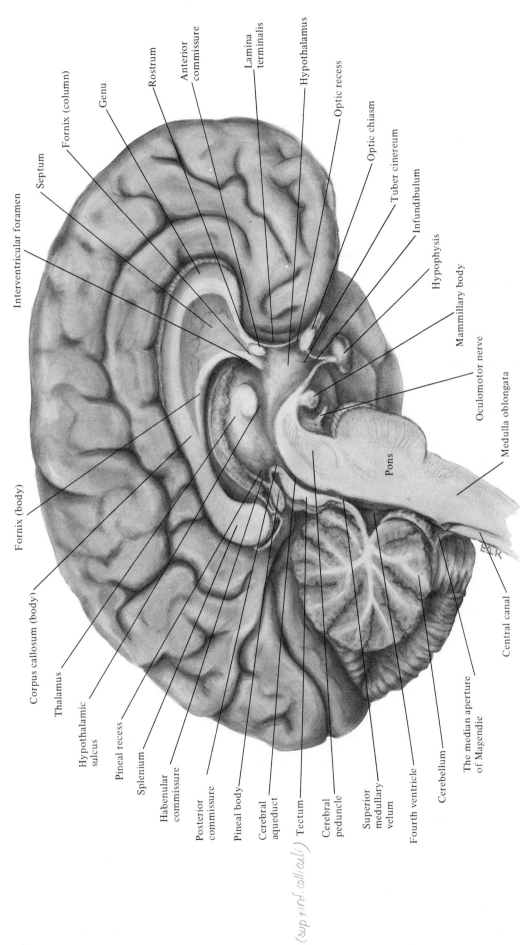

Interventricular foramen

Septum

Fornix (column)

Genu

Rostrum

Anterior commissure

Lamina terminalis

Hypothalamus

Optic recess

Optic chiasm

Tuber cinereum

Infundibulum

Hypophysis

Mammillary body

Oculomotor nerve

Medulla oblongata

Pons

Central canal

The median aperture of Magendie

Cerebellum

Fourth ventricle

Superior medullary velum

Cerebral peduncle

Tectum

(sup + inf. colliculi)

Cerebral aqueduct

Pineal body

Posterior commissure

Habenular commissure

Splenium

Pineal recess

Hypothalamic sulcus

Thalamus

Corpus callosum (body)

Fornix (body)

Fig. 39. Median Sagittal Section of the Brain

Diencephalon

1. *Third ventricle,* whose lateral wall is subdivided by the *hypothalamic sulcus* into an upper part,
2. *Thalamus,* and a lower part,
3. *Hypothalamus,* in which the *tuber cinereum* and the *mammillary body* can be recognized.
4. *Hypophysis* or *pituitary gland* is attached to the hypothalamus through the hypophysial stalk.
5. *Optic chiasm* is located in the rostral part of the hypothalamus. Above the optic chiasm is a recess of the third ventricle, the *optic recess.* Another recess, the *infundibular recess,* extends into the *infundibulum.* Behind the thalamus is the *pineal recess.*
6. *Pineal body* protrudes from the pineal recess over the upper part of the mesencephalon between the two superior colliculi.
7. *Habenular commissure* is located above the pineal recess.
8. *Posterior commissure* is below the pineal recess. The fiber components in the habenular and the posterior commissures connect diencephalic and mesencephalic regions on the two sides. The habenular and posterior commissures, like most commissures in the brain, contain both commissural and decussating fibers.

Telencephalon

1. *Corpus callosum* is the main commissural bundle between the two hemispheres. It is the largest fiber tract in the human brain, and its functions have been enigmatic until recently, when so-called "split brain" experiments (transection of corpus callosum) showed that this massive commissure is important for the transfer of experience from one hemisphere to the other. Corpus callosum consists of
   (a) *Splenium* (the wide caudal part)
   (b) *Body* (the large midportion)
   (c) *Genu* (the anterior part) and
   (d) *Rostrum,* which is continuous with the
2. *Lamina terminalis,* which forms the rostral wall of the third ventricle.
3. *Anterior commissure* contains fibers connecting the two temporal lobes. It is located behind the upper part of the lamina terminalis.
4. *Septum pellucidum,* which stretches between the anterior part of corpus callosum and the fornix, separates the anterior parts of the two lateral ventricles from each other. Its dorsal part is a thin paired lamina that contains fibers and glia cells. Its thicker ventral part, precommissural septum, contains the septal nuclei. Precommissural septum is located in the subcallosal area in front of the anterior commissure (Fig. 42).
5. *Fornix* constitutes a major projection system between the hippocampus in the temporal lobe and the diencephalon. The fornices of the two sides are joined for a short distance underneath the corpus callosum where they form the *body* of the fornix. As the two bundles curve forward and downward, they separate and form on each side a *column* that disappears into the wall of the third ventricle just in front of the *interventricular foramen.* Remove the gray matter of the hypothalamus by blunt dissection and follow the column of fornix to the mammillary body, where most of the fornix fibers terminate (see Fig. 163B, Chapter 15). The posterior part of the fornix, the *crus fornices,* deviates laterally underneath the corpus callosum to reach the temporal lobe. To expose this part of the fornix, the brain stem and cerebellum must be removed from the rest of the brain by a transverse cut close to the mesencephalic–diencephalic border (Fig. 42). If the parahippocampal gyrus is gently pulled down, crus fornices can usually be identified as it sweeps down into the temporal lobe behind the thalamus. When the fornix approaches the parahippocampal gyrus, it appears as a narrow band, the *fimbria hippocampi.* Underneath the fimbria is a very characteristic serrated structure, the *dentate gyrus,* which belongs to the hippocampus formation.
6. *Mammillothalamic tract* can be recognized as it leaves the mammillary body if the hypothalamic gray matter just above and slightly behind the mammillary body is carefully removed (Fig. 163B).

Clinical Notes

Pituitary Tumors

Note the close relationship between the optic chiasm and the pituitary gland. A pituitary tumor that has reached a certain size can dislocate the diaphragma sellae and exert pressure on the optic chiasm, which typically causes bitemporal visual field defects (see Clinical Notes, Chapter 13 and Clinical Example, Chapter 15).

Hydrocephalus

Hydrocephalus, i.e., excessive amount of CSF in the cranial cavity, occurs if the circulation of CSF is obstructed. The obstruction leads to accumulation of fluid proximal to the stoppage, and the increased pressure causes dilation of the ventricular system and even enlargement of the head if the hydrocephalus occurs at birth or an early age before the sutures of the skull have closed. Obstruction in the CSF pathway is often caused by congenital stenosis of the cerebral aqueduct or by a tumor affecting the third or fourth ventricle. Obstruction can also occur at the foramina of Magendie and Luschka as a result of an inflammatory process of the pia–arachnoid, i.e., meningitis, especially if the infection is not properly treated with antibiotics.

LOBES, SULCI, AND GYRI

To increase surface area, the cerebral cortex is heavily folded, and the complicated pattern of ridges, convolutions or *gyri,* and grooves, *sulci,* can be studied in detail following the removal of the pia–arachnoid from the surface of the hemisphere. Although the appearance of the different grooves and ridges varies between different individuals, all brains have basic similarities. The subdivision of the hemisphere into lobes and gyri provides clinicians and students of the brain with a useful anatomic reference system. It may be difficult at times to identify even some of the major landmarks, but it is nevertheless important to know the general position of the main sulci and gyri. One should realize, however, that cortical zones bounded by various fissures and sulci do not usually coincide with specific cytoarchitectonic or functional areas of the cerebral cortex. For example, to localize the motor cortex to the precentral gyrus or the somatosensory cortex to the postcentral gyrus are only rough, but nevertheless useful approximations.

On the basis of some of the major grooves the hemisphere is subdivided into five *lobes:* the frontal, the parietal, the occipital and the temporal lobes, and the insula (Figs. 40 and 41).

The *frontal lobe* occupies the area in front of the *central sulcus* and above the *lateral fissure.* The medial side of the frontal lobe is bounded posteriorly by an imaginary line from the central sulcus to the dorsal surface of the corpus callosum.

The *parietal lobe* is bounded by the central sulcus in the front, and by the lateral fissure and its extension below. An imaginary line between the *parieto-occipital sulcus* and *preoccipital notch* indicates its caudal border.

The *temporal lobe* is situated underneath the lateral fissure and in front of the above mentioned line between the parietooccipital sulcus and the preoccipital notch.

The *occipital lobe* is located behind the arbitrary line joining the parieto-occipital sulcus and the preoccipital notch. On the medial side of the hemisphere, the occipital lobe is bounded anteriorly by the parieto-occipital sulcus.

The *insula,* which is located in the bottom of the lateral fissure, can be seen if the two lips of the lateral fissure are pulled apart. To expose it completely, the covering parts, i.e., the opercula of the frontal, parietal and temporal lobes must be removed (see below), but this should be done only after the surface topography of the other lobes has been studied.

Dorsolateral Surface of the Hemisphere

Frontal Lobe

Through the presence of three main grooves, the precentral sulcus, the superior frontal sulcus, and the inferior frontal sulcus, the frontal lobe is divided into four main gyri:
1. *Precentral gyrus* (primary motor cortex)
2. *Superior frontal gyrus*
3. *Middle frontal gyrus*
4. *Inferior frontal gyrus*

The inferior frontal gyrus is subdivided into an orbital part, a triangular part, and an opercular part by the anterior and ascending ramus of the lateral fissure. The motor speech area (Broca's area) is located in the triangular and opercular parts of the inferior frontal gyrus, usually on the left side.

Parietal Lobe

Parallel to the central sulcus is the postcentral sulcus, and the convolution between these two grooves is the:

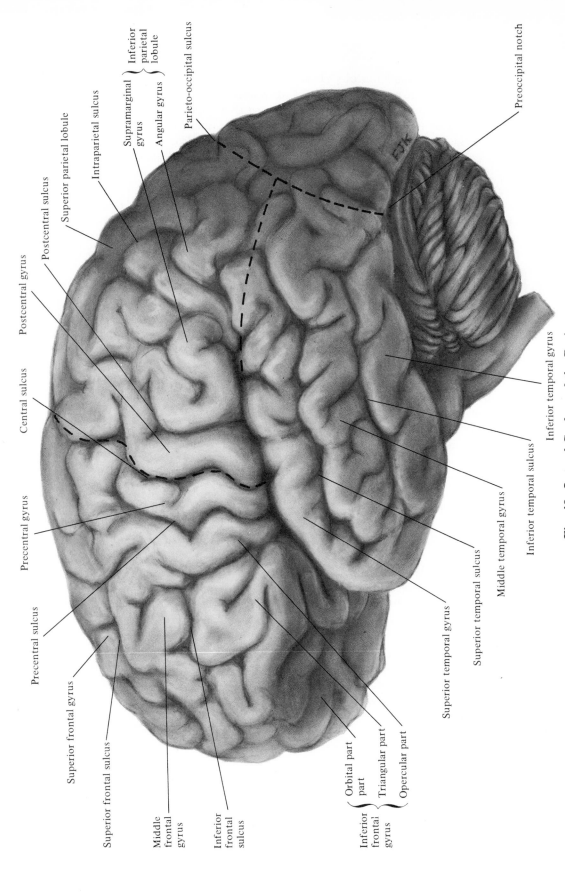

Inferior parietal lobule {
Supramarginal gyrus
Angular gyrus

Parieto-occipital sulcus

Intraparietal sulcus

Superior parietal lobule

Postcentral sulcus

Postcentral gyrus

Central sulcus

Precentral gyrus

Precentral sulcus

Superior frontal gyrus

Superior frontal sulcus

Middle frontal gyrus

Inferior frontal sulcus

Inferior frontal gyrus {
Orbital part
Triangular part
Opercular part

Superior temporal gyrus

Superior temporal sulcus

Middle temporal gyrus

Inferior temporal sulcus

Inferior temporal gyrus

Preoccipital notch

Fig. 40. Lateral Surface of the Brain

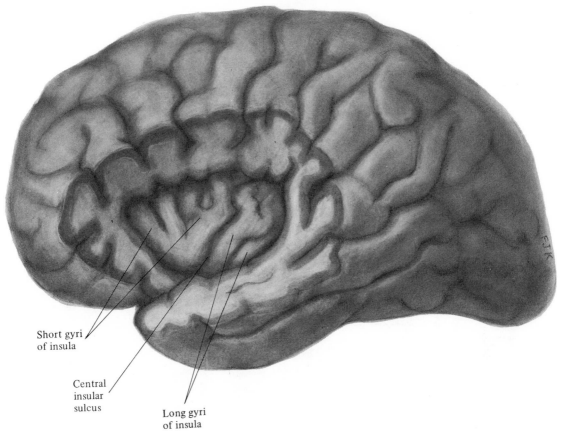

Short gyri
of insula

Central
insular
sulcus

Long gyri
of insula

Fig. 41. Insula
Insula has been exposed by removing the opercular parts of the frontal, parietal, and temporal lobes with a scalpel.

1. *Postcentral gyrus* (primary somatosensory cortex). The intraparietal sulcus separates the
2. *Superior parietal lobule* from the
3. *Inferior parietal lobule*. Two important gyri are located in the last mentioned lobule, namely
4. *Supramarginal gyrus*, which caps the posterior tip of the lateral fissure, and
5. *Angular gyrus*, which caps the posterior tip of the superior temporal sulcus. These two convolutions together with the adjoining parts of the occipital and temporal lobes are of special importance for language functions. They represent the sensory language area, which is usually located in the left hemisphere.

Temporal Lobe

The superior and inferior temporal sulci subdivide the lateral surface of the temporal lobe into:
1. *Superior temporal gyrus*

2. *Middle temporal gyrus* and
3. *Inferior temporal gyrus*
Situated on the extensive dorsal surface of the superior temporal gyrus are several
4. *Transverse temporal gyri*. These small convolutions, which indicate the region of the primary auditory cortex, can be seen in the floor of the lateral fissure if its two borders are pulled apart.

Occipital Lobe

Only a small part of lateral surface of the hemisphere belongs to the occipital lobe. The posterior part of the *calcarine sulcus*, which is the major groove on the medial side (see below), sometimes curves around the occipital pole to the lateral surface. The occipital lobe is primarily related to visual functions.

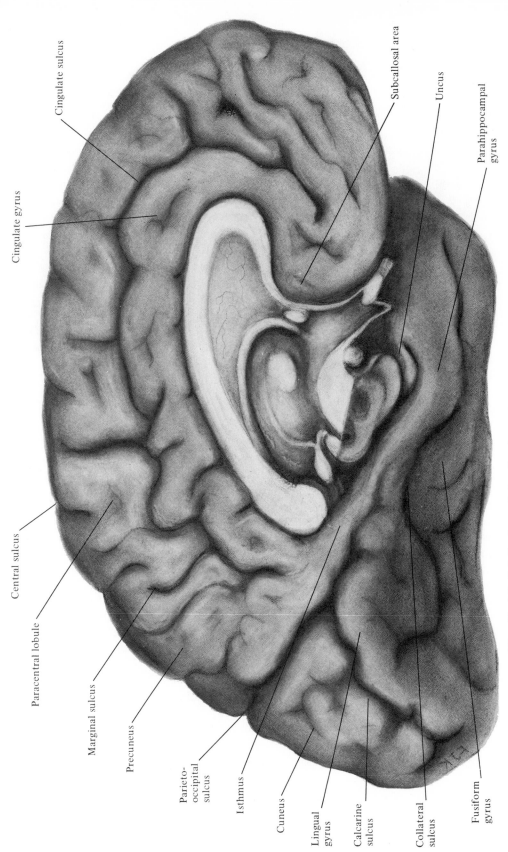

Fig. 42. Medial Surface of the Cerebral Hemisphere
The brain stem has been removed to expose the medial surface of the temporal lobe.

Cingulate sulcus

Subcallosal area

Uncus

Parahippocampal gyrus

Cingulate gyrus

Central sulcus

Paracentral lobule

Marginal sulcus

Precuneus

Parieto-occipital sulcus

Isthmus

Cuneus

Lingual gyrus

Calcarine sulcus

Collateral sulcus

Fusiform gyrus

Insula

Insula can be exposed if the opercular parts of the frontal, parietal, and temporal lobes are removed as illustrated in Fig. 41. Use the side of the brain from which the brain stem and cerebellum were removed. Before the incision is made, however, it is advisable to spread apart the lateral fissure to observe the location and the extent of the insula. Insula is subdivided by a central insular sulcus into several

1. *Short gyri* in front of the sulcus, and one or two

2. *Long gyri* behind the central insular sulcus.

The insula is surrounded by a circular sulcus. The anterior basal part of the insula, which separates the lateral surface of the insula from the anterior perforated space, is known as *limen insulae.*

Medial and Basal Surfaces of the Hemisphere
(Fig. 42)

1. *Cingulate gyrus* begins in the *subcallosal area* underneath the rostrum of the corpus callosum and continues above the corpus callosum into the temporal lobe, where it is continuous with the

2. *Parahippocampal gyrus* through the narrow *isthmus.* The peripheral boundary of the cingulate gyrus is represented by the cingulate sulcus, which gives off a paracentral sulcus on the medial surface of the frontal lobe, and then divides into a marginal and a subparietal sulcus on the medial surface of the parietal lobe. The region between the paracentral sulcus and the marginal sulcus is referred to as

3. *Paracentral lobule.* The anterior part of this lobule is continuous with the precentral gyrus on the lateral side of the hemisphere and the posterior part is an extension of the postcentral gyrus. Behind the marginal sulcus is

4. *Precuneus,* which is continuous with the superior parietal lobule on the lateral surface. The parieto-occipital sulcus separates the precuneus from

5. *Cuneus,* which belongs to the occipital lobe. A deep horizontal fissure, the *calcarine sulcus,* is an important landmark in the occipital lobe. The area surrounding the calcarine sulcus represents primary visual cortex. The calcarine sulcus separates cuneus from

6. *Lingual gyrus,* which extends forward into the temporal lobe, where it is continuous with

7. *Parahippocampal gyrus,* whose rostral part hooks sharply backwards as *uncus.* Part of uncus represents primary olfactory cortex.

8. *Fusiform gyrus* (medial occipitotemporal gyrus) is located on the basal surfaces of the occipital and temporal lobes. It is situated between the lingual and parahippocampal gyri medially, and the *inferior temporal gyrus* (lateral occipitotemporal gyrus) laterally. The collateral sulcus is located on the medial side of the fusiform gyrus.

9. *Gyrus rectus* is located medial to the olfactory sulcus on the basal surface of the frontal lobe. Lateral to the olfactory sulcus are many irregular

10. *Orbital gyri.*

Third Dissection

White Matter, Blunt Dissection of Major Fiber Systems

WHITE MATTER

The massive medullary center of the cerebral hemisphere consists of myelinated fibers, which can be divided into three different groups: *association, commissural,* and *projection fibers.* As an introduction to the blunt dissection of the major fiber bundles of the hemisphere, it is helpful to review and examine the location of the major bundles on a schematic drawing (Fig. 43).

Association Fibers

Association fibers interconnect cortical regions within the same hemisphere. Many of them form bundles, fasciculi, which contain long pathways as well as short fibers that enter and leave the bundles along their course. The main association bundles are summarized below.

1. *Arcuate fibers* (Fig. 44) are short fibers interconnecting adjacent gyri.

2. *Cingulum,* which is located in the cingulate gyrus and the parahippocampal gyrus, connects frontal, parietal, and temporal cortical areas on the medial side of the hemisphere.

3. *Superior longitudinal fasciculus (arcuate fasciculus)* is located in the more lateral parts of the hemisphere above the insula. It interconnects areas within the frontal, parietal, occipital, and temporal lobes. Since many of its fibers form an arch-shaped structure as they sweep down into the temporal lobe behind insula, the bundle is also referred to as the arcuate fasciculus.

4. *Superior occipitofrontal fasciculus* is located in the medial part of the hemisphere underneath the lateral extension of corpus callosum. It runs alongside the dorsal border of the caudate nucleus and interconnects the frontal lobe with more posterior parts of the hemisphere.

5. *Inferior occipitofrontal fasciculus* runs between the occipital and the frontal lobe along the ventral aspect of the insula in the lateral part of the hemisphere. Many of the fibers in the frontal part sweep down into the temporal lobe as the

6. *Uncinate fasciculus* (Fig. 45), which makes a sharp bend around the lateral fissure to interconnect the orbital surface of the frontal lobe with the rostral part of the temporal lobe.

Commissural Fibers (Fig. 39)

The commissural fibers cross the midline and interconnect areas in the two hemispheres with each other. Whereas most of the fibers interconnect similar (homotopic) regions, others link dissimilar (heterotopic) areas on the two sides.

1. *Corpus callosum,* which contains about 300 million fibers, interconnects neocortical areas in all lobes. Although most regions are interrelated through commissural fibers, some regions, notably the primary visual cortex and the hand and foot regions of the somatosensory cortex, do not seem to receive commissural fibers.

2. *Anterior commissure,* which crosses the midline as a compact bundle in front of the fornix column, interconnects areas in the two temporal lobes. A small anterior or olfactory part, which cannot be readily distinguished fron the main posterior part in gross dissections, contains fibers that interconnect the anterior olfactory nucleus at the base of the olfactory tract with the anterior olfactory nucleus and the olfactory bulb on the other side.

3. *Hippocampal commissure* is situated underneath splenium of the corpus callosum, from which it is difficult to separate. Its fibers interconnect the two hippocampus formations. The hippocampal commissure will be exposed during the next dissection.

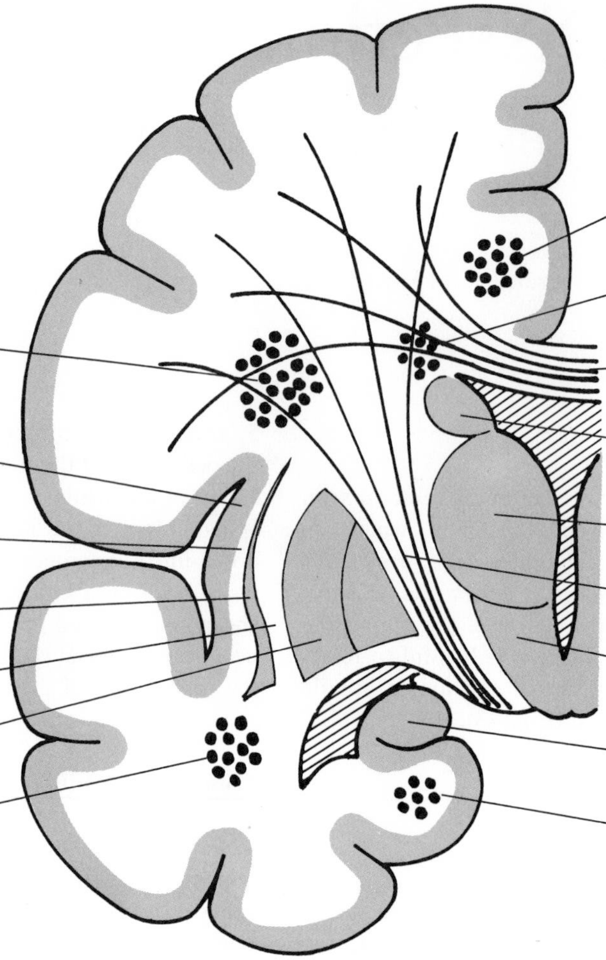

Fig. 43. Major Fiber Bundles
Diagram illustrating the position of some of the major fiber bundles in a frontal section of the brain.

4. *Posterior commissure* is located at the boundary between diencephalon and mesencephalon immediately rostral to the superior colliculus. It is a complex fiber bundle containing different components related to several nearby regions including the pretectal area and part of the oculomotor complex.

5. *Habenular commissure* is located above the pineal recess and contains stria medullaris fibers through which the habenular complex and some other subcortical regions are connected to structures on the opposite side.

Projection Fibers (Fig. 43)

Many of the fibers in the white matter of the hemisphere connect the cerebral cortex with subcortical regions. These are the projection fibers, which to a considerable extent are related to the *internal capsule*. The projection fibers can be divided into *corticopetal* and *corticofugal fibers*, depending on whether they transmit impulses to or from the cortex. The corticopetal fibers come primarily from the thalamus, form part of the internal capsule, and diverge toward the cerebral cortex. The corticofugal fibers, which originate in different parts of the cerebral cortex, converge toward the basal ganglia, the thalamus, and the internal capsule. The large majority of the corticopetal and corticofugal fibers form a fan-shaped fiber mass, *corona radiata*, as they emerge from the internal capsule. Some of the important fiber systems in the internal capsule are:

1. *Thalamic radiation*, which consists of both corticothalamic and thalamocortical projection fibers.

2. *Corticopontine fibers,* which originate in wide areas of the cerebral cortex and project to the pontine nuclei in the basal part of the pons. The pontine nuclei in turn project to the cerebellum.
3. *Corticobulbar and corticospinal fibers,* together often referred to as the pyramidal tract, originate in motor and to a lesser extent in somatosensory cortex, and project to cranial nerve nuclei in the brain stem and to cell groups throughout the length of the spinal cord.
4. *Corticoreticular fibers* originate primarily in motor and somatosensory cortex and project to the brain stem reticular formation.

BLUNT DISSECTION OF MAJOR FIBER SYSTEMS

If the brain substance is peeled away in a methodical fashion from the lateral and the medial sides of the hemisphere, many of the major fiber systems of the white matter can be visualized. By using the blunt end of a scalpel handle on a well-fixed brain, the myelinated fiber bundles can be torn and split apart much like the lamellae of a mushroom. Although the blunt dissection is very useful to gain an appreciation of the structure of the white matter, it is important to realize that information regarding origin and termination of specific fiber tracts cannot be obtained by this type of dissection. Such information is obtained in microscopic analysis of histologic preparations. For the blunt dissection, use the brain half on which the insula was explored, and compare the appearance of the different fiber bundles on your specimen with the location of these bundles in a frontal section through the hemisphere (Fig. 43).

Dissection from the Lateral Side

1. Reveal the *superior longitudinal fasciculus* (arcuate fasciculus) by peeling away the cortex in the circular sulcus surrounding the insula. Expose the whole bundle by extending the dissection into the frontal and occipital lobes, and follow the part that sweeps down behind the insula into the temporal lobe (Fig. 44).
2. Continue the dissection underneath and deep to the basal part of the insula to expose the association system that connects the basal parts of the frontal lobe with the temporal and occipital lobes

(Fig. 45). To do this, the ventral part of the insular cortex must be removed. The dorsal component of this system, the *inferior occipitofrontal fasciculus,* extends in a longitudinal direction between the frontal and the occipital lobes, whereas the more ventral component, the *uncinate fasciculus,* hooks around the lateral fissure to connect the orbitofrontal cortex with the anterior part of the temporal lobe.
3. At this point it is advisable to turn attention to the *optic radiation* or *geniculocalcarine tract,* which is the last link in the optic pathway from the retina to the visual cortex in the occipital lobe. This important projection system is usually exposed in efforts to follow the inferior occipitofrontal fasciculus in a posterior direction underneath the caudal part of the insula.

The optic radiation originates in the lateral geniculate body of the thalamus and proceeds in a more or less lateral direction through the posterior (retrolenticular and sublenticular) part of the internal capsule before its fibers turn in a caudal direction toward the calcarine fissure in the occipital lobe (Fig. 46). It comes into view behind and underneath the caudal part of the insula and sweeps caudally in the form of a broad band, which disappears underneath the arcuate fasciculus (Fig. 45). If the arcuate fasciculus and the lateral part of the occipital lobe are dissected away the radiation can be followed all the way to the primary visual area in the region of the calcarine fissure (Fig. 42).

Although it is usually easy to follow the last part of the optic radiation into the occipital lobe, it is more difficult to appreciate the first part of the radiation, and it may be especially difficult to separate the ventral part of the optic radiation from association fibers in the inferior occipitofrontal fasciculus underneath insula. The more ventrally located fibers in the optic radiation are first directed forward and laterally above the inferior horn of the lateral ventricle before they sweep in a caudal direction toward the occipital lobe. The part of the optic radiation, which makes a rostrolateral detour into the temporal lobe is referred to as *Meyer's loop* (Fig. 46).
4. Remove the rest of the superior longitudinal fasciculus and carefully dissect away the cortical layer of the insula (compare Fig. 43). Underneath the insular cortex is a thin lamella of white matter, the extreme capsule, which is often difficult to identify. Deep to the extreme capsule is a thin

Superior longitudinal fasciculus (Arcuate fasciculus)

Arcuate
fibers

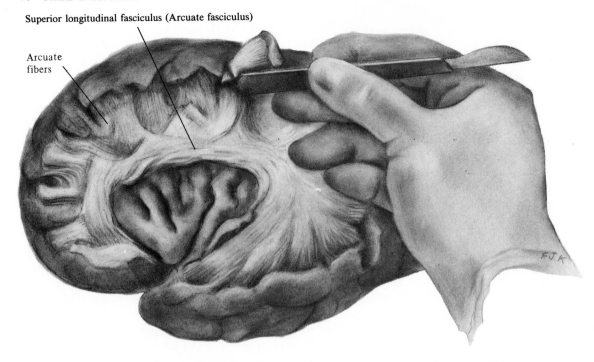

Fig. 44. Blunt Dissection of Superior Longitudinal Fasciculus and Arcuate Fibers

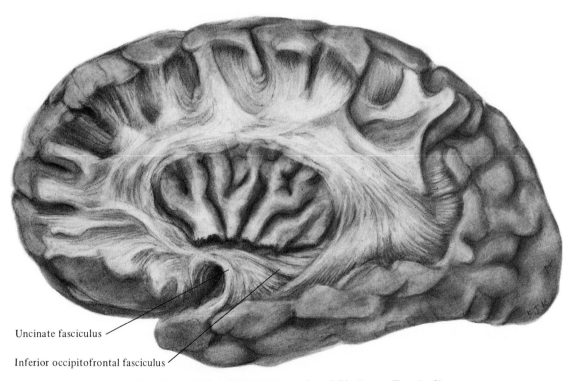

Uncinate fasciculus

Inferior occipitofrontal fasciculus

Fig. 45. Inferior Occipitofrontal and Uncinate Fasciculi

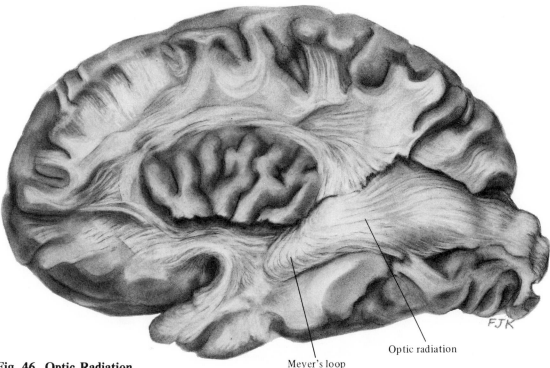

Optic radiation

Fig. 46. Optic Radiation   Meyer's loop

sheet of gray matter, the *claustrum,* which should be carefully stripped away to expose the *external capsule,* which is yet another thin layer of white matter composed of different kinds of fibers, i.e., association fibers, projection fibers and commissural fibers. Although it is sometimes difficult to identify the dorsal part of the claustrum, the more voluminous ventral part can usually be recognized.
5. Carefully strip away the external capsule to expose the lateral surface of the *putamen* (Fig. 47). Putamen can be easily recognized by its gray color. It is the most lateral part of the lentiform nucleus, an important component of the basal ganglia.

Dissection from the Medial Side

1. Expose the *cingulum* by peeling away the cortex of the cingulate gyrus. Follow this association bundle as it arches around the genu of the corpus callosum and continues in the direction of the subcallosal area. Complete the dissection in caudal direction and follow the cingulum as it sweeps down into the parahippocampal gyrus behind the splenium of the corpus callosum (Fig. 48).
2. Strip away the remaining cortex on the medial side and identify numerous U-shaped fibers, i.e., *arcuate fibers,* which interconnect adjacent gyri.

3. Insert the handle of the scalpel between the cingulum and the corpus callosum and remove the cingulum by lifting the scalpel. This exposes the commissural fibers which radiate from *corpus callosum* into the cerebral cortex (Fig. 49).
4. Cut off the free medial part of the corpus callosum as shown in Fig. 50, and remove it together with the septum pellucidum and the main part of the fornix. This can be done by transecting the columns of fornix in front of the interventricular foramen and the crus fornices where it sweeps down behind the caudal part of the thalamus. The removal of the corpus callosum exposes the lateral ventricle. Identify the thalamus in the floor of the lateral ventricle.

If the free edge of the corpus callosum is completely trimmed away, even the more laterally placed caudate nucleus can be identified. By removing also the temporal part of the cingulum together with the parahippocampal gyrus and the hippocampus formation, the whole extent of the lateral ventricle is revealed. Note the highly vascularized *choroid plexus,* which produces the cerebrospinal fluid.
5. Dissect away the gray matter of the caudate nucleus and expose the fibers of the *internal capsule* and the *corona radiata.* The fibers that first come into view belong to the *thalamic radiation,*

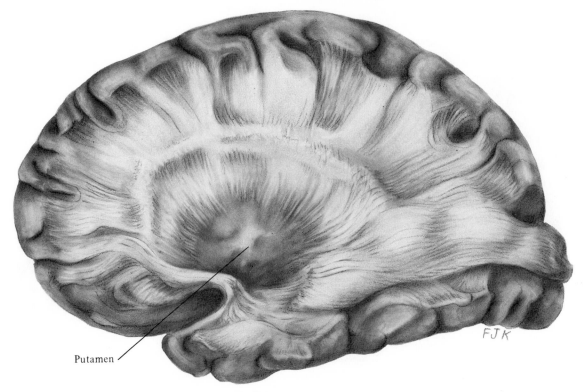

Putamen

Fig. 47. Exposure of Putamen

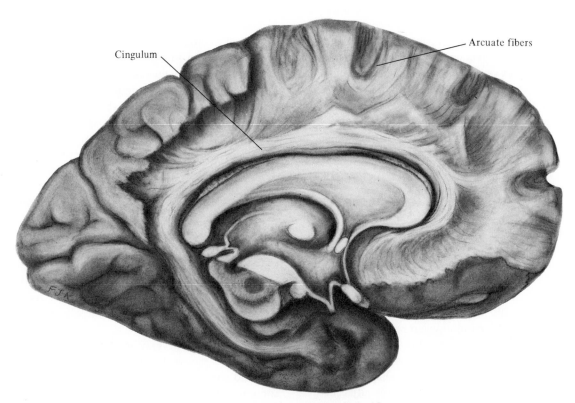

Cingulum

Arcuate fibers

Fig. 48. Cingulum exposed by blunt dissection from the medial side

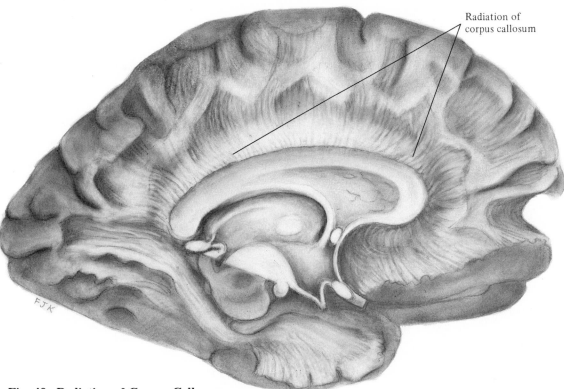

Radiation of
corpus callosum

Fig. 49. Radiation of Corpus Callosum

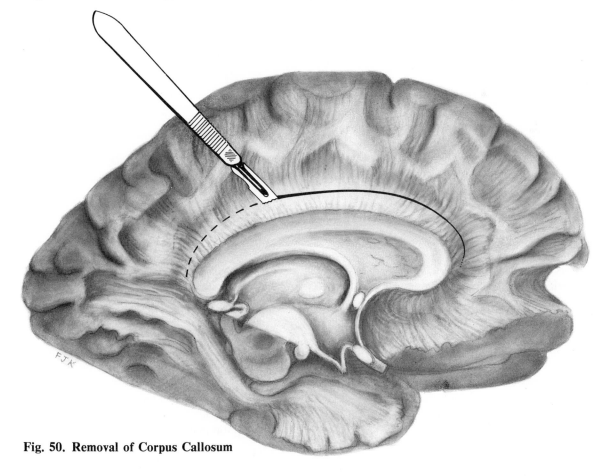

Fig. 50. Removal of Corpus Callosum

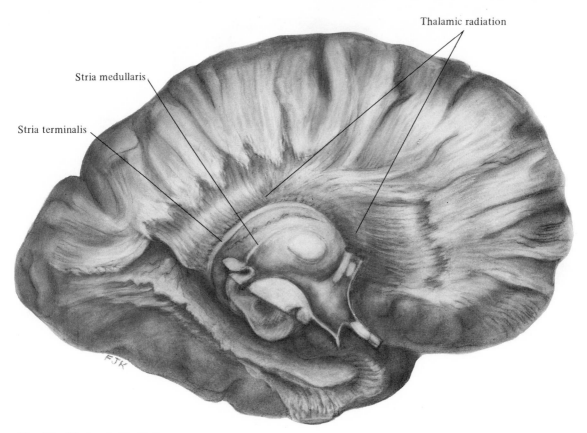

Stria medullaris

Stria terminalis

Thalamic radiation

Fig. 51. Thalamic Radiation

which connect the cortex with the thalamus (Fig. 51).

6. Continue the blunt dissection by removing the thalamus together with the more superficial fibers of the corona radiata. By doing so, other fibers of the corona radiata can be followed as they converge toward the internal capsule, and if the dorsal part of mesencephalon is removed, the projection fibers can be followed all the way to the base of the cerebral peduncle in mesencephalon. This fan-shaped fibersystem (Fig. 52), which bypasses thalamus, contains primarily *corticofugal fibers,* i.e., corticopontine, corticoreticular, corticobulbar, and corticospinal fibers.

7. Locate the cut surface of the *anterior commissure* and expose the string-like commissural bundle by stripping away surrounding tissue. The bundle projects in a lateral direction and gradually curves backwards and downwards to reach the anterior part of the temporal lobe.

Clinical Notes

Cingulotomy

The treatment of mental disorders by brain operations is referred to as psychosurgery. One of the most popular modern psychosurgical operations consists of the stereotaxic destruction, for instance by electrocoagulation, of part of the cingulate gyrus including the cingulum on both sides of the brain. The operation, which is called cingulotomy, is carried out on patients who are tormented and disabled by emotional disorders or who are suffering from intractable pain. The reason for destroying the cingulum is related to the fact that it is one of the main association bundles within the "limbic system," which seems to be of special significance for the emotional aspects of behavior. Patients who have been treated with cingulotomy for chronic pain can still experience pain, but the perception of pain is no longer associated with a disabling emotional experience.

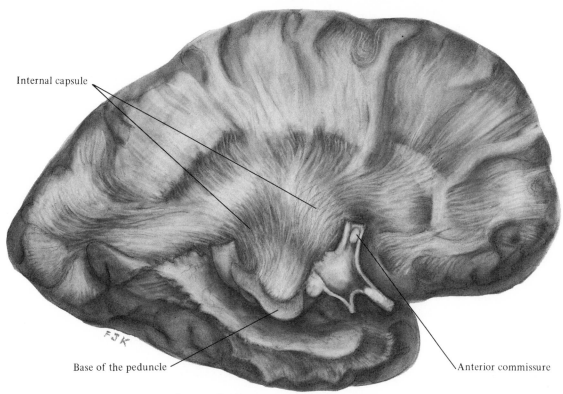

Internal capsule

Base of the peduncle

Anterior commissure

Fig. 52. Internal Capsule and Corona Radiata

The Optic Radiation

The optic radiation has an extensive and somewhat peculiar course, which is of great importance to the clinician. Whereas the fibers in the dorsal part of the bundle proceed more or less directly through the parietal and temporal lobes to the visual cortex in the occipital lobe, the ventral fibers (Meyer's loop) make a rostrally directed detour above the inferior horn of the lateral ventricle before they sweep in a posterior direction on the outside of the lateral ventricle toward the occipital lobe. Some of the fibers in Meyer's loop reach as far forward as the tip of the inferior horn of the lateral ventricle. A lesion in the temporal lobe, e.g., a tumor or an abscess, may destroy part of the fan-like optic radiation even if the lesion is located in the rostral part of the lobe. Such a lesion often results in an incomplete homonymous defect, i.e., a defect affecting the same half of the visual fields of both eyes. For instance, a lesion in the temporal lobe is likely to produce a contralateral upper homonymous defect.

Corpus Callosum and "Split-brain" Patients

Corpus callosum permits the transfer of information and learning from one hemisphere to the other. In patients with severe and disabling epileptic seizures, the corpus callosum was sometimes severed to prevent the spread of the epileptic discharge from one hemisphere to the other. Although such "split-brain" patients can function surprisingly well—there are no obvious changes in intellect or behavior—they are unable to perform certain tasks.

As an example we will assume that the patient's language centers are located in the left hemisphere, which is usually dominant in regard to language. If an object is placed in the patient's right hand (with eyes closed), the patient will be able to name the object, because the sensory information reaches the language centers in the dominant left hemisphere through the ascending somatosensory pathways that cross the midline in the lower part of the brain stem. However, if the object is placed in the patient's left hand, the patient will be unable to name the object, because the right hemisphere does not have access to the memory for language in the left hemisphere.

Fourth Dissection

Ventricular System, Fornix, and Basal Ganglia

VENTRICULAR SYSTEM, FORNIX, AND BASAL GANGLIA

Before starting this dissection, it is useful to study the location of the brain ventricles on Fig. 17C. Afterward, remove the meninges and blood vessels from the dorsal side of the second brain. Then, separate the brain stem and the cerebellum from the rest of the brain by a transverse cut through the mesencephalon.

Exploration of the Lateral Ventricles

1. Pull the two cerebral hemispheres apart gently to study the location of the corpus callosum before cutting a series of horizontal sections down to the level of the corpus callosum (Fig. 53). Remove the medial parts of the cingulate gyri, and expose the dorsal surface of the corpus callosum as shown in Fig. 54. If the anterior cerebral arteries have not been removed they will appear on the dorsal surface of the corpus callosum.

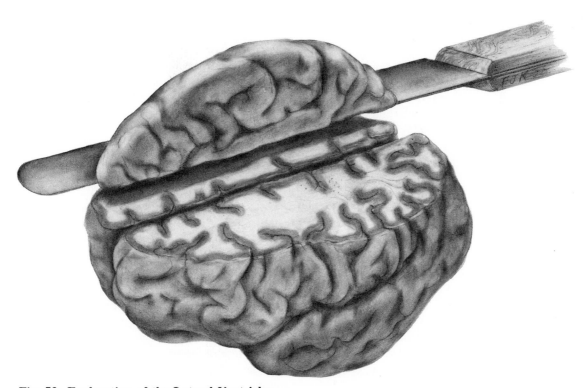

Fig. 53. Exploration of the Lateral Ventricles
To prepare for the exploration of the lateral ventricles, the dorsal parts of the brain are removed by cutting horizontal slices down to to the level of the dorsal surface of the corpus callosum with the aid of a brain knife.

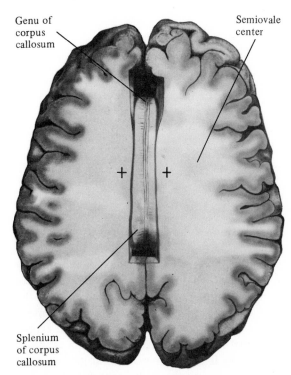

Genu of
corpus
callosum

Semiovale
center

Splenium
of corpus
callosum

Fig. 54. Semiovale Center and Corpus Callosum
The crosses mark the points where access can be gained
to the lateral ventricles. (From Rauber-Kopsch, 1955,
Lehrbuch und Atlas der Anatomie des Menschen, Band
11, 19 Auflage, Georg Thieme Verlag, Stuttgart.)

The white matter in the center of the horizontal
section, the *semioval center,* contains a mixture
of association, commissural, and projection fibers.
The highly convoluted surface of the hemisphere
is covered by a 2–4 mm thick layer of gray matter,
the *cortex cerebri.*
2. Palpate the semioval center just lateral to the
exposed corpus callosum, and localize an area (+
in Fig. 54) where the tissue easily yields to the
pressure of the finger. By cutting a small hole in
the tissue at this point access is gained to the lateral
ventricle.
3. By gradually expanding the hole in a rostral
and caudal direction according to Fig. 55, the
whole roof of the lateral ventricle can be removed.
Repeat the procedure on the contralateral side.
    The most prominent structure related to the *an-
terior horn* of the lateral ventricle is the *caudate
nucleus,* whose massive anterior part, the head of
the caudate nucleus, bulges into the anterior horn
from the lateral side.
    The *central part* of the lateral ventricle is quite
narrow. The *choroid plexus* and the *thalamus* are
the most prominent structures in the floor of the

central part. It may be surprising to realize that
the thalamus, which is a diencephalic structure,
forms part of the floor in the lateral ventricle, a
telencephalic structure. During the development,
however, part of the telencephalon fuses with the
diencephalon. In fact, the dorsal surface of the
thalamus facing the lateral ventricle is covered by
a thin ependymal layer, the *lamina affixa,* which
belongs to the telencephalon (Fig. 18C).
    The *posterior horn* extends for a variable dis-
tance into the occipital lobe. On the medial wall
of the posterior horn is an eminence, *calcar avis,*
which is caused by the calcarine sulcus.
4. Continue the dissection on the right hemisphere
by exposing the *temporal (inferior) horn.* To do
this, cut away the frontal and parietal opercula
covering the insula, and open up the temporal horn
from the lateral side by cutting into the temporal
lobe as indicated in Figs. 55 and 56. Make the
cut in the direction of the superior temporal sulcus
and remove, piece by piece, the superior temporal
gyrus, until the whole extent of the temporal horn
is exposed. The beautifully curved structure in the
medial wall of the temporal horn is the *hippocampus* (Fig. 57).
5. Inspect the location of the choroid plexus and
its extension into the temporal horn. An expanded
portion of the choroid plexus, the *glomus choroideum,* is located in the region of the atrium, i.e.,
where the temporal horn, the posterior horn, and
the central part of the lateral ventricle come together. Localize the *anterior choroidal artery* on
the basal side of the brain and try to identify its
entrance into the temporal horn through the choroid fissure on the medial side of the temporal
lobe (Fig. 34).

Fornix and the Hippocampal Commissure

1. Make a transverse cut behind the genu of the
corpus callosum and continue the cut through the
septum toward the interventricular foramina. As
a consequence, the fornix columns are also transected and the trunk of the corpus callosum together with the body of the fornix can be bent
backward as shown in Fig. 58. This provides a
clear picture of the two *crura fornices* as they diverge laterally, curve around the thalamic nuclei,
and disappear into the temporal horns.
    With the body of the fornix flipped backwards,
it is also easy to appreciate the transversely running fibers between the two crura fornicis. This

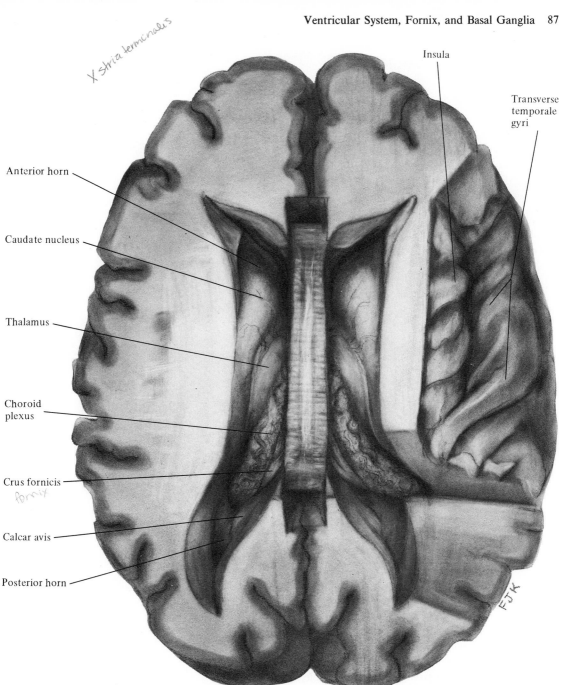

Fig. 55. Lateral Ventricles
The lateral ventricles have been exposed by removing the white substance overlying the ventricles.

is the *hippocampal commissure,* which connects the hippocampus formations on the two sides.
2. Follow the fornix as it sweeps behind the thalamus in a lateral and downward direction into the temporal lobe. The last part of fornix attaches to the hippocampus as a flattened band, *fimbria hippocampi.* If the choroid fissure is carefully widened, the relationships between the fornix and the hippocampus can be more easily appreciated.

Tela Choroidea of the Third Ventricle

The roof of the third ventricle is formed by *tela choroidea* (velum interpositum), which extends between the two thalamic nuclei. The tela choroidea, which is located in the transverse fissure, constitutes a folding of the pia mater, and is continuous underneath the splenium of corpus callosum with the pia–arachnoid on the dorsal surface of the mes-

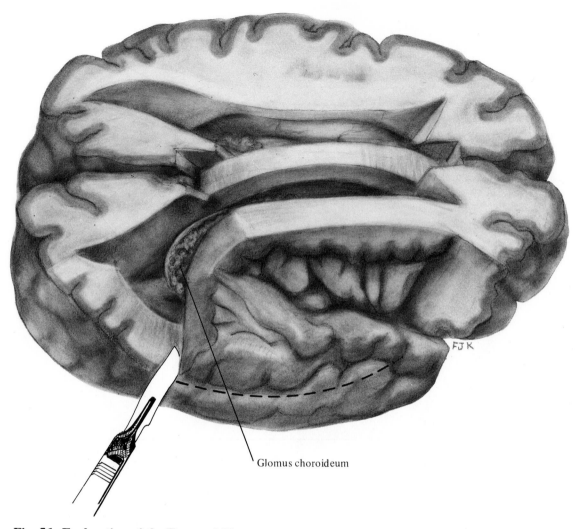

Glomus choroideum

Fig. 56. Exploration of the Temporal Horn
Access to the temporal horn can be gained by making a cut in the direction of the superior temporal sulcus and removing the superior temporal gyrus piece by piece.

encephalon. This highly vascularized part of pia mater, which reaches forward above the two thalamic nuclei to the level of the interventricular foramina, is separated from the third ventricle by a layer of ependymal cells. The choroid plexus, which has penetrated into the lateral ventricle from the tela choroidea, is also covered by a layer of ependymal cells. Two smaller vascular fringes, which project into the third ventricle from the underside of the tela choroidea, are continuous with the choroid plexuses of the lateral ventricles through the interventricular foramina.

The biggest vessels in the tela choroidea are the two *internal cerebral veins,* which unite in the caudal part of tela choroidea to form the *great cerebral vein,* which is continuous with the *straight sinus.* The internal cerebral vein receives blood from the

choroid vein, the *septal vein,* and the *thalamostriate vein* (Fig. 58).

Exploration of the Thalamus, Epithalamus and the Third Ventricle

1. The posterior part of the right hemisphere should be removed before the third ventricle is explored. To do this, transect splenium and the fornix on the left side as indicated in Fig. 59 and free the splenium from the underlying tela choroidea. Then cut a horizontal section between the temporal lobe and the insula on the right side at the level of the limen insulae, and remove the posterior part of the right hemisphere.

2. Remove the roof of the third ventricle by care-

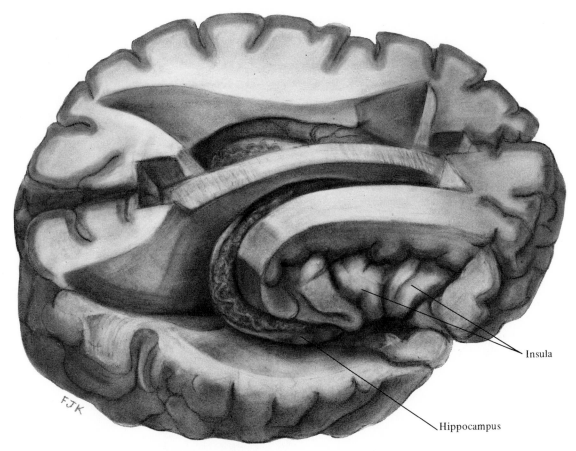

Insula

Hippocampus

Fig. 57. Temporal Horn and Hippocampus
In this lateral view of the brain the temporal horn has been exposed by removing a large part of the temporal lobe.

fully stripping off the tela choroidea with attached choroid plexa from the level of the interventricular foramina and backwards. As a consequence, the ependymal layer that covers the ventricular surface will also be removed. *Tenia choroidea* marks the place where the choroid plexus projected into the lateral ventricle, whereas *tenia thalami* indicates the line where the roof of the third ventricle was attached to the thalamus.

3. Continue the dissection by freeing the posterior part of the tela choroidea to expose the epithalamus, i.e., *habenula* and the *pineal body,* as well as the *quadrigeminal plate* with the *superior* and *inferior colliculi.*

4. Review the remaining walls of the third ventricle on available preparations.

The *anterior wall* is formed by lamina terminalis, the anterior commissure, and the fornix columns.

The *lateral wall* features the medial surfaces on the thalamus and the hypothalamus. Identify the stria medullaris along the mediodorsal edge of the thalamus.

The *posterior wall* of the third ventricle tapers in a funnel-shaped fashion into the cerebral aqueduct. Other formations in the posterior wall are the habenular commissure, the pineal body and the posterior commissure. The *pineal recess* is that part of the third ventricle that bulges into the pineal stalk.

The *floor* is formed by the optic chiasm, the infundibulum, the tuber cinereum and the mammillary bodies. It contains two recesses, the *optic recess* and the *infundibular recess.*

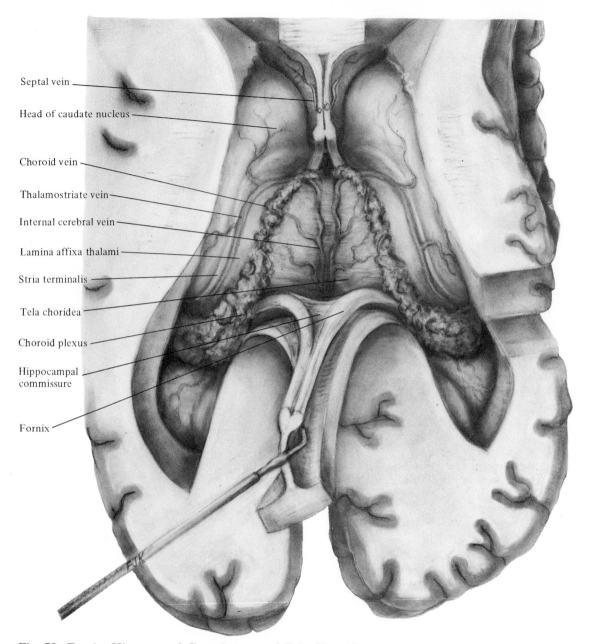

Septal vein

Head of caudate nucleus

Choroid vein

Thalamostriate vein

Internal cerebral vein

Lamina affixa thalami

Stria terminalis

Tela choridea

Choroid plexus

Hippocampal commissure

Fornix

Fig. 58. Fornix, Hippocampal Commissure, and Tela Choroidea
The corpus callosum, septum, and fornix have been transected and flipped backwards to expose the tela choroidea.

Thalamus, Basal Ganglia, and Internal Capsule

At this point it is practical to review the topographic relationships between the major forebrain nuclei and the white matter on the remaining part of the second brain. For this purpose cut a couple of horizontal sections at different levels in the two hemispheres and compare the sections (Figs. 60

A and B) with the picture of a frontal section at rostral or midthalamic level (Fig. 61), and with the drawings in Figs. 21 and 22, Chapter 2. Identify the following structures:

1. *Thalamus* is a collection of nuclei, many of which constitute important "relay" stations for afferent impulses to the cerebral cortex. A vertical lamina of white matter, the *internal medullary lamina,* divides the thalamus into a medial and

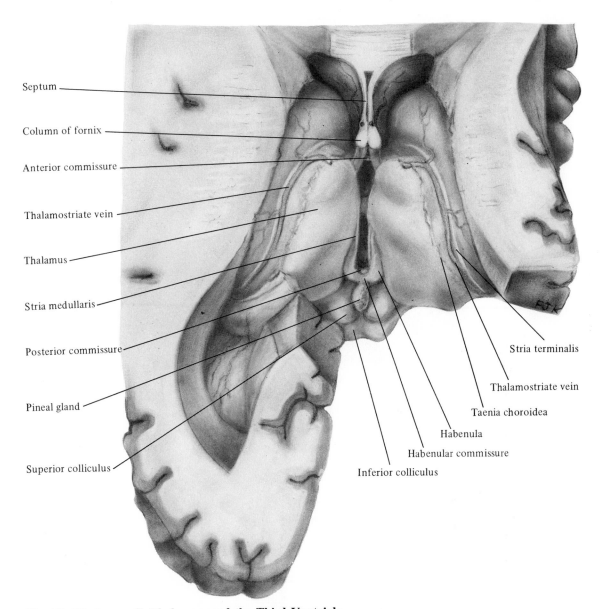

Fig. 59. Thalamus, Epithalamus, and the Third Ventricle
Exposure of the diencephalon and the third ventricle has been accomplished by removing the posterior part of the right hemisphere and the tela choroidea.

a lateral part. Rostrally, the medullary lamina is divided into two layers, which surround a rostral group of nuclei. The extensive caudal part of the thalamus is called *pulvinar,* under which the two geniculate bodies are located. The *medial* and *lateral geniculate bodies* serve as relay nuclei in the auditory and visual pathways.

2. *Caudate nucleus* is an elongated mass of gray matter, whose thick anterior portion, the *head* of the caudate bulges into the anterior horn of the lateral ventricle from the lateral side. At the level of the interventricular foramen the head narrows

into the body of the caudate, which lies adjacent to the thalamus. The body forms part of the floor of the central part of the lateral ventricle. The body of the caudate gradually tapers off and continues behind the thalamus as the *tail* of the caudate, which makes a sweep in a downward and forward direction into the temporal lobe.

3. *Lentiform nucleus,* which is located lateral to the internal capsule, has the form of a short ice cream cone with the broad base facing the insula. However, it is separated from insula by the *external capsule,* the *claustrum,* and the *extreme cap-*

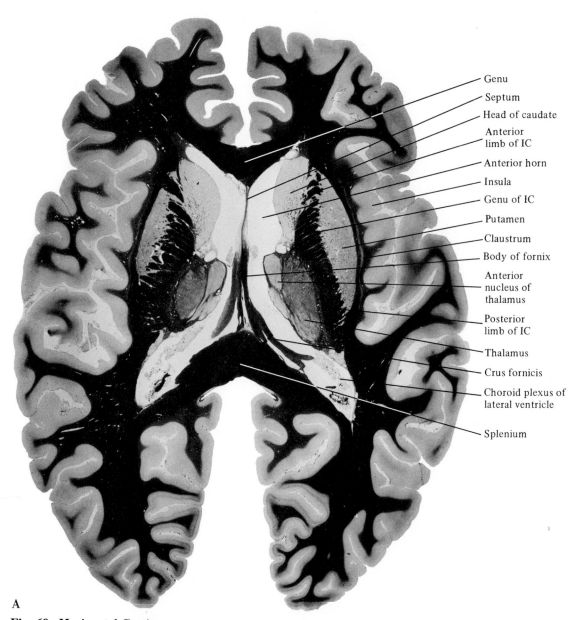

Genu
Septum
Head of caudate
Anterior limb of IC
Anterior horn
Insula
Genu of IC
Putamen
Claustrum
Body of fornix
Anterior nucleus of thalamus
Posterior limb of IC
Thalamus
Crus fornicis
Choroid plexus of lateral ventricle
Splenium

A

Fig. 60. Horizontal Sections
Section **B** is about 2 cm closer to the base of the brain than section **A**. (From the Yakoklev Collection)

sule. The lentiform nucleus is divided into a lateral part, *putamen,* and a medial part, *globus pallidus* (pallidum). Putamen is continuous with the head of the caudate through cell bridges that split apart the white matter, especially in the anterior limb of the internal capsule, giving it a striated appearance. This explains why putamen and caudate nucleus are sometimes referred to as striatum. Putamen and caudate nucleus, furthermore, are characterized by a large number of densely packed, medium-sized neurons that have a similar histologic structure; globus pallidus, on the other hand, contains large cells which lie rather far apart. In addition, it contains many myelinated fibers, which give the structure a pale appearance on a freshly cut brain.

The caudate nucleus and the lentiform nucleus are two of the major components in the basal ganglia, which are well-known for their relationships to motor functions (Chapter 8).

4. *Amygdaloid body* is a large rounded mass of gray matter in the anterior part of the temporal lobe immediately in front of the inferior horn. It can usually be identified on a horizontal section of the temporal lobe just below the level of the limen insulae. The amygdaloid body is continuous

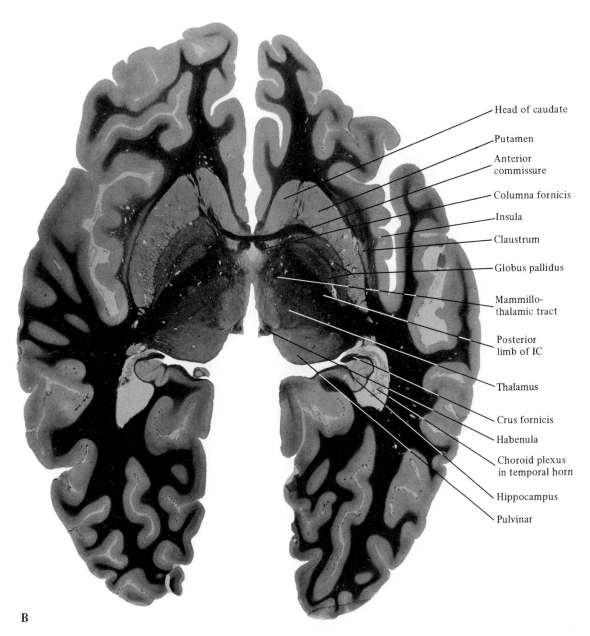

Head of caudate

Putamen

Anterior
commissure

Columna fornicis

Insula

Claustrum

Globus pallidus

Mammillo-
thalamic tract

Posterior
limb of IC

Thalamus

Crus fornicis

Habenula

Choroid plexus
in temporal horn

Hippocampus

Pulvinar

B

with the medial cortex of the temporal lobe in the region of the uncus. Although the amygdaloid body is sometimes included as a part of the basal ganglia, it is not part of the same functional system as the other components of the basal ganglia. Instead, it is one of the key structures in the limbic system and as such it has a close relationship with the hypothalamus (Chapter 17).

5. *Internal capsule*. This massive layer of white matter contains projection fibers connecting the cerebral cortex with various subcortical structures. It is located medial to the lentiform nucleus, where it forms the internal part of the capsule surround-

ing the lentiform nucleus, hence the name internal capsule. The lamina of white matter lateral to the lentiform nucleus is referred to as the external capsule.

The internal capsule has a typical V-form on a horizontal section with the apex of the V pointing medially (Fig. 60). The part of the capsule that is located between the head of the caudate medially, and the lentiform nucleus laterally, is called the *anterior limb*. It is broken up by bands of gray matter which form bridges between the putamen and the head of the caudate nucleus. The anterior limb contains the frontal corticopontine

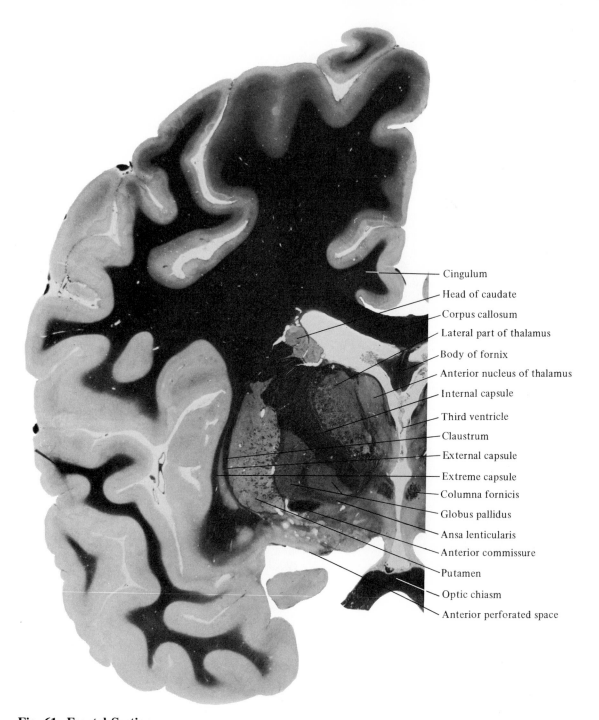

Cingulum
Head of caudate
Corpus callosum
Lateral part of thalamus
Body of fornix
Anterior nucleus of thalamus
Internal capsule
Third ventricle
Claustrum
External capsule
Extreme capsule
Columna fornicis
Globus pallidus
Ansa lenticularis
Anterior commissure
Putamen
Optic chiasm
Anterior perforated space

Fig. 61. Frontal Section
The upper part of the section is tilted somewhat in a posterior direction to cut through both the optic chiasm and the anterior thalamus. (From the Yakoklev Collection)

tract as well as fibers connecting the frontal cortex with the thalamus in both directions, i.e., the anterior thalamic radiation. The angle of the internal capsule is known as the *genu.*

The *posterior limb* of the internal capsule separates the lentiform nucleus on the lateral side from the thalamus on the medial side. The posterior limb consists of the corticospinal tract (pyramidal tract) and the sensory radiation, which carries sensory impulses to the somatosensory cortex in the postcentral gyrus. Other fibers in the posterior limb belong to the corticopontine and corticoreticular systems as well as the thalamic radiation.

Those parts of the posterior limb, which are located behind and underneath the lentiform nucleus, are known as the *retrolenticular* and the *sublenticular* parts of the internal capsule. The optic radiation, which originates in the lateral geniculate body and terminates in the visual cortex, is located in both the retrolenticular and the sublenticular part. The auditory radiation, which comes from the medial geniculate body, projects through the sublenticular part of the internal capsule to the auditory cortex in the superior temporal gyrus.

In a frontal section through the hemisphere at midthalamic level one can usually trace the internal capsule in continuity with the base of the cerebral peduncle in the mesencephalon. The internal capsule fibers that proceed uninterrupted to the base of the cerebral peduncle belong to the corticospinal tract and the corticopontine system.

Clinical Notes

Ventricular System

The ventricular system can be visualized in several radiologic procedures, e.g., *pneumencephalography* and *CAT scan,* and since the shape and the position of the ventricular system are often affected by various pathologic processes, such procedures are important tools in the diagnosis of brain disorders. Except for the posterior horn, which varies greatly in shape, the rest of the ventricular system is quite constant in regard to size, shape, and position, and deformities in its configuration can easily be detected, provided the normal anatomy is known.

Familiarity with the morphology of the ventricular system and with the formation and flow of CSF is also important for understanding one of the most common causes for *increased intracranial pressure.* This serious condition is often seen as a result of obstruction of the CSF circulation through the ventricular system. Narrow passages such as the interventricular foramen, the cerebral aqueduct, or the outlet foramina of the fourth ventricle can readily be obstructed by a pathologic process, e.g., a congenital malformation, a tumor or an inflammatory lesion. Since CSF is continuously produced in the choroid plexus, the obstruction increases the amount of CSF in the cranial cavity, which causes an increase in the intracranial pressure. The cardinal symptoms of increased intracranial pressure are headache, vomiting and papilledema (choked discs). Excessive amount of CSF in the cranial cavity is referred to as *hydrocephalus* (see Clinical Notes, Chapter 3).

Internal Capsule

A pathologic process in the cerebrovascular system is the most common cause of nervous system disease, and the internal capsule, which is supplied by the perforating branches, i.e. striate arteries, of the middle cerebral artery (Fig. 35) is often affected by a cerebrovascular lesion. If bleeding or occlusion affects one of the striate arteries, the most prominent symptom is a sudden weakening or loss of muscle power in the contralateral arm and leg, *capsular hemiplegia.* However, since the internal capsule contains other important fiber tracts besides the descending supraspinal pathways, additional symptoms may appear, especially if the lesion is more extensive. Damage to the ascending somatosensory pathway or the optic radiation, for instance, may result in sensory and visual disturbances.

A capsular hemiplegia is the most classic form of "*stroke*" (sudden appearance of focal neurologic deficits) and it can vary widely in severity from a mild case with transient symptoms to a severe *cerebrovascular accident* (CVA), in which the patient may become unconscious. The main stem of the middle cerebral artery is often involved in severe cases of capsular hemiplegia.

Fifth Dissection

Fourth Ventricle; Cerebellum; Brain Stem

Required for this dissection is one complete brain stem–cerebellum preparation, and one divided by a midsagittal section.

The cerebellum develops from a bilateral expansion of the rhombencephalic alar plate, the rhombic lips, and it is attached to the brain stem by three pairs of compact fiber bundles: the superior, the middle, and the inferior cerebellar peduncles. The cerebellum and the brain stem are thus two closely related structures, which lie in the posterior fossa covered by the tentorium cerebelli. Note that in the normal position in the skull, the cerebellum is behind rather than above the brain stem (Fig. 62A), and a horizontal section through the brain stem–cerebellum preparation would be nearly perpendicular to the long axis of the brain stem (Fig. 67A).

FOURTH VENTRICLE

The fourth ventricle is best studied on a median section through the brain stem and cerebellum (Fig. 62A). The upper part of its tent-shaped roof is formed by the *anterior medullary velum,* a thin plate, which extends between the two superior cerebellar peduncles. Rostrally, where it is attached to the quadrigeminal plate, it contains the decussating fibers of the trochlear nerve, which exits laterally. *Lingula,* a midline part of the cerebellar cortex, is fused to the outer surface of the anterior velum. The lower part of the roof is formed by a thin pia-ependymal membrane, from which the choroid plexus of the fourth ventricle is suspended. Although this membrane is often referred to as the *posterior medullary velum,* its medial part, which is related to the choroid plexus, does not seem to contain any myelinated fibers. The anterior medullary velum is continuous with the posterior velum at the apex of the fourth ventricle, the *fastigium.* The cerebrospinal fluid leaves the fourth ventricle to enter the subarachnoid space through the median aperture, foramen Magendie, and the two lateral apertures, foramina of Luschka. The relatively wide *median aperture,* which opens into the cerebellomedullary cistern, can be seen on the dorsal side of the brain stem in the angle between medulla oblongata and the cerebellum if the two structures are gently parted (Fig. 62B). The *lateral aperture* can be identified on one of the half brain stem–cerebellum preparations by gently probing in the direction of the tubular *lateral recess* of the fourth ventricle as it curves over the dorsal aspect of the brain stem. The lateral aperture, which is located in the *cerebellopontine angle* behind the IXth and Xth cranial nerves, is usually easy to identify from the outside because part of the choroid plexus projects out into the subarachnoid space through the opening.

CEREBELLUM

Although the cerebellum is largely hidden under the caudal parts of the cerebral hemisphere, it is nevertheless an impressive structure of great significance in clinical medicine. The cerebellum receives information from different sensory organs and from many parts of the brain and spinal cord, and on the basis of all this input impulses are sent to other motor centers through which cerebellum exerts its control of posture and movements.

Major Subdivisions

The cerebellum, which weighs about 150 g, is divided into a median part, *vermis,* and two large

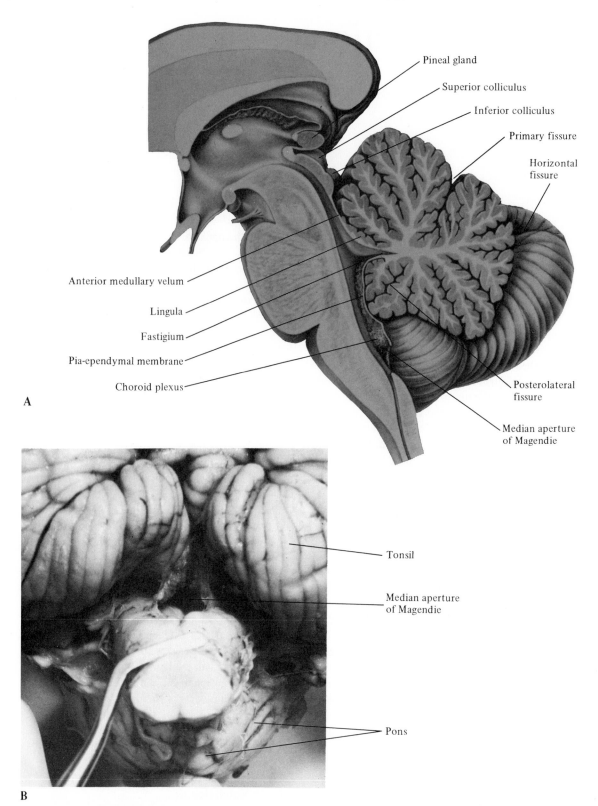

Fig. 62. Fourth Ventricle and Foramen of Magendie

A. Midsagittal section through the brain stem and cerebellum. (From R. Nieuwenhuys, Voogd, J. and Chr. van Huijzen, 1978, The Human Central Nervous System: A Synopsis and Atlas. With permission of the authors and Springer-Verlag, Berlin-Heidelberg.

B. Photograph showing the median aperture of Magendie.

lateral parts, the *cerebellar hemispheres.* The vermis is clearly separated from the hemispheres only on the inferior surface (Fig. 63). The cerebellum is characterized by an extensively folded cortex forming narrow elongated *folia* separated by furrows or *sulci,* which generally run in a transverse direction. Several deep clefts or fissures divide the cortex into various lobes and lobules, which have been given various names by different authors. The many nomenclatures are confusing and of interest only to the specialist. To appreciate the functional anatomy of the cerebellum and its relevance in clinical neurology, the medical student needs to pay attention only to a few major fissures and subdivisions (Figs. 62 and 63). The main subdivisions, which are arranged in a transverse fashion, can best be understood by imagining an unfolded cerebellar surface projected on a flat surface (Fig. 64). Identify the following fissures and lobes:

1. *Primary fissure* on the superior surface separates the *anterior* and *posterior lobes.*
2. *Horizontal fissure,* which extends from one middle cerebellar peduncle to the other within the posterior lobe, lies on the inferior surface close to its junction with the superior surface.
3. *Posterolateral fissure* separates the *posterior lobe* from the *flocculonodular lobe,* which is known for its close relations with the vestibular system. The flocculonodular lobe is located close to the brain stem on the inferior surface of the cerebellum, and it can be properly inspected only if the cerebellum is separated from the brain stem (see below). The main mass of cerebellum, with the exclusion of the flocculonodular lobe, is referred to as *corpus cerebelli.*

Although the vermis is clearly demarcated from the hemispheres on the inferior cerebellar surface, each part of vermis is continuous with a corresponding part of the cerebellar hemisphere, just as on the superior surface. In other words, the *nodule* is continuous with the *flocculus, uvula* with the *tonsil,* and *pyramis* with the *biventer* and *gracile* lobules.

Cerebellar Peduncles

The cerebellum is attached to the brain stem by three pairs of compact fiber bundles: the superior, the middle, and the inferior cerebellar peduncles.
1. *Inferior cerebellar peduncle* contains both cerebellopetal and cerebellofugal fibers. It approaches

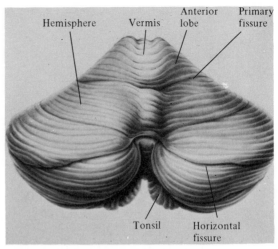

Fig. 63. Dorsal View of Cerebellum
(From Nieuwenhuys, R., Voogd, J, and van Huijzen, Chr., 1978. The Human Central Nervous System. With permission of the authors and Springer-Verlag, Berlin-Heidelberg.)

the cerebellum from the posterolateral surface of the medulla oblongata.
2. *Middle cerebellar peduncle* (brachium pontis) is the largest of the peduncles. It occupies the most lateral position of the three peduncles, and can easily be identified as it extends laterally into the cerebellum from the base of the pons. It contains fibers that originate in the pontine nuclei in the contralateral basilar part of pons.
3. *Superior cerebellar peduncle* (brachium conjunctivum) contains most of the efferent pathways that come from the intracerebellar nuclei and project to structures in the brain stem and diencephalon.

Blunt Dissection of the Cerebellar Peduncles

The blunt dissection of the cerebellar peduncles should be done only if there are extra brain stem–cerebellum preparations available, in which case it is well suited for a prosection. It can be properly performed only after some practice. If carefully done, however, the dissection reveals beautifully the topographic relations between the different peduncles. It is most practical to use a brain stem–cerebellum preparation cut in half by a median section.

Start from the lateral side of the middle cerebellar peduncle by removing the different cerebellar lobules, including the vermis until the core of white

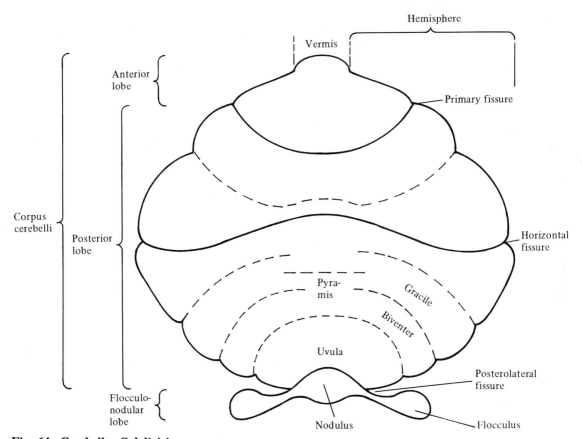

Fig. 64. Cerebellar Subdivisions
A highly schematic diagram of the exposed surface of the cerebellum showing the major fissures and subdivisions of the cerebellar cortex.

matter is exposed (Fig. 65A). Identify the vestibulocochlear nerve and its attachment to the dorsolateral side of the brain stem and pull it gently in a dorsal direction. By doing so the ridge of gray matter, i.e., the cochlear nuclei, which extends from the attachment of the nerve transversely across the lateral aspect of the brain stem, is stripped away. This exposes the *inferior cerebellar peduncle.* Push a probe upward alongside the lateral aspect of the inferior cerebellar peduncle until the probe becomes visible on the opposite side between the superior and the middle cerebellar peduncles (Fig. 65A). Cut through the fibers of the *middle cerebellar peduncle* lateral to the probe and remove the group of fibers that have just been cut. This exposes the intracerebellar part of the inferior cerebellar peduncle, whose fibers sweep on the outside of the *superior cerebellar peduncle* and fan out toward the cerebellar cortex. The relationship between the inferior and the superior peduncles is best studied by pushing a probe in a superior direction alongside the medial aspect of

the inferior cerebellar peduncle, and then separating the fibers of the two peduncles by forcing the probe in a posterior direction (Fig. 65B). The capsule of fibers that forms the "paddle," of the superior cerebellar peduncle (Fig. 65C) surrounds the largest of the intracerebellar nuclei, the dentate nucleus. By lifting the "paddle" in a posterior direction, the superior cerebellar peduncle is also lifted from its bed, because its fibers arise to a large extent in the dentate nucleus. The characteristic corrugated form of this nucleus can be observed by cutting a section through the fiber capsule.

Flocculonodular Lobe

The flocculonodular lobe can best be appreciated on the whole cerebellum following its separation from the brain stem (Fig. 66). This will also provide a brain stem preparation on which the floor of the fourth ventricle, the rhomboid fossa, can

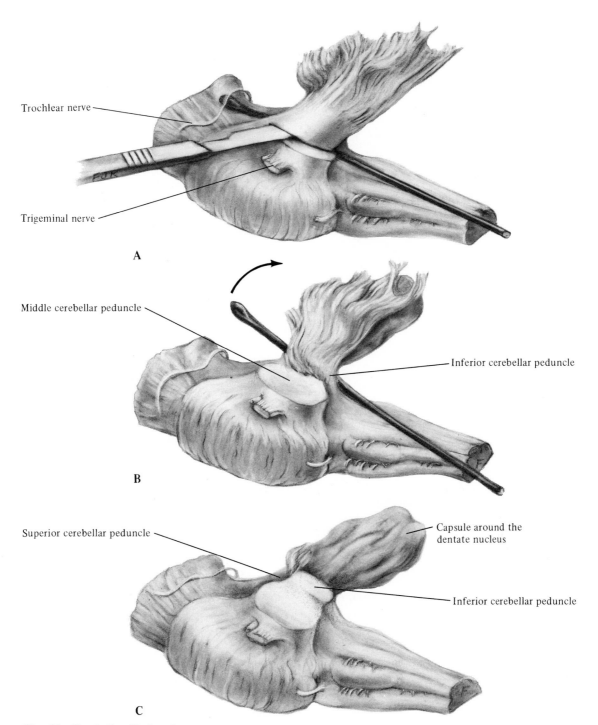

Fig. 65. Cerebellar Peduncles

A. After removal of the cerebellar lobules, a probe is pushed upwards alongside the inferior cerebellar peduncle until it becomes visible between the superior and middle cerebellar peduncles. The fibers of the middle cerebellar peduncle is then transected.

B. The relationships between the inferior and superior cerebellar peduncles can be studied by pushing the probe upwards alongside the medial aspect of the inferior cerebellar peduncle whereupon the fibers of the two peduncles are separated by forcing the probe in a posterior direction.

C. The inferior cerebellar peduncle has been transected to reveal the capsule of fibers around the dentate nucleus.

Lingula and
anterior
medullary   Superior   Inferior   Middle
velum   cerebellar   cerebellar   cerebellar
             peduncle   Vermis   peduncle   peduncle

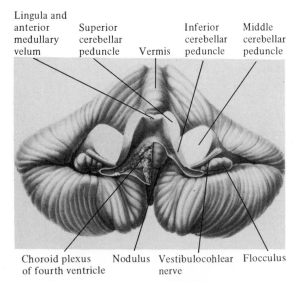

Choroid plexus   Nodulus Vestibulocohlear Flocculus
of fourth ventricle   nerve

Fig. 66. Ventral View of Cerebellum
(From Nieuwenhuys, R., J. Voogd, and Chr. van Huijzen, 1978. The Human Central Nervous System. With
permission of the authors and Springer-Verlag, Berlin-
Heidelberg.)

be inspected (see below). To separate the cerebellum from the brain stem, cut at right angle through
the middle cerebellar peduncle posterior to the
trigeminal nerve, and extend the cut toward the
lateral aperture just in front of the flocculus. Now,
lift up the inferior surface of the cerebellum from
the brain stem, identify the inferior cerebellar peduncle by removing the tela choroidea of the
fourth ventricle, and transect the peduncle. Likewise, lift carefully the anterior lobe of the cerebellum from the brain stem and cut through the superior cerebellar peduncle. Repeat the same
procedure on the other side and remove the cerebellum.

The flocculonodular lobe, which constitutes
only a small part of the whole cerebellum, consists
of two divisions, the *nodule* in the vermis, and
the laterally located *flocculus* which resembles a
small fragment of cauliflower. Nodulus is tucked
away under the main part of cerebellum, whereas
flocculus lies adjacent to the vestibulocochlear
nerve. The flocculonodular lobe, which receives
its main input from the vestibular system, is a
center for various vestibular reflexes.

Intracerebellar Nuclei

The intracerebellar nuclei, in which the efferent
cerebellar projections arise, can usually be identified by gross anatomic inspection if suitable sections are cut through the cerebellum. Use the half
brain stem–cerebellum preparation and cut a
nearly horizontal section along a line stretching
from the horizontal fissure to slightly above the
fastigium (Fig. 67A). This plane of sectioning,
which displays all four nuclei within the centrally
located medullary substance, is sometimes used
by neuropathologists at autopsies, because it produces a good overview of the intracerebellar nuclei
and the vermis. Identify the nuclei from lateral
to medial (Fig. 67B):
1. *Dentate nucleus* (red)
2. *Emboliform nucleus* (yellow)
3. *Globose nucleus* (yellow)
4. *Fastigial nucleus* (blue)

The large irregularly folded bag-shaped dentate
nucleus,[1] with its hilus directed medially, is easy
to identify. The round fastigial nucleus close to
the midline can usually be identified, whereas the
emboliform nucleus, which partially covers the hilus of the dentate nucleus, may be difficult to identify. The globose nucleus is composed of one or
more small cell groups not easily seen in macroscopic examination. The extent of the intracerebellar nuclei, especially the dentate nucleus, can be
appreciated by cutting a series of sagittal sections
through the still unused cerebellum from the second brain.

Clinical Notes

Tonsillar Herniation (Cerebellar Pressure Cone)

Herniation of parts of the cerebellar hemisphere,
primarily the tonsils, through the foramen magnum can occur as a result of increased pressure
in the posterior fossa, usually because of an expanding lesion in the infratentorial compartment

---

1. As the name indicates, the dentate nucleus appears as a
wrinkled band of gray matter in the human. In nonprimates,
where the nucleus is not folded, it is simply referred to as
the lateral nucleus. Emboliform and globose nuclei are together
referred to as the intermediate or interposed nuclei, and fastigial
nucleus is called the medial nucleus.

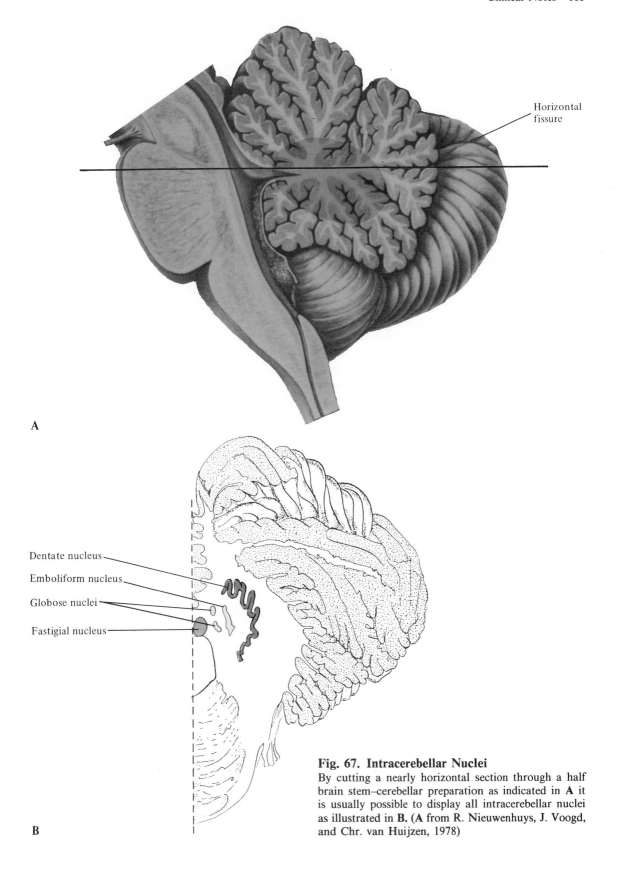

Horizontal
fissure

A

Dentate nucleus

Emboliform nucleus

Globose nuclei

Fastigial nucleus

B

Fig. 67. Intracerebellar Nuclei
By cutting a nearly horizontal section through a half
brain stem–cerebellar preparation as indicated in **A** it
is usually possible to display all intracerebellar nuclei
as illustrated in **B**. (**A** from R. Nieuwenhuys, J. Voogd,
and Chr. van Huijzen, 1978)

or as a result of a general brain swelling that can occur in many disorders of the brain. One should also remember that a tonsillar herniation can be precipitated by a lumbar puncture in a patient who is suffering from increased intracranial pressure. A tonsillar herniation causes pressure on vital centers in medulla oblongata, and can easily result in respiratory failure.

Medulloblastom

Almost two-thirds of all brain tumors in children are located in the infratentorial cavity. One of the most important tumors is the rapidly growing and very malignant medulloblastoma, which usually is located in the inferior vermis. Due to its strategic location in the main course of exit of the CSF from the fourth ventricle, the symptoms of increased intracranial pressure (papilledema, vomiting and headache) usually occur early as a result of obstructive hydrocephalus. Also, the tumor may occasionally spread throughout the subarachnoid space to the surface of the rest of the CNS, especially the spinal cord.

BRAIN STEM

Rhomboid Fossa

The floor of the fourth ventricle is shaped more or less like a rhombus and is accordingly referred to as the rhomboid fossa (Fig. 68). On each side of the *median sulcus*, which divides the fossa into two symmetrical halves, is a longitudinally running ridge, the *medial eminence*. The medial eminence is bounded laterally by the somewhat ill-defined sulcus limitans. The small medullary fold that overhangs the opening of the central canal at the inferior end of the rhomboid fossa is called the *obex*. Identify the following structures in the rhomboid fossa:

1. *Striae medullares,* group of medullated fiber bundles that connect the arcuate nuclei adjacent to the pyramis, with the cerebellum. The pronounced elevation on the medial eminence rostral to the striae medullares is
2. *Facial colliculus,* which overlies the abducens nucleus and the genu of the facial nerve.
3. *Locus ceruleus,* a bluish gray area rostral to the facial colliculus in the area of the sulcus limitans. The area overlies the nucleus of the locus

ceruleus, the cells of which contain melanin pigments and give rise to noradrenergic pathways, which are distributed widely in the brain and the spinal cord.
4. *Hypoglossal trigone* behind the striae medullares is formed by the underlying nucleus of the hypoglossal nerve.
5. *Vagal trigone,* lateral and posterior to the hypoglossal trigone, overlies the dorsal nucleus of the vagus nerve.
6. *Vestibular area* overlies the vestibular nuclei in the lateral part of the rhomboid fossa.

Cross-sections Through the Brain Stem

The structure of the brain stem is complicated, and many of its nuclear groups and pathways can be studied only in properly stained microscopic sections. However, the general topographic features and some of the main nuclei and fiber systems can be identified with the naked eye in transverse sections cut during the brain dissection. The brain stem contains the cranial nerve nuclei and several other specific nuclei, many of which are embedded in the reticular formation (see Chapter 10). It also contains many ascending and descending pathways, through which impulses to and from the forebrain, the cerebellum, and the spinal cord are being transmitted.

Mesencephalon (Fig. 69)

Mesencephalon is divided into *tectum* (quadrigeminal plate) and the two *cerebral peduncles* by an imaginary plane through the cerebral aqueduct. Each cerebral peduncle in turn consists of the *tegmentum* dorsally and the *basis pedunculi* ventrally.

Tectum. The roof of the midbrain is composed of the *superior* and *inferior colliculi,* which contain important reflex centers for visual and auditory impulses. The inferior colliculus, furthermore, serves as a relay center in the auditory pathway from the cochlear nuclei to the medial geniculate body and the auditory cortex. *Periaqueductal gray* surrounds the cerebral aqueduct.

Tegmentum. The *nuclei* for the *oculomotor* (III) and *trochlear* (IV) *nerves* are located in the tegmentum at the border of the central gray sub-

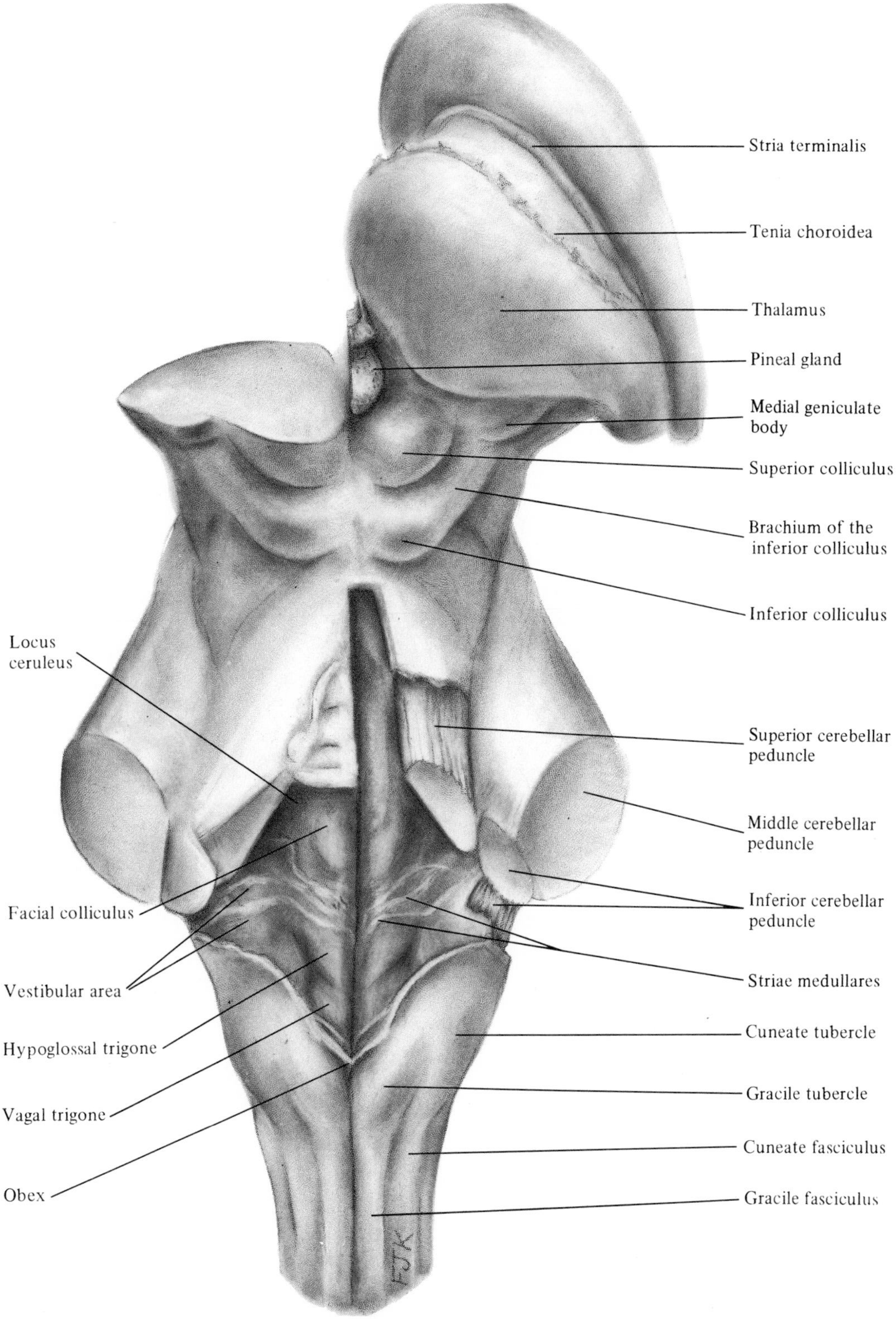

Stria terminalis

Tenia choroidea

Thalamus

Pineal gland

Medial geniculate
body

Superior colliculus

Brachium of the
inferior colliculus

Inferior colliculus

Locus
ceruleus

Superior cerebellar
peduncle

Middle cerebellar
peduncle

Inferior cerebellar
peduncle

Facial colliculus

Striae medullares

Vestibular area

Cuneate tubercle

Hypoglossal trigone

Gracile tubercle

Vagal trigone

Cuneate fasciculus

Obex

Gracile fasciculus

Fig. 68. Rhomboid Fossa
The floor of the fourth ventricle, the rhomboid fossa, has been exposed by removing the cerebellum.

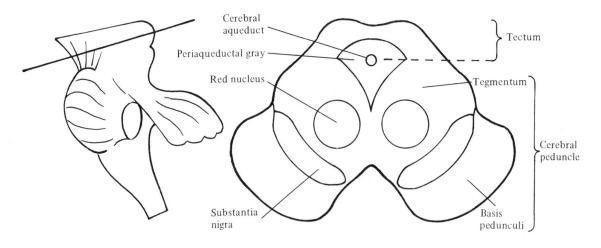

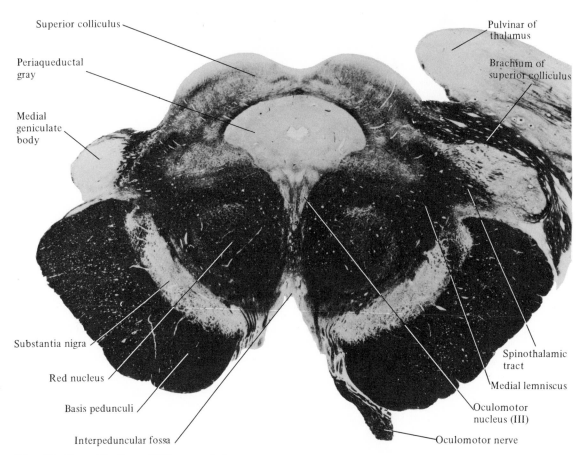

Fig. 69. Cross-Section of Mesencephalon
(From DeArmond, S. J., M. M. Fusco, and M. M. Dewey, 1976. Structure of the Human Brain, 2nd ed. With permission of Oxford University Press.)

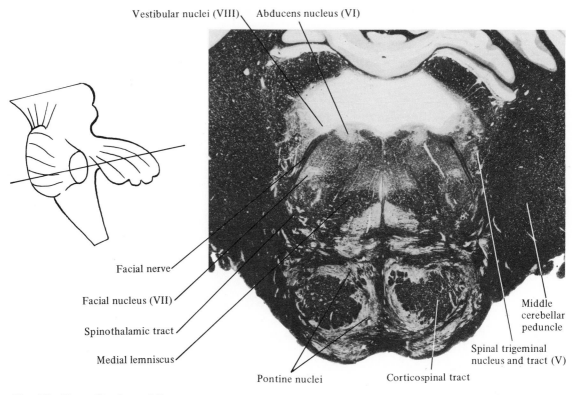

Vestibular nuclei (VIII)   Abducens nucleus (VI)

Facial nerve

Facial nucleus (VII)

Spinothalamic tract

Medial lemniscus

Pontine nuclei

Corticospinal tract

Middle
cerebellar
peduncle

Spinal trigeminal
nucleus and tract (V)

Fig. 70. Cross-Section of Pons
(From DeArmond, S. J., M. M. Fusco, and M. M. Dewey, 1976. Structure of the Human Brain, 2nd ed. With permission of Oxford University Press.)

stance. The oculomotor complex is located at the level of the superior colliculus, and the trochlear nucleus at the level of the inferior colliculus. The oculomotor centers cannot be recognized with certainty in the gross anatomic preparations. However, the most conspicuous structure in the tegmentum, the *red nucleus* (nucleus ruber), can usually be recognized as a round grayish-brown area (7–8 mm in diameter) surrounded by a capsule of white matter. The red nucleus is part of the motor system (Chapter 7).

The central part of the tegmentum throughout the brain stem is occupied by the *reticular formation,* which is characterized by a mixture of different cell aggregations separated by a wealth of nerve fibers running in all directions. The brain stem reticular formation influences a variety of functions; it controls motor activities and it is concerned with such basic activities as sleep and consciousness. The reticular formation in lower pons and medulla contains important respiratory and cardiovascular centers. The somatosensory fiber systems, the *medial lemniscus* and the *spinothalamic tract,* are located in the lateral half of the tegmentum.

The Base of the Peduncle. The dorsal part of the basis pedunculi is characterized by a black or dark brown area, the *substantia nigra,* which gets its color from the presence of melanin-containing cells. Many of the cells in the substantia nigra project to the caudate nucleus and the putamen. This is the dopaminergic nigrostriatal pathway, which is of special importance for the control of involuntary coordinated movements (Chapter 8).

The ventral portion of the basis pedunculi, which is referred to as *pes pedunculi,* contains descending pathways, which carry impulses from the cerebral cortex to the brain stem and the spinal cord.

Pons (Fig. 70)

Pons consists of a large ventral or basal part and a smaller dorsal part, the pontine tegmentum.

The Ventral Part. This part contains a large collection of cellgroups, the *pontine nuclei,* as well as many transversely and longitudinally running myelinated fiber bundles, which gives the basal

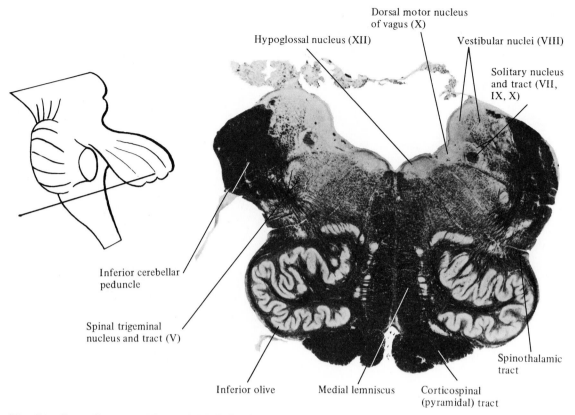

Fig. 71. Cross-Section of Rostral Medulla Oblongata
(From DeArmond, S. J., M. M. Fusco, and M. M. Dewey, 1976. Structure of the Human Brain, 2nd ed. With permission of Oxford University Press.)

part a white color. The transverse fiber bundles, the *pontocerebellar tracts,* originate in the pontine nuclei on one side, cross the midline, and enter the cerebellum as the middle cerebellar peduncle. The pontocerebellar fibers form the second link in an important corticopontocerebellar pathway, through which cortical regions in one cerebral hemisphere can communicate with the opposite half of the cerebellum. The first link in this system is represented by longitudinally running fibers, the *corticopontine tracts,* which descend through the base of the cerebral peduncle, and terminate in the pontine nuclei. The longitudinally running fiber bundles of the *corticospinal tract* come together at the lower end of pons to form the two pyramids of the medulla oblongata (see below).

Tegmentum. The *pontine tegmentum* is continuous with the tegmentum of the midbrain and the medulla. Embedded in the pontine reticular formation are many fiber tracts and several cranial nerve nuclei, namely those of the Vth, VIth, VIIth, and VIIIth cranial nerves. The *medial lemniscus* is situated close to the midline in the ventral part of tegmentum, whereas the *spinothalamic tract* and the *lateral lemniscus* (secondary auditory fibers) are located more laterally in the tegmentum.

Medulla Oblongata (Figs. 71 and 72)

Medulla oblongata, which is the most caudal part of the brain stem, decreases in thickness as it approaches the spinal cord, and its boundary toward the spinal cord cannot be easily appreciated since the distinctive external features of the medulla gradually disappear in its lower part. The area of transition, however, is usually indicated on the ventral side by fibers crossing the median fissure. These fibers, which come from the pyramids, form part of the *pyramidal* or *corticospinal decussation* (Fig. 72B). This is the most conspicuous feature of the spinomedullary transition area.

One of the most characteristic structures in a cross-section through the upper half of medulla oblongata is the *inferior olivary nucleus,* which

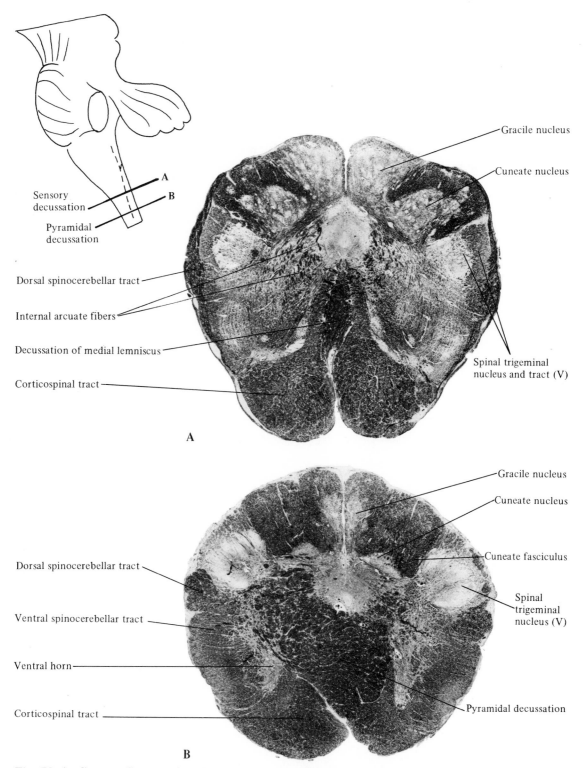

Fig. 72–A. Sensory Decussation (Decussation of medial lemniscus)

These cross-sections of caudal medulla oblongata were kindly provided by Dr. T. H. Williams. (From Gluhbegovic, N. and T. H. Williams, 1980. The Human Brain and Spinal Cord. With permission from Harper and Row Hagerstown.)

Fig. 72–B. Pyramidal Decussation

These cross-sections of caudal medulla oblongata were kindly provided by Dr. T. H. Williams. (From Gluhbegovic, N. and T. H. Williams, 1980. The Human Brain and Spinal Cord. With permission from Harper and Row Hagerstown.)

looks like the dentate nucleus, i.e., like a crumpled bag with its hilus directed medially. It projects through the *inferior cerebellar peduncle* to the contralateral half of cerebellum. The corticospinal tract forming the *pyramid* is located ventromedially to the inferior olive. The *medial lemniscus* is located close to the midline. Embedded in the gray matter underneath the floor of the fourth ventricle are several of the cranial nerve nuclei, namely those of the VIIIth, IXth, Xth, and XIIth cranial nerves.

The cross-section through the lower half of the medulla below the obex (Fig. 68), is similar to that of the spinal cord primarily because the dorsally located fourth ventricle has been replaced by the narrow *central canal.* The *dorsal funiculi* (posterior columns) represent additional spinal cord features. If the section was stained and examined in the microscope, however, one would immediately recognize some major departures from the typical spinal cord appearance. In contrast to the situation in the spinal cord, where the dorsal funiculi contain ascending somatosensory pathways in the form of heavy myelinated fiber bundles, i.e., the *gracile* and *cuneate fasciculi,* the dorsal funiculi in the lower half of the medulla oblongata are composed primarily of large nuclear masses, the *gracile* and *cuneate nuclei* (dorsal column nuclei), which form the *gracile* and *cuneate tubercles* on the dorsal surface of the bulb. These nuclei represent relay stations for the ascending somatosensory fibers in the dorsal funiculi. Fibers arising in the gracile and cuneate nuclei on one side cross over to the opposite side anterior to the central canal to form the medial lemniscus. The crossing fibers are referred to as *internal arcuate fibers,* and the crossing itself as the *decussation of the medial lemniscus* (sensory decussation, Fig. 72A). The *pyramidal decussation* (Fig. 72B) is situated immediately below the sensory decussation.

Sixth Dissection

Atlas of the Brain: Frontal, Sagittal, and Horizontal Brain Sections; Anatomical Correlation of Computerized Brain Tomography

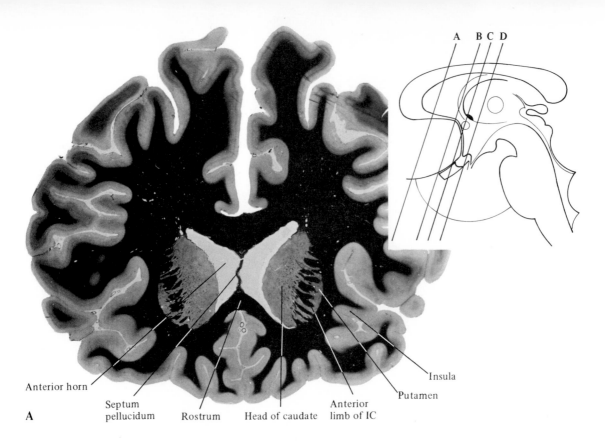

Insula

Putamen

Anterior horn

Septum
pellucidum

Rostrum

Head of caudate

Anterior
limb of IC

A

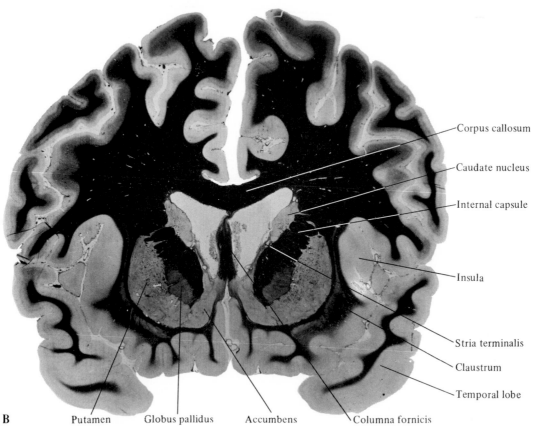

Corpus callosum

Caudate nucleus

Internal capsule

Insula

Stria terminalis

Claustrum

Temporal lobe

B

Putamen

Globus pallidus

Accumbens

Columna fornicis

Fig. 73 A–H. Frontal Sections of the Brain
(From the Yakovlev Collection)

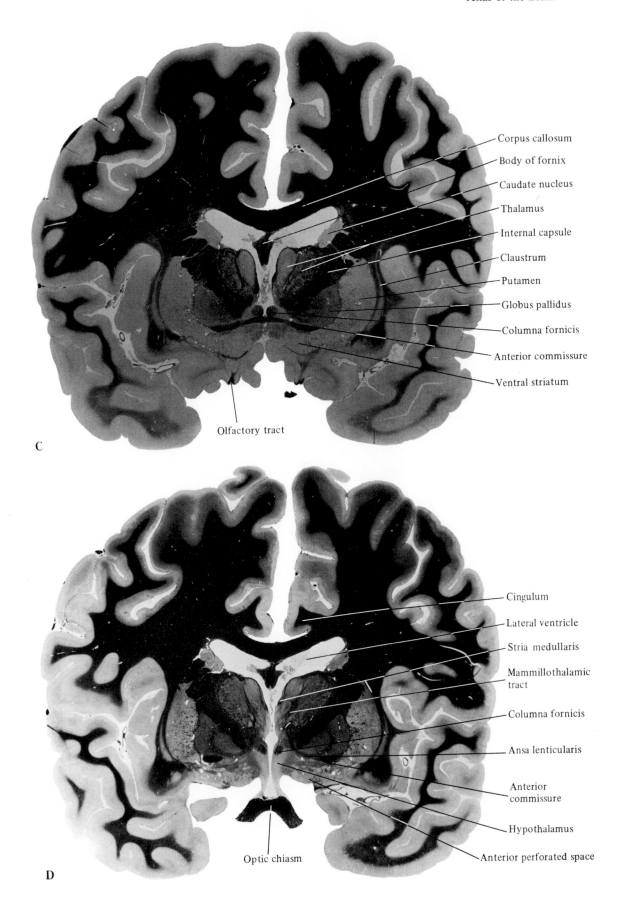

Corpus callosum

Body of fornix

Caudate nucleus

Thalamus

Internal capsule

Claustrum

Putamen

Globus pallidus

Columna fornicis

Anterior commissure

Ventral striatum

Olfactory tract

C

Cingulum

Lateral ventricle

Stria medullaris

Mammillothalamic tract

Columna fornicis

Ansa lenticularis

Anterior commissure

Hypothalamus

Anterior perforated space

Optic chiasm

D

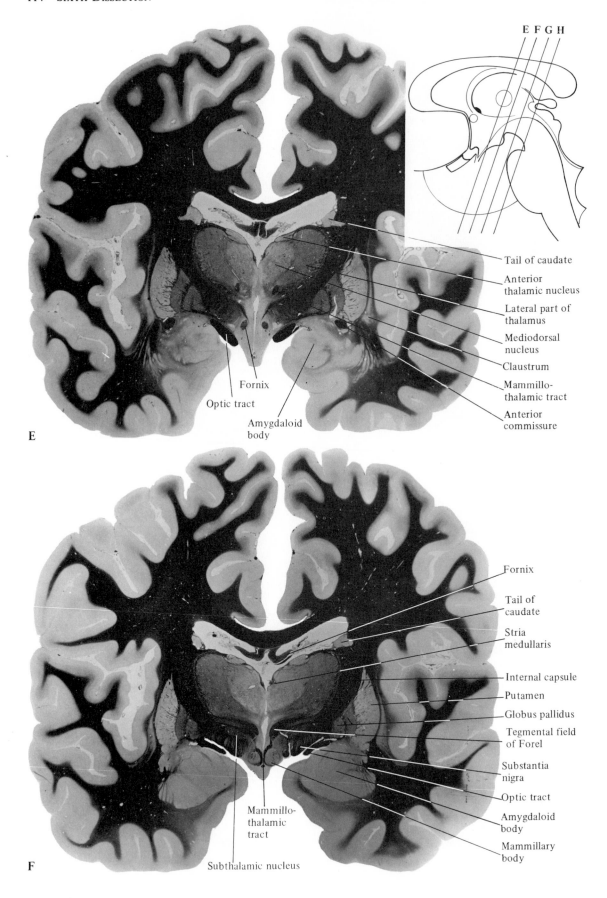

E F G H

Tail of caudate

Anterior
thalamic nucleus

Lateral part of
thalamus

Mediodorsal
nucleus

Claustrum

Mammillo-
thalamic tract

Anterior
commissure

Fornix

Optic tract

Amygdaloid
body

E

Fornix

Tail of
caudate

Stria
medullaris

Internal capsule

Putamen

Globus pallidus

Tegmental field
of Forel

Substantia
nigra

Optic tract

Amygdaloid
body

Mammillary
body

Mammillo-
thalamic
tract

Subthalamic nucleus

F

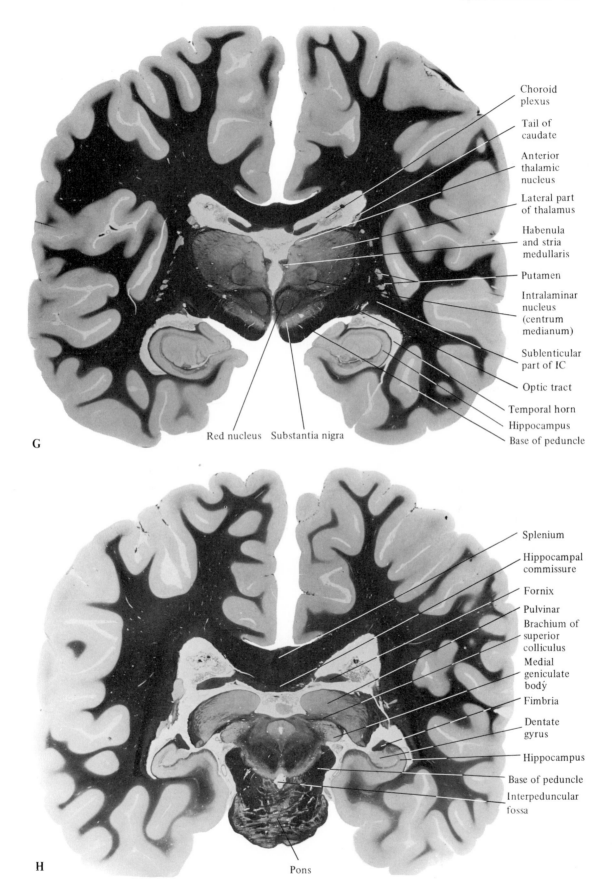

Choroid
plexus

Tail of
caudate

Anterior
thalamic
nucleus

Lateral part
of thalamus

Habenula
and stria
medullaris

Putamen

Intralaminar
nucleus
(centrum
medianum)

Sublenticular
part of IC

Optic tract

Temporal horn

Hippocampus

Base of peduncle

Red nucleus   Substantia nigra

G

Splenium

Hippocampal
commissure

Fornix

Pulvinar

Brachium of
superior
colliculus

Medial
geniculate
body

Fimbria

Dentate
gyrus

Hippocampus

Base of peduncle

Interpeduncular
fossa

Pons

H

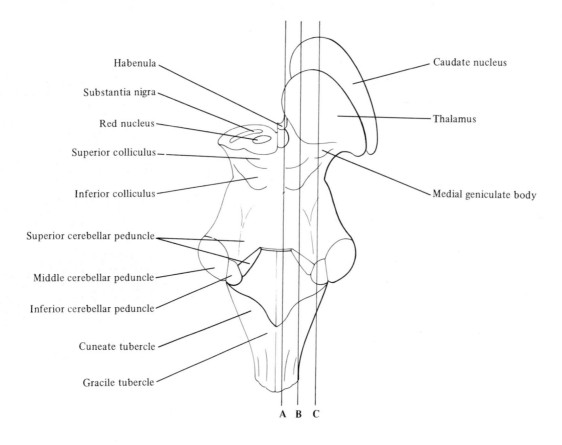

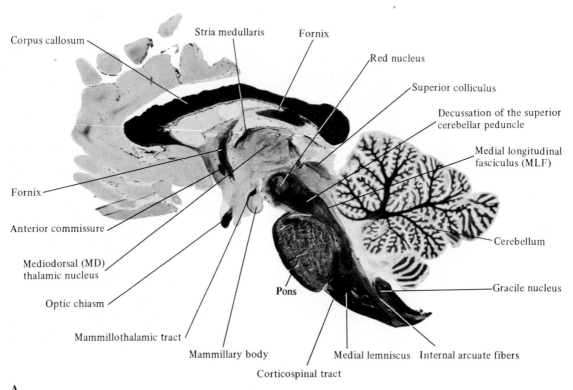

Habenula

Substantia nigra

Red nucleus

Superior colliculus

Inferior colliculus

Superior cerebellar peduncle

Middle cerebellar peduncle

Inferior cerebellar peduncle

Cuneate tubercle

Gracile tubercle

Caudate nucleus

Thalamus

Medial geniculate body

A B C

Corpus callosum

Stria medullaris

Fornix

Red nucleus

Superior colliculus

Decussation of the superior cerebellar peduncle

Medial longitudinal fasciculus (MLF)

Cerebellum

Fornix

Anterior commissure

Mediodorsal (MD) thalamic nucleus

Optic chiasm

Mammillothalamic tract

Mammillary body

Pons

Gracile nucleus

Corticospinal tract

Medial lemniscus

Internal arcuate fibers

A

Fig. 74 A–C. Sagittal Sections of the Brain
(From the Yakovlev Collection)

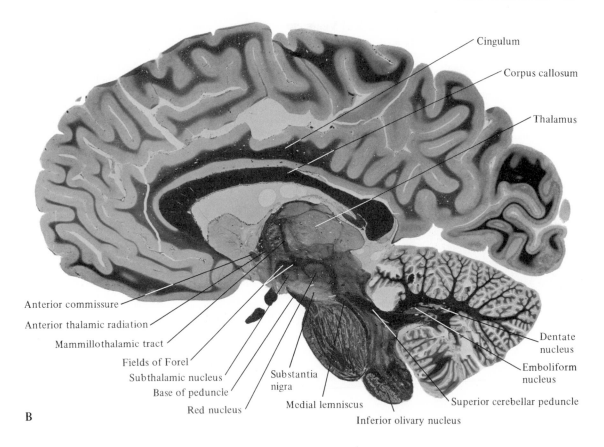

Cingulum

Corpus callosum

Thalamus

Anterior commissure

Anterior thalamic radiation

Mammillothalamic tract

Fields of Forel

Subthalamic nucleus

Base of peduncle

Red nucleus

Substantia nigra

Medial lemniscus

Inferior olivary nucleus

Dentate nucleus

Emboliform nucleus

Superior cerebellar peduncle

B

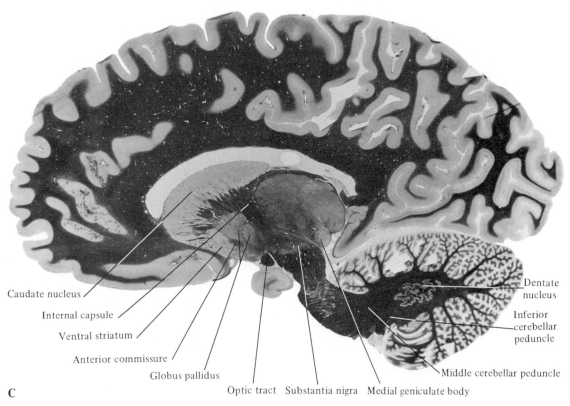

Caudate nucleus

Internal capsule

Ventral striatum

Anterior commissure

Globus pallidus

Optic tract   Substantia nigra   Medial geniculate body

Dentate nucleus

Inferior cerebellar peduncle

Middle cerebellar peduncle

C

Fig. 75. 30° Section Dorsal to the Lateral Ventricle   ▷

The sections in Figures 75–79 are angled at 30° to the anatomic baseline of Reid (infraorbital margin to the top of the external auditory meatus). This plane of section corresponds to an angle of 20° from the cantomeatal line. By choosing an angle of 25°–30° to the anatomic baseline the eye does not become involved and the whole brain can be scanned with a minimal amount of radiation. (The brain sections in Figures 75–79 have been borrowed from Matsui, T., and A. Hirano, 1978. An Atlas of the Human Brain for Computerized Tomography. With permission from the authors and the publisher. Igaku-Shoin, Tokyo–New York. The matching CT scans in Figures 75, 76 and 77 were provided by Dr. V. Haughton, whereas the scans for Figures 78 and 79 were provided by Dr. L. Morris.)

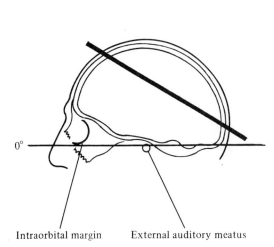

Intraorbital margin   External auditory meatus

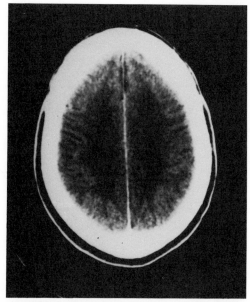

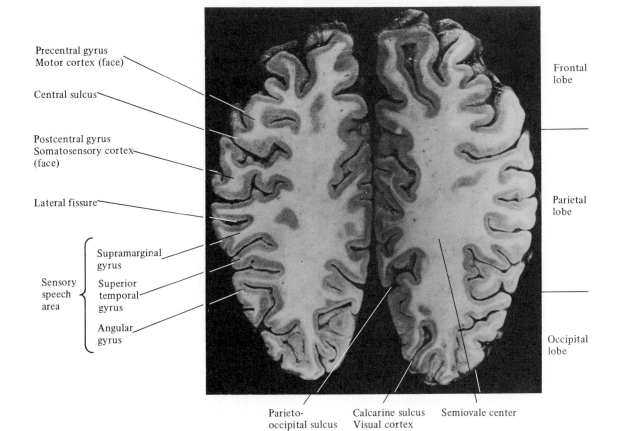

Precentral gyrus
Motor cortex (face)

Central sulcus

Postcentral gyrus
Somatosensory cortex
(face)

Lateral fissure

Sensory
speech
area

Supramarginal
gyrus

Superior
temporal
gyrus

Angular
gyrus

Frontal
lobe

Parietal
lobe

Occipital
lobe

Parieto-
occipital sulcus

Calcarine sulcus
Visual cortex

Semiovale center

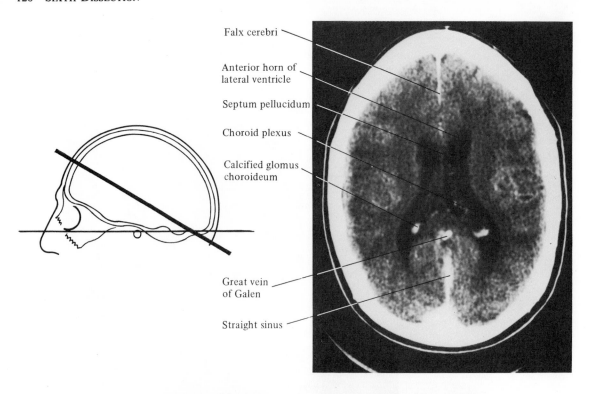

Falx cerebri

Anterior horn of lateral ventricle

Septum pellucidum

Choroid plexus

Calcified glomus choroideum

Great vein of Galen

Straight sinus

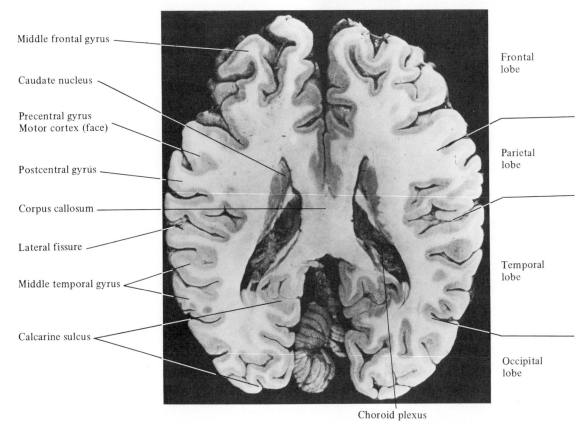

Middle frontal gyrus

Caudate nucleus

Precentral gyrus Motor cortex (face)

Postcentral gyrus

Corpus callosum

Lateral fissure

Middle temporal gyrus

Calcarine sulcus

Frontal lobe

Parietal lobe

Temporal lobe

Occipital lobe

Choroid plexus

Fig. 76. 30° Section Through the Central Parts and Posterior Horns of the Lateral Ventricles
Note that the CT scan is somewhat closer to the base of the brain than the corresponding brain section. This
is most easily appreciated by the fact that the body of the corpus callosum has disappeared in the CT scan.

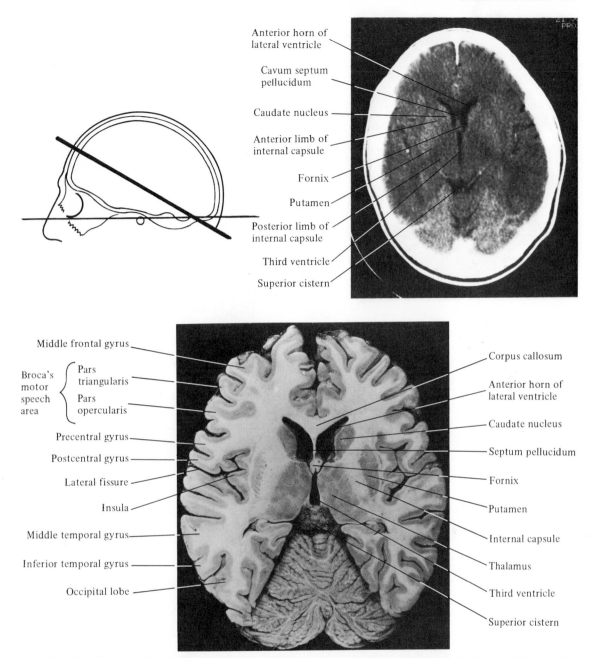

Fig. 77. 30° Section Through the Third Ventricle and the Anterior Horn of the Lateral Ventricles

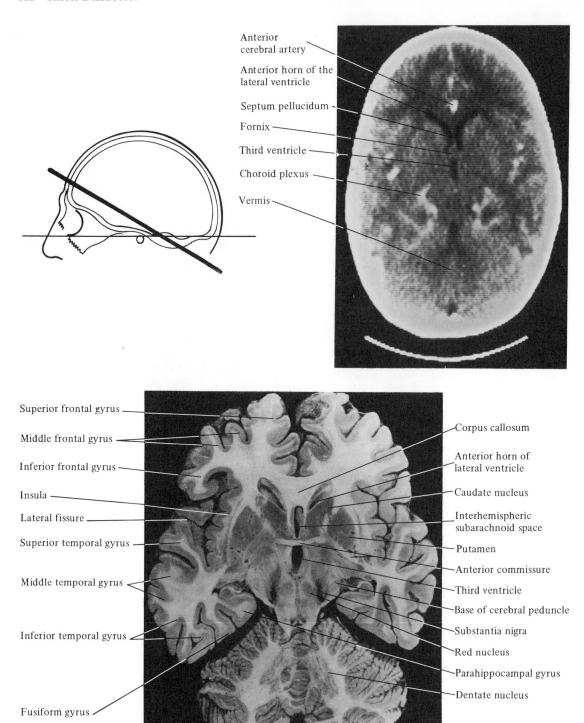

Anterior
cerebral artery

Anterior horn of the
lateral ventricle

Septum pellucidum

Fornix

Third ventricle

Choroid plexus

Vermis

Superior frontal gyrus

Middle frontal gyrus

Inferior frontal gyrus

Insula

Lateral fissure

Superior temporal gyrus

Middle temporal gyrus

Inferior temporal gyrus

Fusiform gyrus

Corpus callosum

Anterior horn of
lateral ventricle

Caudate nucleus

Interhemispheric
subarachnoid space

Putamen

Anterior commissure

Third ventricle

Base of cerebral peduncle

Substantia nigra

Red nucleus

Parahippocampal gyrus

Dentate nucleus

Fig. 78. 30° Section Through the Basal Forebrain and Mesencephalon

Note that the anterior half of the CT scan is somewhat more dorsal than the corresponding brain section. This is indicated by the fact that the anterior horns of the lateral ventricles are more extensive in the CT scan than in the brain section. Furthermore, part of the interhemispheric subarachnoid space, which is located behind the corpus callosum in the brain section, is not present in the CT scan.

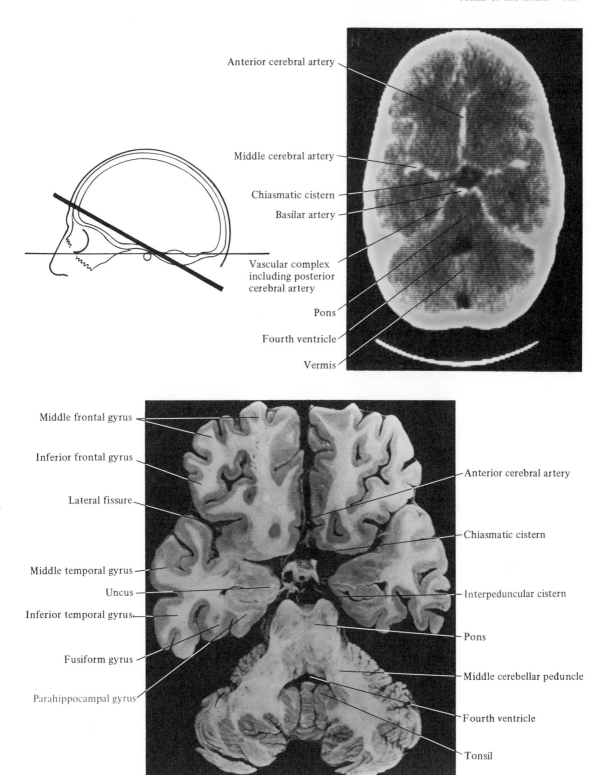

Anterior cerebral artery

Middle cerebral artery

Chiasmatic cistern

Basilar artery

Vascular complex
including posterior
cerebral artery

Pons

Fourth ventricle

Vermis

Middle frontal gyrus

Inferior frontal gyrus

Lateral fissure

Middle temporal gyrus

Uncus

Inferior temporal gyrus

Fusiform gyrus

Parahippocampal gyrus

Anterior cerebral artery

Chiasmatic cistern

Interpeduncular cistern

Pons

Middle cerebellar peduncle

Fourth ventricle

Tonsil

Fig. 79. 30° Section Through the Circle of Willis, Pons and Fourth Ventricle

PART 3
Functional Neuroanatomy

4

Neurohistology and Neuroanatomic Techniques

THE NEURON
  Cell Body
  Cell Processes
  Axonal Transport

THE SYNAPSE
  Synaptic Vesicles
  Classification of Synapses
  Neuron Doctrine

NEUROGLIA
  Astroglia
  Oligodendroglia
  Microglia
  Ependyma

NEUROANATOMIC TECHNIQUES
  Nissl and Golgi Methods
  Reduced Silver Impregnation Methods
  Axonal Transport Methods
  Histochemical Methods

CLINICAL NOTES
  Multiple Sclerosis
  Myasthenia Gravis
  Parkinson's Disease
  Regeneration and Plasticity
  Spread of Virus and Toxin
  Blood–Brain Barrier

SUGGESTED READING

One of the most prominent characteristics of nervous tissue is the great flexibility with which it responds to various stimuli. This unique feature of the nervous system can easily be appreciated in light of its histology. Basically, the nervous system is built up of billions of neurons that are connected to each other by means of processes—dendrites and axons—of variable length and arrangement. The nervous tissue thus forms a complicated network of pathways and neuronal circuits for the transmission of chemoelectric impulses.

Although knowledge of the pathways in the brain and spinal cord cannot in itself explain how the nervous system works, the mapping of the central nervous connections is a prerequisite for such understanding. The study of neuronal connections and synaptic relationships, therefore, is one of the most active areas of research in the nervous system, and the modern neuroscientist is fortunate enough to have a large number of sophisticated light and electron microscopic techniques available.

Although basic information about the gross anatomic features of the brain and the spinal cord has accumulated through centuries of observation, it was not until the *light microscope* was refined in the 19th century that a successful study of the histologic structure of the nervous system was begun. At this same time, techniques for the preparation and staining of histologic sections were developed that made it possible to visualize the different components of the nervous tissue and to study the distribution of neurons and the relationships between their processes.

Another great step forward in defining the structure of the nervous system occurred in the mid-20th century with the introduction of the *electron microscope*. In contrast with the light microscope, which shows only a few components of nervous tissue, the electron microscope displays, with a high degree of magnification and resolution, all the different structures present in a section.

The Neuron

In spite of great variability in size and configuration, all neurons have in common certain morphologic features, which reflect the fact that nervous tissue functions as a communication system. To provide for efficient communication, the neurons have processes, *dendrites* and *axons*. The dendrites and axons usually receive input from specialized terminals of axons. The axon, of which there is one per neuron, is specialized to conduct nerve impulses (Fig. 2, Chapter 1). Transmission of the signal from one neuron to another neuron, or to an effector organ (muscle or gland), occurs at specialized contact regions called synapses.

Cell Body

The cell body consists of a *large nucleus* and the surrounding cytoplasm, the *perikaryon*. It is the trophic center of the neuron and the function and survival of the axon and dendrites are dependent on the integrity of the cell body.

The classic light microscopic method for the study of the cell body is the *Nissl method*, which relies on the use of basic dyes such as cresyl violet. Besides showing the form of the cell body, the Nissl method selectively stains the nucleus and one of the most characteristic cell components of

the neuron, the *Nissl bodies* (Fig. 80). The Nissl bodies are basophilic and in the light microscope appear as dust-like material or as small or large granules. The Nissl substance is present in the cell body and the proximal dendrites, but it is conspicuously absent from the axon as well as from the axon hillock, which is the pale, conical shaped region from which the axon extends. Electron microscopic studies show that the Nissl substance (Fig. 80A) consists of concentrations of granular or *rough endoplasmic reticulum* (*RER*) and free *polyribosomes* (Fig. 80B). The ribosomes are important organelles for the synthesis of proteins, which are in great demand for the maintenance of the elaborate neuronal processes. In neurons, some of the cisterns of the endoplasmic reticulum have an unusually narrow lumen and are closely opposed to the plasma membrane (subsurface cisterns).

The appearance of the Nissl substance is one of the most valuable features for the identification and evaluation of neurons in both normal and pathologic materials because the Nissl patterns vary between different types of neurons. Motor neurons, for instance, have large Nissl bodies (Fig. 80A), whereas sensory neurons have smaller ones (Fig. 80C), and small neurons often contain dust-like Nissl substance. The appearance of the Nissl substance also varies with the activity of the cell. The Nissl bodies gradually diminish in neurons subjected to functional stress, and they disintegrate when the axon is injured or sectioned. The latter phenomenon, known as *chromatolysis,* is often part of a general cell change in response to axonal injury. Besides chromatolysis, such *retrograde cell reaction* generally includes swelling of the cell and displacement of its nucleus to the periphery of the perikaryon (Fig. 80D).

Neurons impregnated with one of the classic silver methods, e.g., the Bielschowsky method, display another characteristic structure, the *neurofibril.* The neurofibrils apparently represent bundles of 10-nm thick *neurofilaments* and *microtubules* on which silver has been deposited. Neurofibrils are usually seen in the perikaryon between the Nissl bodies and in the large dendrites and axons.

In addition to Nissl substance, neurofilaments, and microtubules, the nerve cell body contains other organelles that are commonly found in cells, e.g., *Golgi apparatus, mitochondria,* and various *inclusions* (Figs. 81A and B). The electron micrograph reveals that the chromatin-rich nucleus,

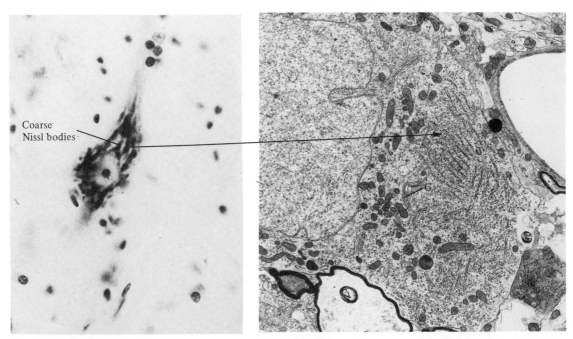

Coarse Nissl bodies

A. Motor neuron

B. Perinuclear region

Small Nissl bodies

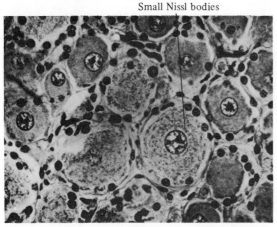

C. Sensory neurons

D. Chromatolysis

Fig. 80. Neuronal Cell Bodies Stained with the Nissl Method

A. Motor neuron from the spinal cord.

B. Electron micrograph from the perinuclear region of a neuron shows that the Nissl substance consists of rough endoplasmic reticulum and free polyribosomes.

C. Sensory neurons from dorsal root ganglion.

D. Retrograde cell reaction with chromatolysis, cellular swelling, and peripheral displacement of the nucleus.

(A. Photograph courtesy of H. Schroeder. C. from Bargman, W., 1977: Histologie und Mikroskopische Anatomie des Menschen. With permission of Thieme, Stuttgart. D. from Escourolle, E. and J. Poirier, 1978. Manual of basic neuropathology. W. B. Saunders Company. With permission of Masson et Cie, Paris.)

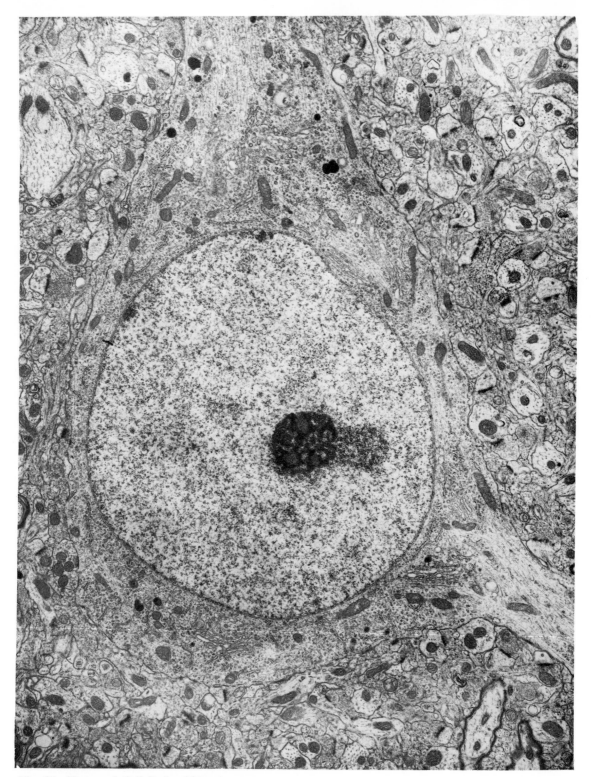

Fig. 81. Neuronal Cell Body: Ultrastructure
A. A pyramidal neuron of the cerebral cortex has been enlarged 10,000 times in this electron micrograph. The map in **B** identifies the various organelles. Mitochondria are colored blue, and boutons from other neurons red. (Micrograph courtesy of A. Peters.)

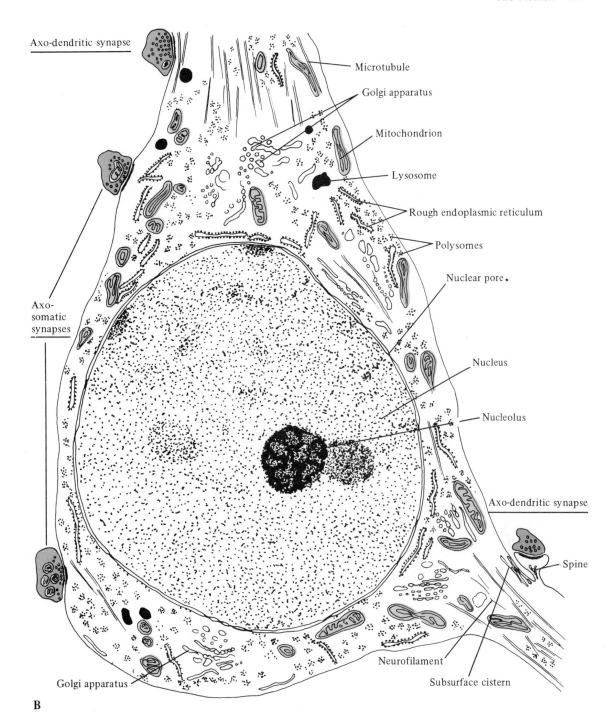

Axo-dendritic synapse

Microtubule

Golgi apparatus

Mitochondrion

Lysosome

Rough endoplasmic reticulum

Polysomes

Nuclear pore

Axo-somatic synapses

Nucleus

Nucleolus

Axo-dendritic synapse

Spine

Golgi apparatus

Neurofilament

Subsurface cistern

B

which contains a conspicuous *nucleolus,* is separated from the cytoplasm by a double-layered envelope. The two membranes of the *nuclear envelope* come together periodically to form *nuclear pores,* which are bridged by a diaphragm.

Cell Processes

With the use of the *Golgi method* the configuration of the cell processes can be studied in detail. A seemingly random and as yet unexplained impregnation of only a few out of hundreds of neurons has made the Golgi silverchromate method and its modifications an extraordinarily valuable technique. Because of the relatively small number of nerve cells stained, the sections can be 100–300 μm thick, and it is often possible to obtain a three-dimensional view of the cell and its processes (Figs. 82A and D). If all the nerve cells with their processes were impregnated in the section, the details would be lost in a dense tangle of fibers. In recent years it has also become possible to stain single neurons in a Golgi-like fashion by *intracellular dye injections.* A much practiced approach is to inject horseradish peroxidase, which can be visualized by a specific staining reaction (Fig. 83A). The Purkinje cells (Fig. 83B) in the cerebellum have one of the most remarkable dendritic arborizations in the CNS. The dendritic tree, which arises from one or several trunks at the apical pole of the cell body, is spread out in a vertical plane at a right angle to the longitudinal axis of the cerebellar folium.

According to the number of their processes, neurons can be classified as *multipolar, bipolar,* or *unipolar.* Most cells in the CNS are multipolar. Bipolar cells are found in a few locations, including the retina (Fig. 149, Chapter 13) and the olfactory bulb as well as in the cochlear and vestibular ganglia. Unipolar cells are present in most sensory ganglia and have a single process, which divides in a T-like manner close to the cell body; one branch projects to the periphery and the other enters the CNS through the posterior root. These cells are sometimes referred to as *pseudounipolar* because they develop from bipolar neurons, in which the initial part of the two processes move toward each other and eventually fuse.

Another classification of neurons is based on the length of their axons. Cells with long axons are referred to as *Golgi type I neurons* and those with short axons, *Golgi type II neurons.*

Dendrites

The dendrites constitute protoplasmic extensions of the cell body. They gradually taper off as they arborize in a tree-like manner in the vicinity of the cell body (Figs. 82A and D). The profuse branching explains why most of the neuronal surface area usually is associated with the dendrites, which are eminently suited for the reception of a large number of axon terminals. Further, the dendrites of many neurons are studded with thorn-like processes, *dendritic spines,* or gemmules, which are structures specialized for synaptic contact (Figs. 82B and C). The cytoplasm of the dendrites resembles that of the cell body. Large dendrites can usually be recognized in electron micrographs on the basis of their lack of a myelin sheath and the presence of a large number of *microtubules* (Fig. 82C) and of scattered polyribosomes. Small dendritic branches, on the other hand, are often difficult to distinguish from small unmyelinated axons.

The shape of the dendritic trees and their spines are often among the most characteristic morphologic features of a neuron. *Pyramidal cells,* which are found in all areas of the cerebral cortex, have cell bodies that are pyramidal or conical in shape (Fig. 82A). A pyramidal cell is characterized by two systems of spiny dendrites: a long and branched apical dendrite, which is directed toward the surface, and several basal dendrites, which emerge from the angles formed by the base and the walls of the pyramid. The dendritic tree of the *Purkinje cell* in the cerebellar cortex arises from the apex of the cell and is characteristically spread out in one plane and is laden with thousands of spines (Fig. 83B). The *stellate cells,* which appear in many parts of the CNS, have the dendrites extended about equally in all directions (Fig. 82D), and certain types of stellate cells are nearly devoid of spines.

Axon

The axon arises from the cell body (Fig. 84) or from one of the main dendrites. Whereas the dendrites usually taper off gradually as they extend from the cell body, the axon acquires a relatively small diameter near its point of emergence at the axon hillock, and the rest of the axon has a rather uniform diameter. The first segment of the axon, the *initial axon segment,* is usually somewhat thin-

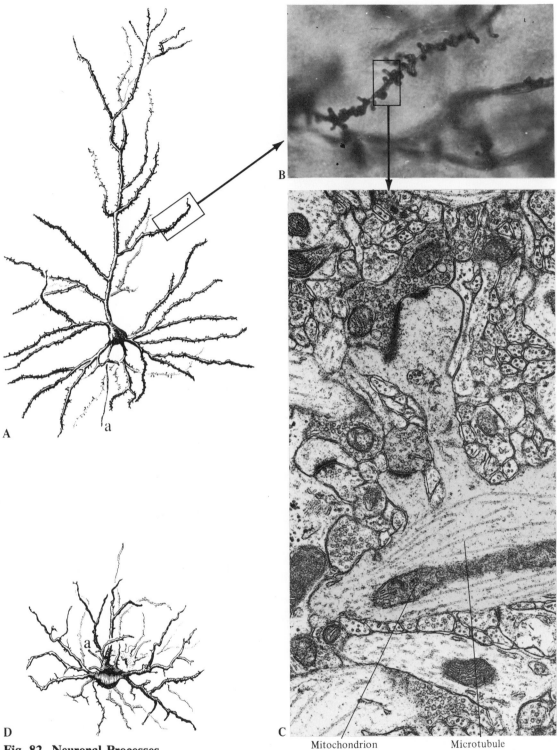

Mitochondrion   Microtubule

Fig. 82. Neuronal Processes

A. Pyramidal cell from the cerebral cortex stained with the Golgi method.

B. Enlargement of a dendritic spine.

C. The electron microscope reveals that the dendritic spines are specialized for synaptic contacts. Dendrite and dendritic spines, *yellow;* boutons, *red.*

D. Stellate cell from the dentate nucleus of the cerebellum. (A and D from Peters, A., S. L. Palay and H de F. Webster, 1976. The fine structure of the nervous system. With permission of the authors and W. B. Saunders Company, Philadelphia.)

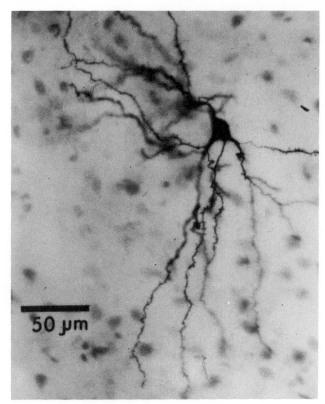

A. Neuron in striatum

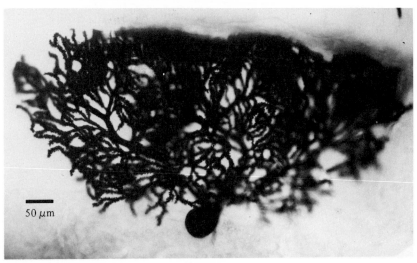

B. Purkinje cell

Fig. 83. Neuronal Processes

A. Neuron from the striatum visualized by a specific staining reaction following intracellular injection of horserad-ish peroxidase. (Micrograph courtesy of S. T. Kitai.)

B. Purkinje cell from the cerebellum stained with the Golgi method. (Micrograph courtesy of S. Palay. From Palay, S. L. and V. Chan-Palay, 1974. Cerebellar Cortex. With permission of Springer-Verlag, New York–Heidel-berg-Berlin.)

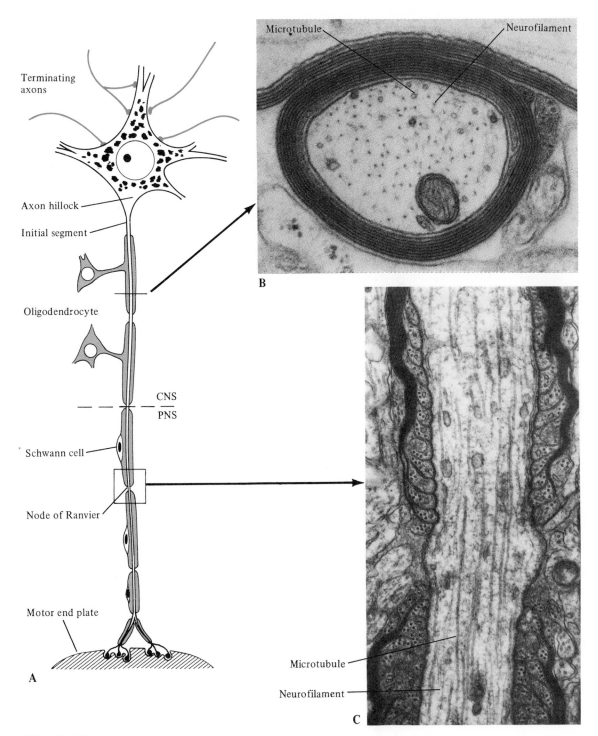

Fig. 84. The Axon

A. Schematic drawing of a motor neuron. The myelin sheath surrounding the axon is interrupted at regular intervals, and appears as a series of tubes in the light microscopic preparation.

B. Electron micrograph of a transversely sectioned axon indicates that the myelin sheath consists of thin lamellae, which form a regular pattern of concentric thin and thick lines.

C. Electron micrograph of a longitudinally cut axon at a node of Ranvier. When the myelin sheath approaches the node, it becomes increasingly thinner as successive lamellae terminate. Note that the axon contains both microtubules and neurofilaments. (C from Peters, A., S. L. Palay and H de F. Webster, 1976. The fine structure of the nervous system. With permission of the authors and W. B. Saunders Company. Philadelphia, London, Toronto.)

ner than the rest of the axon. This is the site where the nerve impulse or action potential is initiated. Distinctive features of the initial axon segment are bundles of microtubules interconnected by tiny cross-bridges, and the undercoating of the plasma membrane by electron-dense, granulo-fibrillar material (Fig. 88B). If the axon is myelinated, the myelin sheath begins just distal to the initial segment.

The length of the axon and its number of collateral branches vary widely. The large motor neurons that innervate the striated muscles have long axons; some of them reach from the lower end of the spinal cord to the muscles of the foot. The neurons that coordinate the activity within a specific region of the CNS, the interneurons or local circuit neurons, usually have short axons that arborize in the vicinity of their cell bodies. Some axons proceed from one region of the CNS to another without emitting collateral branches, whereas the collateralization and branching pattern in other axons is more elaborate than in the most profusely branching dendritic tree.

Near its point of termination, the axon forms terminal branches, whose distal ends are enlarged to form *axon terminals* or *boutons*. The bouton constitutes the presynaptic part of the synapse (see below) and it is here that the nerve impulses cause the release of a neurotransmitter, which in turn affects another neuron or muscle. Terminal axonal branches may also form a series of terminals along their course, the *bouton en passant* (Fig. 85).

Neurofilaments (Figs. 84B and C) are common in axons and rare in dendrites. Ribosomes, on the other hand, are not present in the axoplasm, so that the proteins needed for the turnover of axonal components and for interactions with other cells must be transported from the cell body.

Myelin Sheath.   This lipid-rich spiralling sheath serves as an electric insulator that considerably increases conduction velocity. Large axons are usually myelinated, and they are easily recognized in electron micrographs (Fig. 84B), in which the myelin sheath is seen to consist of a regular pattern of concentric thinner and thicker lines. The myelin sheath, which is formed by oligodendrocytes in the CNS and by Schwann cells in the PNS, is interrupted at regular intervals by gaps, the *nodes of Ranvier* (Fig. 84). The length and the thickness of the myelin segment between two nodes vary with the thickness of the axon. The largest fibers

have the thickest and longest internodal segments. Since the nerve impulse jumps from node to node (saltatory conduction) in myelinated fibers, the length of the myelin segment is of considerable importance. The largest fibers, which may have a conduction velocity of up to 100 m/sec, have myelin segments of more than 1 mm length.

At its point of termination, a myelinated axon gradually loses its myelin sheath to form an axon terminal (Fig. 85). The peripheral motor neurons terminate on specialized parts of the muscle fiber known as motor end plates (Chapter 7).

In peripheral nerves, each Schwann cell forms a single myelin segment. In the CNS, a single oligodendrocyte forms several myelin segments around different axons, which vary in thickness and may even belong to different pathways.

Axonal Transport

Because the axoplasm does not contain ribosomes, protein synthesis cannot take place in the axon. All axonal proteins, therefore, must come from the cell body, and their passage along the axon is accomplished by a perpetual somatofugal movement. The proteins are transported as components of intact cytologic structures and not as individual protein molecules. The microtubule–neurofilament network and proteins needed for the continuous renewal of the axonal matrix move at a rate of less than 4 mm/day, referred to as *slow axonal transport.* Membrane-bound structures, e.g., vesicles and the agranular reticulum, are transported in a somatofugal direction at a rate of 200–400 mm/day, i.e., *fast axonal transport.* The fast component is bidirectional. Membrane material targeted for replacement is engulfed by lysosomes and transported in a retrograde direction back to the cell body for degradation and recycling.

Although the axonal transport mechanisms are not yet fully understood, the discovery of the axoplasmic transport phenomenon has greatly improved our understanding of many fundamental neurobiologic events, and it has served as a powerful stimulus for research on neuronal functions. Further, some of the most useful techniques for the tracing of neuronal pathways are based on the use or anterograde and retrograde axonal transport (see below).

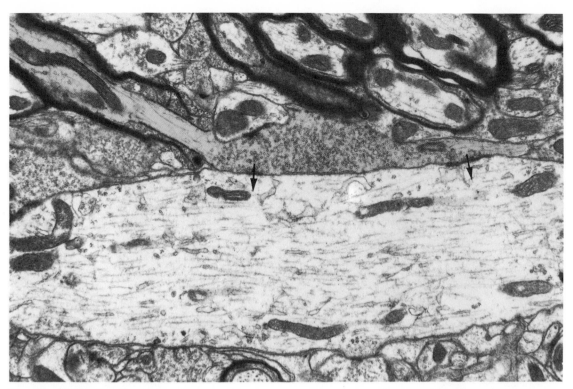

Fig. 85. Bouton en Passant
Axon (*red*) losing its myelin sheath and forming en passant bouton on dendrite with synaptic junctions (*arrows*). (Micrograph courtesy of E. Mugnaini.)

THE SYNAPSE

The synapse consists of a *presynaptic membrane,* a *synaptic gap* (cleft), and a *postsynaptic membrane.* The most characteristic feature of the synapse is the accumulation of a large number of *synaptic vesicles* in the presynaptic element, the bouton (Fig. 86). Some of the vesicles cluster on the presynaptic aspect of the synaptic junction. The presynaptic and the postsynaptic membranes can easily be identified by the presence of electron-dense material, which forms a grid of spoke-like projections presynaptically, and a thickening, or plaque, postsynaptically. Dense material is also present in the 10–30 nm wide synaptic cleft.

Synaptic Vesicles

Synaptic vesicles usually are clustered close to the presynaptic membrane (Fig. 86A) and may have different sizes and shapes. They contain a chemical substance, the neurotransmitter. The cholinergic boutons at the neuromuscular junction, as well as the boutons in many other regions of the nervous system for which the transmitter has not been established, are characterized by the presence of small spherical vesicles that have a diameter of 40–50 nm and a clear center, i.e., *agranular vesicles.* The shape of the vesicles is to some extent dependent on the fixative used. Vesicles of certain inhibitory fibers, e.g., those containing γ-aminobutyric acid (GABA), have a tendency to become flattened in aldehyde-fixed material (Fig. 87). Vesicles containing catecholamines (noradrenaline, adrenaline, dopamine) have a dense core, i.e., *granular vesicles,* and may be somewhat larger than the agranular vesicles.

When the nerve impulse reaches the bouton, the synaptic vesicles fuse with the presynaptic membrane in the intervals between the spokes of the presynaptic grid and, via exocytosis, release definite amounts (quanta) of the transmitter. The neurotransmitter diffuses across the synaptic gap to combine with specific receptor proteins on the surface of the postsynaptic membrane, and the activation of the receptors triggers a response in the postsynaptic neuron or in the muscle cell.

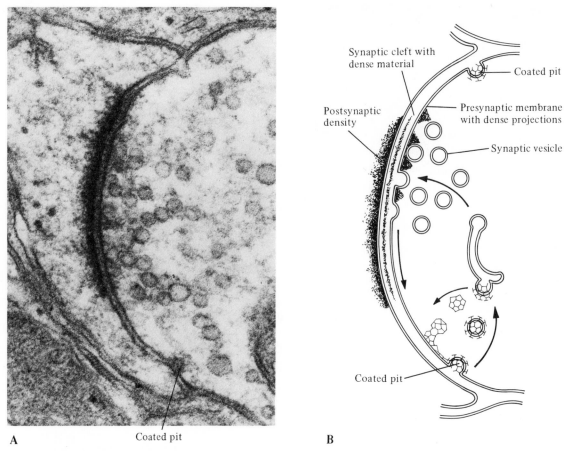

A   Coated pit   B

Fig. 86. The Synapse and the Synaptic Vesicles
A. The synapse consists of a presynaptic component, a synaptic gap, and a postsynaptic component. The presynaptic component is characterized foremost by the accummulation of synaptic vesicles, which contain the neurotransmitter. **B.** Idealized drawing of the synapse in **A** illustrating the recycling of synaptic vesicle membrane. (Diagram modified after Heuser, J. E. and J. S. Reese, 1973. Evidence for recycling of synaptic vesicle membrane during transmitter release at the frog neuromuscular junction. J. Cell. Biol. 57:315–344.)

Recycling of Synaptic Vesicle Membrane

The synaptic vesicle membrane can apparently be used several times, and the path of synaptic membrane recycling is schematically illustrated in Fig. 86B. The synaptic vesicle membrane is added to the presynaptic membrane during the process of exocytosis. An equal amount of membrane, however, is retrieved by *coated vesicles,* which arise from nearby regions of the plasma membrane. The coated vesicles subsequently lose their coat and coalesce to form cisternae, which divide to form new synaptic vesicles.

Classification of Synapses

Most synapses can be divided into *symmetric* and *asymmetric* types (Fig. 87) according to the amount of dense material on the cytoplasmic face of the postsynaptic membrane. In the symmetric synapse, the dense material associated with the two opposing synaptic membranes are of more or less equal density. The asymmetric synapse is characterized by a prominent *postsynaptic density.* In aldehyde-fixed material, asymmetric synapses are usually associated with spherical vesicles whereas symmetric synapses are associated with a mixture of flattened and spherical vesicles. It has been proposed that the two types of synapses may serve

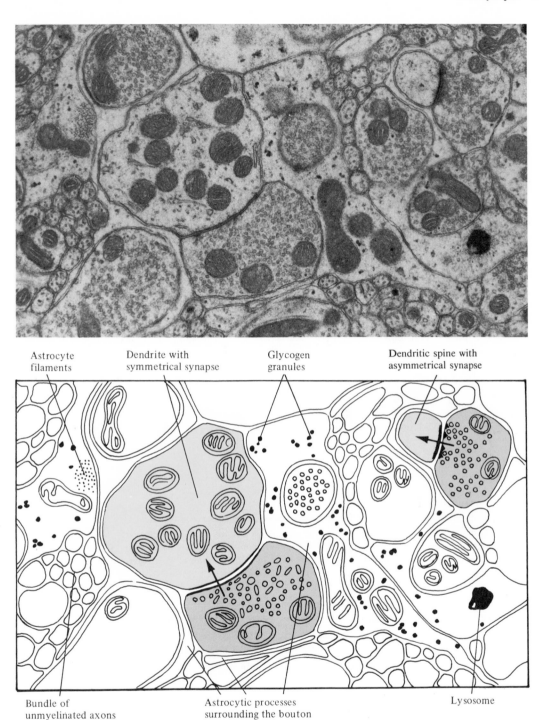

Astrocyte
filaments

Dendrite with
symmetrical synapse

Glycogen
granules

Dendritic spine with
asymmetrical synapse

Bundle of
unmyelinated axons

Astrocytic processes
surrounding the bouton

Lysosome

Fig. 87. Symmetric and Asymmetric Synapses

The symmetric synapse is characterized by a mixture of flattened and spherical vesicles, and the pre- and postsynaptic membranes are of about equal density. The asymmetric synapse is characterized by spherical vesicles and a prominent postsynaptic density. (The micrograph, which shows the neuropil in the dorsal cochlear nucleus of the rat, was kindly provided by E. Mugnaini.)

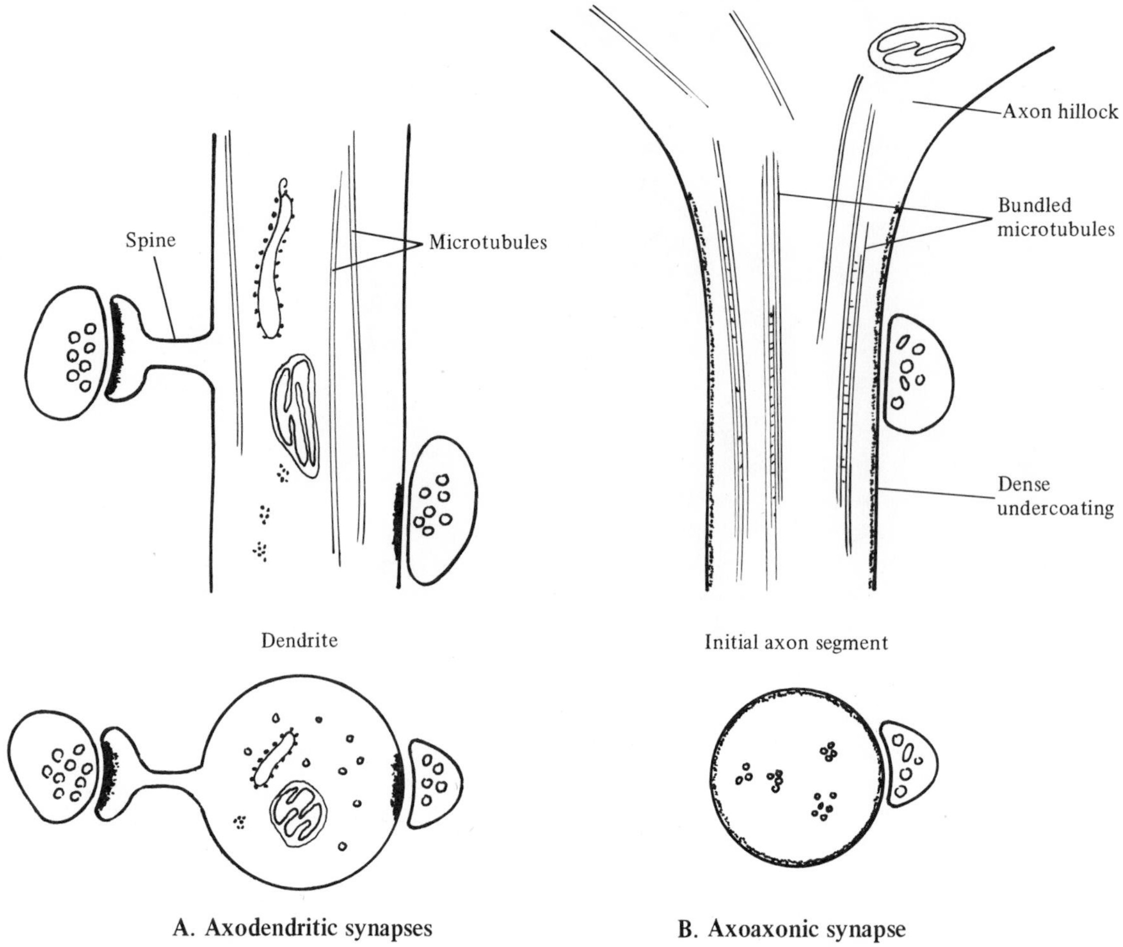

Spine — Microtubules

Dendrite

A. Axodendritic synapses

Axon hillock

Bundled microtubules

Dense undercoating

Initial axon segment

B. Axoaxonic synapse

Fig. 88. Axodendritic and Axoaxonic Synapses
A. The postsynaptic element of an axodendritic synapse can be either a spine or a dendritic shaft.
B. The postsynaptic component of an axoaxonic synapse is usually the initial segment or another bouton. The initial segment of an axon can usually be distinguished from a dendrite by a characteristic undercoating, or dense layer, beneath the cell membrane and the presence of microtubules that are bundled together into fascicles.

different functions, i.e., the asymmetric synapses would be excitatory and the symmetric ones inhibitory. This seems to be the case in many instances, although the correlation may not be universal. The functional characteristics of a synapse are dependent not only on the presynaptic organelles but also on the properties of the postsynaptic component.

A useful anatomic classification of synapses is based on the position of the bouton on the postsynaptic neuron. Depending on the character of the postsynaptic component, the synapse can be *axodendritic, axosomatic,* or *axoaxonic.* The postsynaptic element of an exodendritic synapse is either a dendritic shaft or a spine (Fig. 88A), whereas the postsynaptic component in an axo-

axonic synapse is usually the initial segment of the axon (Fig. 88B) or one of its boutons. The termination of a bouton on another bouton is likely to constitute the morphologic substrate for presynaptic inhibition and facilitation.

Neuron Doctrine

It is now accepted that the nervous system is composed of a large number of individual neurons that are related to each other by means of *synapses.* That the nervous system consists of cellular units (the neuron theory) rather than a continuous protoplasmic network (the reticular theory) was finally established by the aid of the electron microscope, in which the detailed structure of the synapse can be studied.

According to the neuron theory, neurons are anatomic, functional, and trophic units. The theory, however, also implies that the neurons are dynamically polarized in the sense that the dendrites and the cell body receive impulses, whereas the axon carries the impulses away from the cell body to other neurons or to the effector organs. Although this is generally true, it has recently been shown that dendrites or even cell bodies may in certain situations act as effectors in the sense that they establish specialized contacts with other neurons. Such atypical neurons are found in the retina, the olfactory bulb, and the thalamus. Further, some neurons communicate with one another via ultramicroscopic channels formed by special proteins in regions referred to as *gap junctions*. These intercellular channels provide electrotonic coupling and synchronized firing of neurons, and the gap junctions are often referred to as *electrical synapses* to distinguish them from the *chemical synapses* discussed above. Therefore, it is difficult to uphold the neuron theory in its classic form; the interactions between neurons seem to be highly differentiated.

NEUROGLIA

The neuroglial cells, which are more numerous than the nerve cells, are not directly involved in the transmission of nerve impulses, but they assist the neurons in various ways. Neuroglial cells in the CNS are of four different types: *astrocytes, oligodendrocytes, microglia cells,* and *ependyma* (Fig. 89). Schwann cells and satellite cells in the peripheral ganglia are referred to as peripheral neuroglia.

Astroglia

The astrocytes seem to provide structural support for the neurons. Some of them have irregular and profusely branching processes, i.e., *protoplasmic astrocytes* (Fig. 89A), whereas others have straight and fibrous processes, i.e., *fibrous astrocytes* (Fig. 89B). Astrocytic processes form end-feet that cover the basal lamina around blood vessels and at the pia, where they form an almost continuous sheath. Astrocytes are easily recognized in electron micrographs (Fig. 87) because of their relatively clear cytoplasm and the presence of small dense glycogen granules and filaments.

Because astrocytic processes are often seen to encircle individual synapses or groups of synapses, they are thought to isolate the receptive surface of neurons and to buffer it against sudden ionic changes. Astroglia, finally, help form the scar tissue in response to lesions of the central nervous tissue, and, like the other types of neuroglia, can under certain circumstances serve as phagocytic cells.

Oligodendroglia

As the name indicates, these cells have few although somewhat branched processes arising from their cell bodies (Fig. 89C). They are the myelin-forming cells in the CNS, and they also have the capacity to become involved in phagocytosis of degenerating neurons.

Microglia

The microglial cells (Fig. 89D) are small cells with delicate processes that give off spine-like projections. The microglial cells undergo rapid proliferation in response to tissue destruction, and they migrate toward the site of injury where they act as scavengers by phagocytosis and removal of tissue debris. As already indicated, other glial cells may also become phagocytic in response to injury, and there may in addition be an influx into the nervous tissue of phagocytic cells from the blood, especially if the lesion has involved blood vessels.

Ependyma

These epithelial cells (Fig. 89E) line the brain ventricles and the central canal of the spinal cord. The ventricular surface of most ependymal cells is covered with cilia, which seem to facilitate the movement of the cerebrospinal fluid. Special types of ependymal cells, the *tanycytes,* line the floor of the 3rd ventricle; such cells have an apical process extending to the pial membrane and terminating with an end-foot, like that of astrocytes in other parts of the brain.

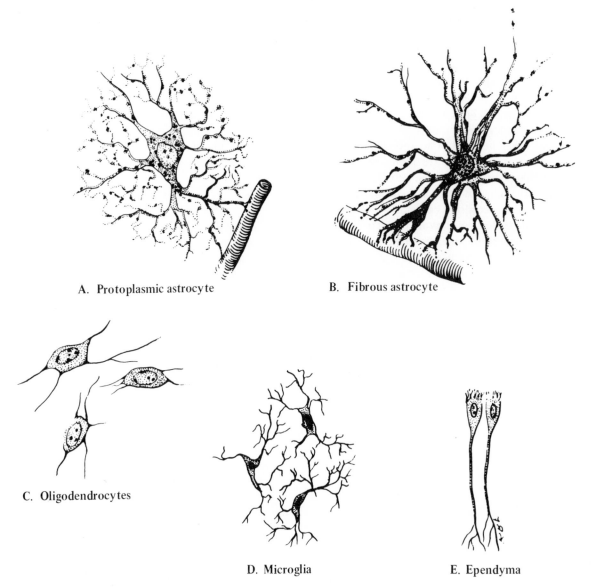

A. Protoplasmic astrocyte

B. Fibrous astrocyte

C. Oligodendrocytes

D. Microglia

E. Ependyma

Fig. 89. Neuroglia
Schematic drawings of the different types of glial cells. (From Jenkins, T. N., 1978. Functional Mammalian Neuroanatomy, 2nd Edition. With permission of the author and Lea and Febiger, Philadelphia.)

NEUROANATOMIC TECHNIQUES

For more than a century, scientists have devised a variety of light microscopic techniques for mapping fiber connections. A big step forward was taken in the 1950s with the introduction of the *electron microscope,* which made it possible to analyze in detail the synaptic contacts between individual neurons. It is in the specific arrangement of these specialized contacts that the flexibility and the potentials of the nervous system appear to reside.

During the last decade a number of tracing methods, based on the principle of axonal transport, have revolutionized neuroanatomy, and a rapidly increasing number of neuroscientists are using light and electron microscopic techniques in various combinations to chart previously unexplored regions and circuits with great success and with a precision unthinkable only a few years ago. Only the most important neuroanatomic techniques can be mentioned within the framework of this textbook.

Nissl and Golgi Methods

The usefulness of these two classic neuroanatomic techniques has already been highlighted. Like all other light microscopic techniques, the Nissl and Golgi methods are selective in the sense that they display a specific component or demonstrate certain characteristics of a neuron.

The Nissl method, which is based on the staining with basic aniline dyes, reveals the cell body (Fig. 80). In particular, these dyes stain the nucleus and the chromophilic substance in the perikaryon. It was introduced almost 100 years ago, but is still one of the most widely used techniques for studying the cytology of the nervous system. The Nissl method provides the scientist with a map of cell assemblies and other cytoarchitectonic landmarks (see Fig. 161, Chapter 15), which can be correlated with the staining pattern obtained in nearby sections by the aid of experimental techniques.

The Golgi method, which is also more than 100 years old, is especially valuable for studying the distribution of dendrites, axons, and axon collaterals, which appear pitch black (Figs. 82 and 83B). The Golgi method is based on a pretreatment of the tissue with dichromate, followed by exposure to silver nitrate. The method is often used as a correlate to neurophysiologic and ultrastructural studies of neurons.

Reduced Silver Impregnation Methods

Most nerve fibers are argyrophilic, i.e., they can be impregnated with silver if the material is treated in a silver solution followed by a reduction of the silver in a reducing solution. Silver methods based on this principle have been used since the beginning of this century. At the outset they were appreciated primarily for their remarkable capacity to reveal normal histology and fiber architecture. However, it proved to be difficult to trace individual fiber bundles arising in specific neuron populations through the complex meshwork of axons impregnated in normal material, and it was not until scientists discovered that degenerating nerve fibers could be selectively stained by silver that these methods became widely used in tract-tracing.

An axon that is severed from its cell body (Fig. 90A) or an axon whose cell body is destroyed, undergoes a gradual disintegration which is re-

ferred to as *Wallerian degeneration*[1] By transecting a pathway or producing a surgical or chemical lesion in the area where a pathway originates, this phenomenon can be used to "mark" the pathway of interest, thus facilitating its recognition as it meanders through the nervous system. The *Nauta-Gygax silver method* and many of its modern variations impregnate degenerating axons and boutons with a high degree of selectivity and sensitivity, and by studying the Wallerian degeneration in silver-impregnated sections, the precise course and distribution of the degenerating nerve fibers (Fig. 90B) and their terminals can be determined (Figs. 90C and D).

Since it is not possible to identify precisely the synaptic contacts in light microscopic sections, silver impregnation studies of pathways are often complemented by *electron microscopic studies,* in which the degenerating boutons and their postsynaptic structures can be identified by the changes they undergo (Fig. 90D).

The cell body's response to transection of its axon is called a *retrograde reaction*. This usually consists of chromatolysis, swelling of the cell, and peripheral displacement of the nucleus (Fig. 80D). Although this acute retrograde response can be used to identify the neurons of origin for well delimited pathways, the modern tract-tracing methods based on retrograde axonal transport are considerably more effective (see below).

Axonal Transport Methods

These methods are based on the principle of axonal transport, and two such methods have particularly wide application, namely the autoradiographic technique and the horseradish peroxidase technique.

In an *autoradiographic tract-tracing study,* a highly concentrated solution of a radioactively labeled essential amino acid, e.g., [3H]leucin, is injected into the area of presumed origin of the pathway. The labeled precursor is taken up by the cell bodies, incorporated into newly synthesized proteins, and transported in an anterograde direction to the axon terminals, where their radioactivity can be detected by the process of autoradiogra-

---

1. The phenomenon was discovered by Augustus Waller in 1850.

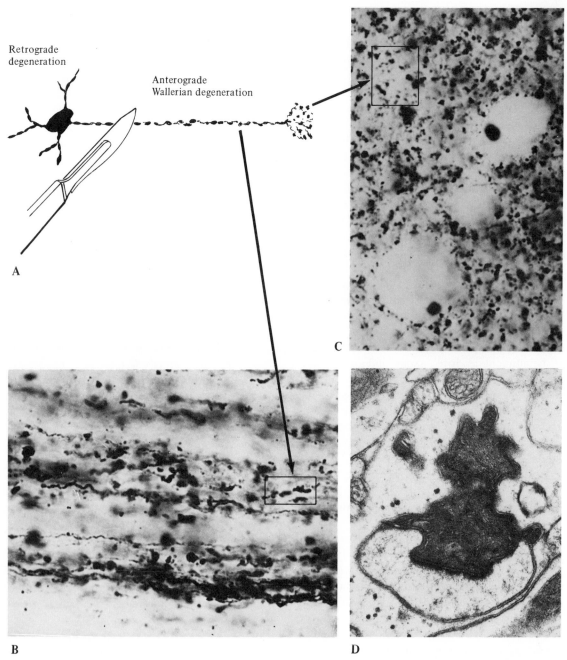

Fig. 90. The Study of Anterograde Degeneration with the Silver Method and Electron Microscopy
Following an experimental lesion **(A)** the reduced silver method can be used to reveal degenerating axons **(B)** en route to their destination **(C)**. A silver impregnation study is often complemented by an electron microscopic investigation, in which the degenerating boutons and their postsynaptic structures can be identified **(D)**. (A–C from de Olmos, J. S., S. O. E. Ebbesson and L. Heimer, 1981. Silver methods for the impregnation of degenerating axoplasm. In Heimer, L. and M. Y. Robards (Eds.) Neuroanatomical Tract-Tracing Methods. With permission of Plenum Press, New York.)

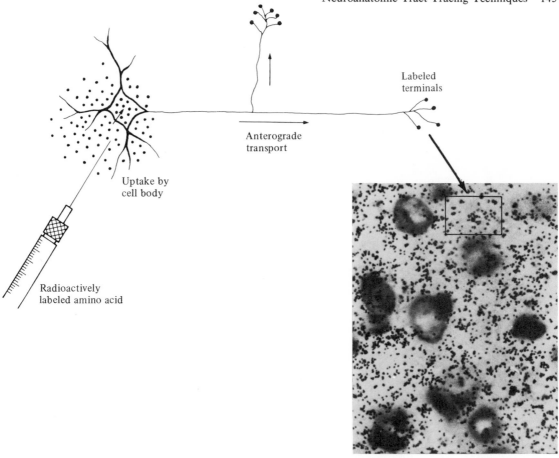

Fig. 91. The Autoradiographic Tract-Tracing Method
If a highly concentrated solution of radioactively labeled amino acid is injected into a presumed origin of a pathway, the tracer is taken up by the cell bodies in the vicinity of the injection and transported through the axons to their terminals, where the label can be detected with the aid of the autoradiographic technique. (From Edwards, S. B. and A. Hendrickson, 1981. The autoradiographic tracing of axonal connections in the central nervous system. In Heimer, L. and M. J. Robards. Neuroanatomical Tract-Tracing Methods. With permission of Plenum Press, New York)

phy in animals sacrificed 1 or 2 days following the injection (Fig. 91).

The most important advantage of the autoradiographic tracing method is based on the fact that only neuron cell bodies and not axons take up the injected precursor. This selective uptake by the cell bodies makes it possible to demonstrate axonal projections arising from cells surrounded by passing fibers.

The *horseradish peroxidase (HRP) method* probably symbolizes the success of the modern tracer techniques better than any other method. Although it was introduced as a retrograde tracing technique in the early 1970s, it is now used effectively in both retrograde and anterograde tracing experiments. In other words, if an HRP solution is injected into a region of the nervous system, HRP is taken up by both cell bodies and axon terminals in the region of injection. In the neurons, whose axon terminals have incorporated HRP, the enzyme is carried by retrograde axonal transport to the cell bodies, where it can be detected by a simple staining procedure, usually less than a day after the injection (Fig. 92). The HRP that has been taken up by cell bodies in the area of the injection is transported in an anterograde direction to the axon terminals. Therefore, both pathways that project to the injection area and axonal projections that arise in the area of injection can be studied in one and the same experiment.

HRP can also be injected into individual neurons through a micropipette, in which case the whole neuron, including its dendrites and axonal projections, can be stained in a Golgi-like fashion (Fig. 83A). By the aid of this technique, scientists can study the morphology of a neuron whose func-

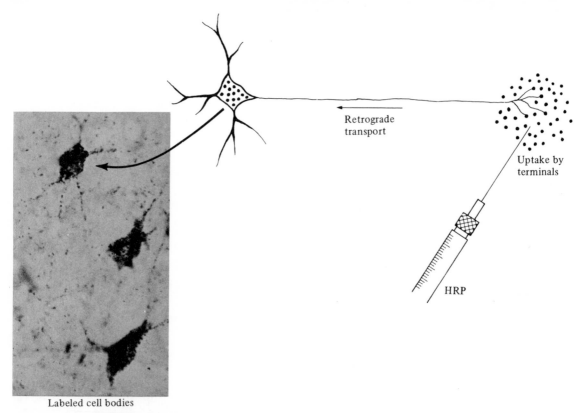

Labeled cell bodies

Fig. 92. The Horseradish Peroxidase Method
Although horseradish peroxidase (HRP) is readily transported both in retrograde and anterograde direction, it is most often used in retrograde tracing experiments. The enzyme is injected into the terminal area of a projection, where it is taken up by boutons. It is subsequently transported in retrograde direction to the cell bodies, where it can be detected by a simple staining procedure.

tional characteristics have first been investigated by electrophysiologic recording techniques.

The search for better and more effective tracers has resulted in the introduction of *fluorescent substances,* which hold great promise, especially as retrograde tracers. Fluorescence microscopy has the capacity to reveal substances in very low concentrations, and if two substances are chosen so that each fluoresces in a different color at a different excitation wavelength, it is possible to double-label cells in a single preparation following injections of the two substances in different projection regions of long branching axons (Fig. 93). The introduction of such double-labeling procedures has demonstrated that the axonal projections of many cell groups in the CNS are characterized by long branching axons.

Histochemical Methods

Whereas the above-mentioned neuroanatomic techniques can usually be used successfully for the study of pathways everywhere in the nervous system, other methods are used for the selective demonstration of neurons containing a known neurotransmitter. The *fluorescence histochemical method* for the demonstration of monoamine-containing neurons, for instance, is based on the fact that biogenic amines tend to fluoresce if the tissue is reacted with formaldehyde or glyoxylic acid. Three different monoamines, i.e., dopamine, noradrenaline, and serotonin (5-hydroxytryptamine), serve as transmitters in the CNS, and the cell groups that give rise to the monoaminergic systems are located primarily in the brain stem (Chapter 10). The fluorescence histochemical method has a restricted application because it can be used only for demonstrating monoamine-containing neuronal systems, which account for a small proportion of all pathways in the brain.

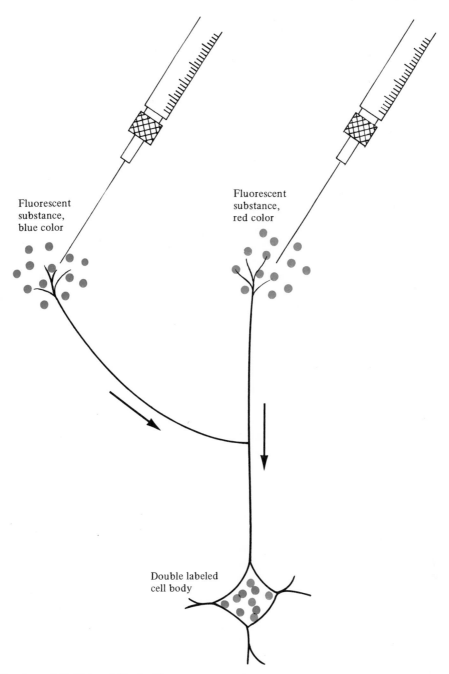

Fig. 93. Tracing of Collateral Projections
Two substances that fluoresce with different colors are injected in different projection areas of long branching axons. The fluorescent substances are transported in a retrograde direction to the same cell body, which thus becomes double-labeled. (From Steward, O. Horseradish peroxidase and fluorescent substances and their combination with other techniques, 1981. In: Heimer, L. and M. J. Robards. Neuroanatomical Tract-Tracing Methods. With permission of Plenum Press, New York.)

The *immunohistochemical methods* can be more widely used for the demonstration of chemically distinct pathways. The immunocytochemical methods are based on the immunologic concept of antigen–antibody reaction, and specific antibodies are now available for many neuron-specific antigens, including neurotransmitter-synthesizing enzymes and a series of neuroactive peptides (e.g., enkephalin, substance P, and neurotensin). The power of the immunocytochemical techniques is demonstrated in Fig. 122, Chapter 9, which demonstrates GABAergic neurons in the cerebellum. The production of GABA, the main inhibitory transmitter in the brain, is dependent on the presence of a catalyzing enzyme, glutamic acid decarboxylase (GAD), which can be identified with the immunocytochemical technique. The immunocytochemical methods have opened up new exciting avenues for the neuroscientist, and the detailed light and electron microscopic localization of chemically identified neuron systems has rapidly advanced our understanding of many brain mechanisms. It is hoped that such knowledge will lead to the development of a more goal-directed therapy for certain nervous or mental disorders, e.g., the application of specific drugs for the treatment of disorders related to dysfunction in specific neuronal systems.

The functional organization of specific systems can be studied with the *2-deoxyglycose method.* For this method, a radioactively labeled substance, $[^{14}C]$2-deoxyglucose (2DG), is injected into the animal. Since 2DG is an analogue of glucose, it is taken up by the neurons as a source of energy. Unlike glucose, however, 2DG forms a metabolite that cannot cross the cell membrane and therefore accumulates in the cell. If the cells of a specific neuronal system are being stimulated, they increase their uptake of glycose and 2DG. This results in an increased intracellular accumulation of the radioactively labeled metabolite, which can be visualized by the aid of the autoradiographic technique (Fig. 154B).

CLINICAL NOTES

Multiple Sclerosis

The importance of the myelin sheath in the conduction of nerve impulses is well illustrated in cases of *demyelinative diseases,* i.e., conditions in which the destruction of the myelin sheaths is the most striking feature. Of the many demyelinative disorders, multiple sclerosis (MS) is the most well-known. It is a rather common neurologic disease that often affects young adults in their prime. As the name indicates, multiple sclerotic (scar-like) plaques appear in the white matter of the CNS. The symptoms vary according to the localization of the sclerotic plaques in the brain and the spinal cord.

Unfortunately, there is little potential for repair of the demyelinated fibers, since the oligodendrocytes do not possess the remarkable capacity to reform myelin sheaths, as do Schwann cells. Therefore, although there may be striking remissions, the disease usually causes a gradual deterioration of the patient's condition over many years.

Myasthenia Gravis

Myasthenia gravis is a serious disorder characterized by an excessive fatigability of striated musculature, especially the extraocular muscles, the levator palpebrae, and the muscles of facial expression. Although the etiology of myasthenia gravis is still unclear, the disease is apparently caused by a postsynaptic defect of neurotransmission at the neuromuscular junction. The fact that muscle power can be improved by treating the patient with a cholinesterase inhibitor, e.g., physostigmine, is in line with this hypothesis.

Parkinson's Disease

This is a relatively common disorder characterized by a deficiency in a specific transmitter, i.e., dopamine, as a result of degeneration of the dopamine-synthesizing cells in the substantia nigra. The disease is discussed in more detail in Chapter 8.

Regeneration and Plasticity

To what extent a patient recovers following an injury to peripheral or central nervous pathways depends in large measure on the regenerative capacity of the damaged neurons. The capacity for regeneration in the PNS is quite impressive in the sense that useful function can be restored following successful nerve repair of a transected peripheral nerve. Regeneration in the CNS, on the other hand, is quite limited. Indeed, there is little evidence for the regrowth of damaged axons and the subsequent reestablishment of the original pattern of connections in the human brain or spinal cord. This, however, does not necessarily mean a lack of repair and recovery following lesions in the CNS. On the contrary, there is a high degree of *plasticity* in the CNS, and the destruction of a central nervous pathway may well induce so-called *collateral sprouting* in nearby intact axons (*see below*). Further, if the regrowing axons are helped to bypass the glial scar that forms at the site of the lesion, for instance by grafting Schwann's cells, regrowth can also occur in the CNS.

Regeneration of Peripheral Nerve Fibers

The degenerative changes that occur in a neuron whose axon has been transected are most pronounced in the part of the nerve fiber that is separated from the perikaryon. As mentioned previously, this part undergoes Wallerian degeneration, i.e., it breaks up into fragments and finally disappears, while the cell body generally undergoes chromatolytic changes.

If the cell body survives, reparative processes take place and sprouts appear at the distal end of the intact part of the axon. This regenerative process can be quite effective in peripheral nerves, where some of the growing tips may find their way into endoneurial tubes in the peripheral part of the degenerating nerve and eventually reinnervate the denervated target organ. If the gap between the proximal and the distal stump is too long, the growing axonal tips will not be able to cross the scar, in which case the sprouts and the scar tissue may form a painful *neuroma*. To prevent this from happening it is important that the two ends of a nerve that has been interrupted by an injury are approximated as closely as possible, if necessary with the help of nerve transplants, which can provide chains of Schwann cells capable of guiding the regrowing fibers through the gap.

Plasticity and Functional Reorganization in the CNS

Reinnervation following lesions in the CNS is quite limited, not only because the guiding function provided by endoneurial tubes in the peripheral nerves is lacking, but because the structure of the CNS is infinitely more complicated than the peripheral nerves. Nevertheless, some late recovery of function is usually seen following traumatic and vascular lesions of the CNS, and it is possible that the recovery in some cases is due to reinnervation of the denervated synaptic sites by collateral sprouts from nearby intact fibers.

The phenomenon of *collateral sprouting* is generally considered to be one of the main reasons for *functional reorganization* in the CNS. However, to what extent the sprouting fibers establish synaptic connections with denervated neurons is not known; nor do we know to what extent the specificity of the connection is reestablished. Whatever the role of collateral sprouting, it is generally recognized that an active training program facilitates recovery.

Brain Transplantations

Recently, transplantations in experimental animals have proven remarkably successful in the sense that transplanted embryonic or neonatal central nervous tissues have survived transplantation to brains of adult recipients. More importantly, the grafted neurons have been shown to form functionally relevant connections in the host brain. This indicates that it may be possible in some cases to repair nervous pathways that have been destroyed by a lesion, or to replace certain tissue defects in the CNS. Some type of "reconstructive" brain surgery, therefore, may become a reality within the not too distant future.

Spread of Virus and Toxin

Although viral infection of the nervous system is relatively uncommon, it may have serious consequences. Often viruses spread to the nervous system through the blood vessels. Sometimes, however, the spread can occur through retrograde axonal transport. *Herpes* and *rabies* viruses are especially likely to use this route to travel from the periphery to the CNS. *Tetanus* toxin can also reach the CNS through retrograde transport in nerve fibers.

Blood–Brain Barrier

The endothelial cells of the capillaries in the brain are joined by tight junctions that provide an effective barrier, the blood–brain barrier, to passage of some substances, especially large protein molecules. Other substances, such as water, oxygen, and carbon dioxide, diffuse easily through the endothelial plasma membrane as do highly lipid-soluble substances including some anesthetics and ethyl alcohol.

The blood–brain barrier is of great functional importance, because it protects the CNS from many undesirable substances and from gross variations in the bodily environment. The permeability of the barrier varies for different medications, a factor of importance in drug therapy.

SUGGESTED READING

1. Escourolle, R. and J. Poirier, 1978. Manual of Basic Neuropathology, 2nd ed. W. B. Saunders: Philadelphia, pp. 1–17.
2. Heimer, L. and M. J. Robards (eds.), 1981. Neuroanatomical Tract-Tracing Methods. Plenum Press: New York.
3. Jones, E. G. and W. M. Cowan, 1977. Nervous tissue. In L. Weiss and R. O. Greep (eds.): Histology, 4th ed. McGraw-Hill: New York, pp. 283–372.
4. Morell, P. and W. T. Norton, 1980. Myelin. Scientific American 242(5): 88–117.
5. Peters, A., S. L. Palay, and H. de F. Webster, 1976. The Fine Structure of the Nervous System. W. B. Saunders: Philadelphia.
6. Schwartz, J. H., 1980. The Transport of Substances in Nerve Cells. Scientific American 242(4): 152–171.
7. Shepherd, G. M., 1979. The Synaptic Organization of the Brain: An Introduction, 2nd ed. Oxford University Press: New York.
8. Stevens, C. F., 1979. The Neuron. Scientific American 241(3): 49–59.

5

The Spinal Cord

THE SPINAL CORD AND ITS RELATIONSHIP TO
THE VERTEBRAL COLUMN
    Gross Anatomic Features
    Spinal Nerves
    Segmental Innervation of the Body

INTERNAL ORGANIZATION OF THE SPINAL CORD
    Gray Matter
    White Matter

CLINICAL NOTES
    Segmental Signs and Symptoms in Diseases of
        the Spinal Nerves or the Nerve Roots
    Disc Prolapse
    Herpes Zoster
    Spinal Cord Disorders

CLINICAL EXAMPLE
    Disc Prolapse

SUGGESTED READING

The spinal cord has a unique role as a conductor of impulses between the brain and the various peripheral nerves; it also serves many important reflex functions.

The frequency with which the vertebral column and its associated structures are damaged underscores the clinical importance of the spinal cord. Spinal cord disorders are often serious in nature, and their treatment presents a great challenge to the clinical staff. Although such disorders cannot always be cured, they can be understood and properly managed by people who are familiar with the functional anatomic features of the spinal cord and its structural relationships to the vertebral column.

Although the vertebral canal and its contents are seldom dissected in medical school courses, the anatomy of the spinal cord is of great importance in medical theory and practice. The gross anatomic features of the spinal cord and its particular relationship to the surrounding vertebral column is a subject of immediate interest for the practicing physician, and a basic knowledge of the internal organization of the spinal cord is a prerequisite for further inquiry into the functional anatomic systems of the CNS.

THE SPINAL CORD AND ITS RELATIONSHIP TO THE VERTEBRAL COLUMN

Gross Anatomic Features

The spinal cord has several distinctive gross anatomic features. It forms a nearly cylindrical column that is almost 0.5 m long in the adult; its diameter varies between 1 and 1.5 cm. Two continuous rows of nerve roots emerge on each side of the cord (Fig. 94). The roots join distally to form 31 pairs of spinal nerves, which exit through the intervertebral foramina. The spinal nerves distribute sensory and motor axons to all parts of the body.

The thickness of the spinal cord varies with the number of outgoing and incoming peripheral nerve fibers at different levels. The parts of the spinal cord that innervate the upper and lower limbs form spindle-shaped enlargements, the *cervical enlargements,* which extend between C3 and T1, and the *lumbar enlargement,* segments L1–S2 (see Fig. 96).

A cross-section of the spinal cord shows a characteristic division between the centrally placed gray substance and the surrounding white substance. The latter is formed by the long ascending and descending fiber tracts as well as intraspinal pathways. The cell groups seen in cross-sections actually form columns of cells that in some instances extend throughout the length of the spinal cord.

Spinal Nerves

The gray matter and white matter of the spinal cord are not segmented. However, the innervation of the body is orderly in the sense that one part of the spinal cord supplies a limited segment of the body with sensory and motor axons. This occurs through the distribution of 31 pairs of segmentally arranged spinal nerves, which give the impression of a segmental organization of the spinal cord.

A ventral root and dorsal root come together in the intervertebral foramen and form a *spinal nerve* (Fig. 94). The *ventral root,* which emerges as a series of root filaments along the ventrolateral sulcus, contains efferent somatic and, at specific levels, efferent visceral (sympathetic and parasympathetic) fibers.[1] These axons originate in motor nuclei of the spinal cord. A *dorsal root,* likewise, consists of several root filaments, which are attached to the spinal cord in the region of the dorsolateral sulcus. It contains primary afferent somatic and visceral fibers from cells in the *dorsal root ganglion* (spinal ganglion). The dorsal root ganglion appears as an oval swelling along the dorsal root close to its junction with the ventral root.

After the third fetal month, the vertebral column grows faster than the spinal cord. This results in a relative displacement of especially the lower parts of the spinal cord to higher levels of the vertebral column. The spinal nerves emerge from the vertebral canal before this unequal growth commences, and the dorsal and ventral roots, in particular the lumbosacral ones, are stretched out between their point of attachment to the cord and their entry into the intervertebral foramina. This growth or lengthening of the roots occurs within the vertebral canal, and the large collection of nerve roots below the first lumbar vertebra is called the *cauda equina* (Fig. 6, Chapter 2).

Segmental Innervation of the Body

The peripheral distribution of the spinal nerves reflects an original segmental organization in which each spinal nerve is composed of fibers that are related to the region of the skin, muscles, or the connective tissue that develops from one body segment (somite).

---

1. It has recently been shown that certain ventral roots do contain a significant number of unmyelinated sensory fibers. Their function is unknown, but they may account for the occasional lack of success of dorsal rhizotomy in relieving pain.

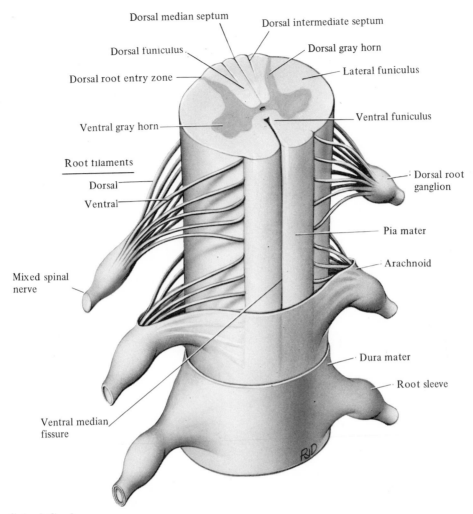

Fig. 94. Spinal Cord
The spinal cord forms a nearly cylindrical column surrounded by dura mater, arachnoid, and pia mater, all of which are continuous with the corresponding membranes of the brain. A series of dorsal and ventral rootlets emerges on each side of the cord. (Photograph courtesy of M. B. Carpenter. From Carpenter, M. B., 1978. Core Text of Neuroanatomy. 2nd. ed. With permission of the Williams & Wilkins Company, Baltimore.)

Innervation of the Skin: Dermatomes

The segmental organization is most pronounced in regard to the sensory innervation of the skin. The area of the skin that is supplied by sensory fibers of an individual spinal nerve is called a *dermatome*. Charts of the different dermatomes (Fig. 95) are important aids in the diagnosis and localization of pathologic processes that affect the spinal nerves or the spinal cord. However, one should be aware of the fact that there is considerable overlap between neighbouring dermatomes. It is useful to remember a few key dermatomes (Fig. 95B):

C3: Neck
C5: Deltoid region
C6: Radial forearm and thumb
C8: Ulnar border of hand and little finger
T4–T5: Nipple
T10: Umbilicus
L1: Groin
L3: Knee region
L5: Dorsal side of foot and great toe
S1: Lateral side of foot and little toe
S3–S5: Genito-anal region

It is important to try to distinguish a spinal nerve or root lesion from a peripheral neuropathy.

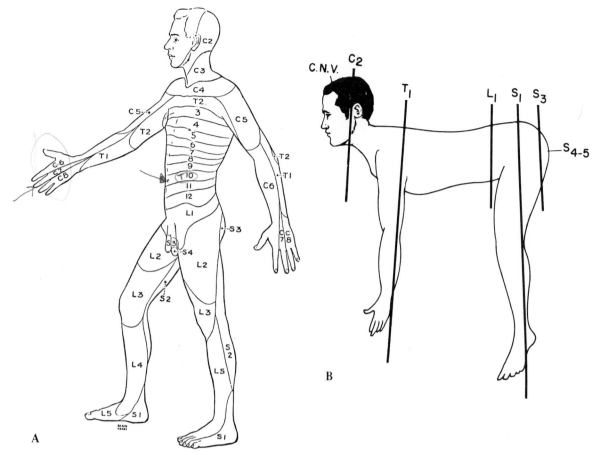

Fig. 95. Dermatomes
A. The segmental innervation of the skin, i.e., the dermatomes, from a lateral view.
B. Key dermatome boundaries (A. After Foerster 1933, B. From Curtis, B. A., S. Jacobson and E. M. Marcus. 1972. An Introduction to the Neurosciences. With permission of W. B. Saunders Company, Philadelphia.)

To do so one must know the cutaneous distribution of the peripheral nerves. The cutaneous areas supplied by the various nerves are illustrated in the appendix.

Innervation of the Muscles

Although the segmental organization is less obvious in regard to the motor innervation, the muscles deep to a certain area of the skin are usually innervated by approximately the same segments as the overlying skin. The nerve supply of the individual muscles are illustrated in the appendix. A summary of the spinal cord levels for the motor neurons that innervate various muscle groups is presented below.

C1–C4: Neck muscles
C3–C5: Diaphragm
C5–C6: Biceps
C5–C8: Muscles of the shoulder joint
C7–C8: Triceps and long muscles of the forearm
C8–T1: Muscles for movements of the digits and the small intrinsic muscles of the hand
T2–T12: Axial musculature, intervertebral muscles, muscles of respiration, and abdominal muscles
L1–L2: Flexors of the thigh
L2–L3: Quadriceps femoris
L5–S1: Gluteal muscles
S1–S2: Plantar flexors of the ankle
S3–S5: Muscles of the pelvic floor, bladder, sphincters, and external genital organs.

INTERNAL ORGANIZATION OF THE SPINAL CORD

The pattern of gray and white matter seen in transverse sections through the cord varies according to the level of the cord (Fig. 96). The largest cross sections are present in the cervical and the lumbar enlargements. Here the dorsal and especially the ventral horns of the gray substance are particularly well developed. A characteristic feature of the gray matter in the thoracic and upper lumbar segments is the presence of a lateral horn, in which the autonomic preganglionic motor neurons are located. The amount of white substance decreases in progressively caudal sections because the long ascending and descending pathways contain fewer axons at successively more caudal levels of the spinal cord.

Gray Matter

The gray matter has a characteristic butterfly appearance in cross-sections. It consists of a large number of neurons and their processes, in addition to an even larger number of neuroglial cells. The apex of the dorsal horn, the substantia gelatinosa, is characterized by a large number of small neurons, and one generally gets the impression that the neurons increase in size as one moves from the apex of the dorsal horn in the direction of the ventral horn, where the large motor neurons appear (Fig. 96). A more detailed analysis, however, reveals that all parts in front of substantia gelatinosa contain neurons of various sizes.

Although the different parts of the gray matter are usually referred to as the *ventral* and *dorsal horns,* and the *intermediate gray* between the two horns, it is important to realize that the horns in reality represent columns of gray matter that extend throughout the entire length of the spinal cord. Likewise, the various cell groups, which one can recognize in cross-sections through the spinal cord, form longitudinal columns of cells for shorter or longer distances. Some of the more characteristic cell columns have special designations.

Cell Groups (Fig. 96)

Nucleus Posteromarginalis.   This nucleus consists of a thin layer of cells that caps the tip of the dorsal horn. The axons of many of the large and medium-sized cells join the spinothalamic pathway (Chapter 6), which also receives contributions from other cell groups, including the nucleus proprius and the intermediate gray.

Substantia Gelatinosa.   Most of the apex of the dorsal horn or column is formed by a cup-shaped area, the substantia gelatinosa, which acquires its gelatinous appearance from a wealth of small neurons and unmyelinated or thinly myelinated fibers. It typically is unstained in myelin stained preparations. The small cells, whose axons arborize within the substantia gelatinosa, have attracted much attention in recent years in connection with the gate control theory (see Clinical Notes, Chapter 6).

Nucleus Proprius.   This cell column is located in the head of the dorsal horn and consists of nerve cells of various sizes. The anatomic affiliations and functional properties of the nucleus proprius neurons are many. Some of the cells project to the thalamus as part of the long ascending spinothalamic system; neurons at the base of the dorsal horn are the source of spinocerebellar pathways; still others belong to the propriospinal system. Many of the small neurons are interneurons in spinal reflexes or targets for descending pathways from the brain.

Lateral Cervical Nucleus.   This nucleus is located on the ventrolateral aspect of the dorsal horn in the 1st and 2nd cervical segments. It is a relay nucleus in one of the ascending pathways for touch-pressure sensitivity (see Fig. 106, Chapter 6).

Nucleus Dorsalis (Clarke's Column).   The cells in the nucleus dorsalis form a cell column that is located at the base of the dorsal horn in segments about C8–L3. Axons from large and medium-sized cells in the column of Clarke form the dorsal spinocerebellar tract (Chapter 9).

Intermediolateral and Intermediomedial Nuclei. The middle portion of the gray substance between the ventral and dorsal horn is referred to as the intermediate gray. It is a heterogeneous region with small and medium-sized cells. Two prominent cell columns in the intermediate gray are the *intermediolateral* and *intermediomedial cell columns,* which are present from T1 to L2, where the inter-

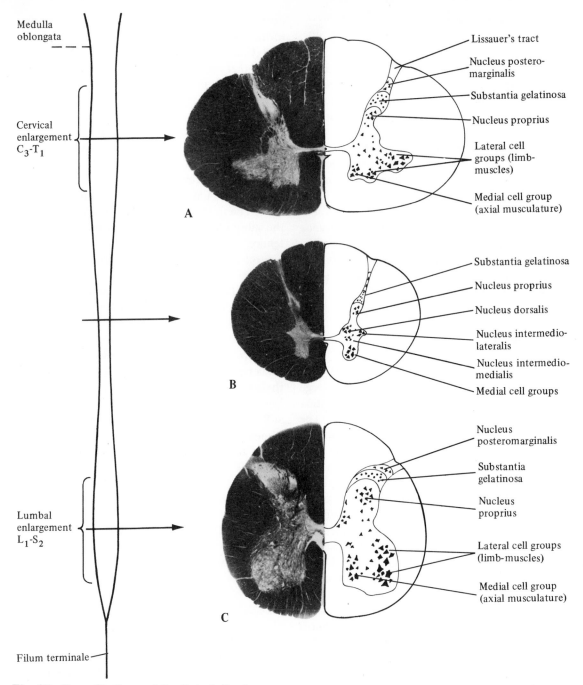

Fig. 96. Cross-Sections of the Spinal Cord

The cross-sections of the spinal cord are wider at the level of the cervical and lumbar enlargements than elsewhere. Note that the relative amount of gray and white matter is also different at different levels. The amount of white matter decreases gradually in caudal direction, since the long ascending and descending fiber tracts contain fewer axons at successively more caudal levels of the spinal cord. The main nuclear groups in the gray matter have been indicated in the schematic drawings of the right halves of the spinal cord sections. (The myelin stained left halves of the spinal cord are reprinted from Gluhbegovic, N. and T. H. Wiiiliams, 1980. The Human Brain and Spinal Cord. With permission from the authors and from Harper and Row, Hagerstown.)

mediolateral column is responsible for the formation of a lateral horn. The columns contain preganglionic visceral motor neurons for the sympathetic part of the autonomic nervous system. Corresponding cell columns are located at levels S2–S4 for the sacral part of the parasympathetic division.

Motor Cell Columns in the Ventral Horn. Cross-sections through cell stained preparations of the spinal cord reveal several groups of large somatic motor neurons in the ventral horn. The cell groups are especially prominent in the spinal cord enlargements, wherein prominent lateral and medial cell groups can be distinguished. These cell groups belong to longitudinally arranged cell columns of varying length. One of the medial cell columns, which innervates trunk and neck muscles, is present throughout the spinal cord, whereas the lateral columns, which supply the muscles of the limbs are present only in the cervical and lumbar enlargements. Within the lateral groups of motor neurons there is a further pattern of *somatotopic localization* in the sense that the neurons that innervate the distal limb musculature are located dorsal to those supplying the proximal limb muscles.

The large motor neurons that innervate the striated muscles are referred to as alpha (α) motor neurons. Scattered among the large motor neurons are many small neurons called gamma (γ) motor neurons; they send their axons to intrafusal muscle fibers, which are attached to special receptors in the muscles called muscle spindles.

Rexed's Laminae

Rexed divided the spinal cord gray substance into a series of 10 zones or laminae (Fig. 97) on the basis of cytoarchitectonic features. Rexed's map is used often in descriptions of scientific experiments, where the location of cellular elements is indicated according to Rexed's laminae.

The first six laminae subdivide the dorsal horn into horizontal zones. The posteromarginal nucleus is represented by Rexed's lamina I, whereas the substantia gelatinosa is most often equated with laminae II and III. The ill-defined nucleus proprius corresponds to cell groups in laminae IV and V. A large part of lamina VII corresponds to the intermediate gray, where nucleus dorsalis as well as the intermediolateral and interme-

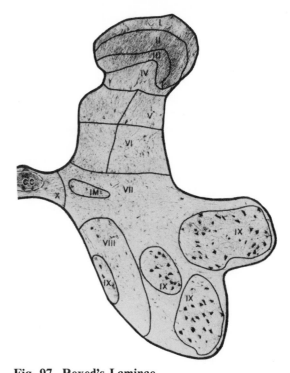

Fig. 97. Rexed's Laminae
Human spinal cord segment L5 stained with the Nissl method. On the basis of cytoarchitectonic features, the gray substance of the spinal cord can be subdivided into 10 zones or laminae (From Truex and Carpenter, 1969. Human Neuroanatomy. With permission of Dr. Carpenter and the Williams & Wilkins Company.)

diomedial cell columns are located. The motor neuron cell groups in the ventral horn form lamina IX.

Interneurons

The majority of the neurons in the gray substance of the spinal cord as well as in the rest of the CNS are *interneurons* (association neurons, intercalated neurons), which serve important integrative functions. The interneurons in the spinal cord have short axons or axons of medium length, which remain in the same segment (intrasegmental interneurons), or project to neighboring segments (intersegmental interneurons), or proceed to the opposite side of the spinal cord (commissural interneurons). Neurons that connect different segments within the spinal cord are also referred to as *propriospinal neurons.*

It is hardly possible to overestimate the importance of the interneuronal system. The number of interneurons in the spinal cord by far outnumber the motorneurons and the long-axoned neurons that represent the origin for ascending pathways. The interneurons are intercalated in various reflex loops and intrinsic neuron circuits; they also serve as intermediaries in relationships between long descending pathways and spinal motor and sensory mechanisms, or between peripheral afferent fibers and spinal cord neurons giving rise to long ascending pathways. The multitude of interneurons provide an almost infinite number of circuits and synaptic contacts, where messages can be modified or fundamentally altered. In short, the interneuronal net is largely responsible for the amazing readiness and flexibility with which we respond to various stimuli.

Spinal Reflexes

A reflex is a preprogrammed stereotyped reaction that occurs in response to a stimulus. Many of the somatic and autonomic functions mediated by the spinal cord are reflexogenic in nature.

A reflex consists of five elements: (1) A *receptor* receiving the stimulus; (2) an *afferent fiber* constituting the input to the CNS; (3) a *reflex center* in the CNS, where the stimulus can be influenced in various ways; and (4) an *efferent fiber* carrying the impulse to the fifth element, the *effector organ*. The nature of the reflex center determines to a large extent the complexity of the reflex. The simplest form of reflex is composed of only two neurons, in which case it is called a *monosynaptic reflex*. An example of a monosynaptic reflex is the stretch (myotatic) reflex, e.g., the quadriceps reflex (patellar reflex or knee jerk). Usually, the reflex center consists of one or more interneurons, in which case the reflex is referred to as a *polysynaptic reflex*. Examples of polysynaptic reflexes are the flexor withdrawal reflex and the crossed extensor reflex.

Stretch Reflex. The most famous stretch reflex is the quadriceps reflex (Fig. 98), produced by tapping the patellar tendon, which in turn stretches the quadriceps. The reflex is initiated by special muscle receptors called muscle spindles (Chapter 7), which are sensitive to stretch. The impulses generated by the receptors are transmitted through primary afferent fibers (blue in Fig. 98) to the spi-

nal cord, where the fibers establish synaptic contacts with motor neurons (red), which in turn produce contraction of quadriceps and extension of the leg at the knee. At the same time as the quadriceps contracts there is a reciprocal inhibition of the antagonistic muscles, the flexors of the knee. The inhibition of the flexors is mediated by polysynaptic reflex arcs, and since the motor neurons for the flexors are located in more caudal segments than the motor neurons for quadriceps, the inhibitory reflex is intersegmental, in contrast with the stretch reflex, which is intrasegmental.

Some stretch reflexes are routinely tested in neurologic examinations. The most commonly tested stretch reflexes have the following segmental reflex center:

1. *The Biceps reflex* (flexion of the elbow by tapping the biceps tendon) = C5–6.
2. *The brachioradial reflex* (flexion of the elbow and supination of the forearm by tapping the styloid process of the radius) = C5–6.
3. *The Triceps reflex* (extension of the elbow through a tap on the triceps tendon) = C7–8.
4. *Quadriceps (patellar) reflex* (extension of the knee by tapping the ligamentum patellae) = L3–L4.
5. *Triceps surae (Achilles) reflex* (plantar flexion of the foot by tapping the Achilles tendon) = S1.

Although there are stretch reflexes in all muscles, they are especially prominent in antigravity muscles, where they form the basis for postural reflexes.

Flexor Reflex and Crossed Extensor Reflex. The polysynaptic flexor reflex serves important protective functions. One of its purposes is to achieve a rapid withdrawal of a limb in response to painful cutaneous stimuli. This is referred to as a withdrawal reflex. To maintain balance, a flexor withdrawal reflex is usually accompanied by extension of the opposite limb through the action of the crossed extensor reflex.

The examples mentioned above include only some of the most well known spinal reflexes, which have been studied extensively by neurophysiologists. The many functions of the spinal cord are dependent on a multitude of other less well-known reflexes, whose reflex arcs and reflex centers are often little known. However, the situation is changing rapidly. Aided by intracellular recording and staining of neurons and by other modern

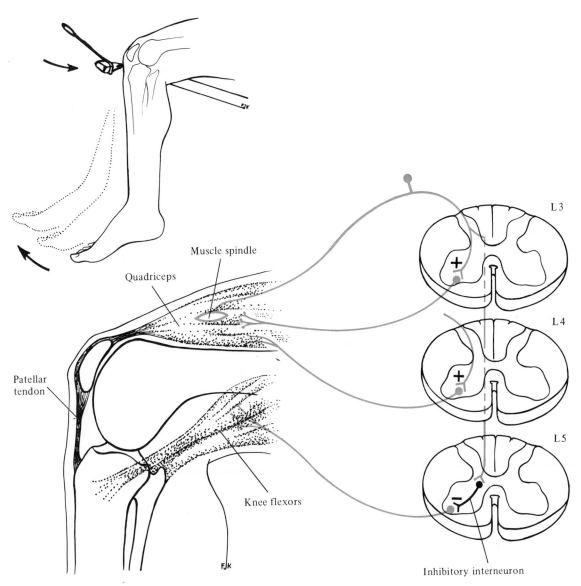

Fig. 98. The Quadriceps Reflex

Diagram of the pathways involved in a well known stretch reflex, the quadriceps reflex. If the quadriceps is suddenly stretched, usually by tapping the patellar tendon with a reflex-hammer (*inset*), the muscle spindles generate impulses that are transmitted in primary afferent fibers (*blue*) to the spinal cord, where they establish contact directly with motor neurons (*red*) innervating the quadriceps. This monosynaptic reflex results in extension of the leg at the knee. For this to occur, there must be a reduction of tension in the antagonists, the knee flexors, which is accomplished by the aid of a polysynaptic intersegmental reflex using an inhibitory interneuron (*black*).

tracer techniques, present-day neuroscientists are successfully mapping interneuronal pathways and polysynaptic circuits with a precision unthinkable a few years ago.

White Matter

The white matter on each side of the spinal cord can be divided into a *dorsal, lateral* and *ventral*

funiculus (Fig. 99A). The fibers are arranged functionally in more or less well defined ascending and descending pathways, which are given names implying their origin and termination (Fig. 99B). There are also association pathways which connect different segments within the spinal cord. These pathways, the *fasciculi proprii,* are found in all three funiculi and they are usually located adjacent to the gray substance. *Lissauer's tract,* which is wedged between the dorsal horn and the surface

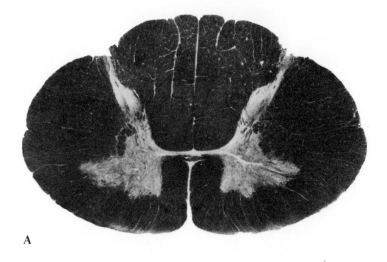

A

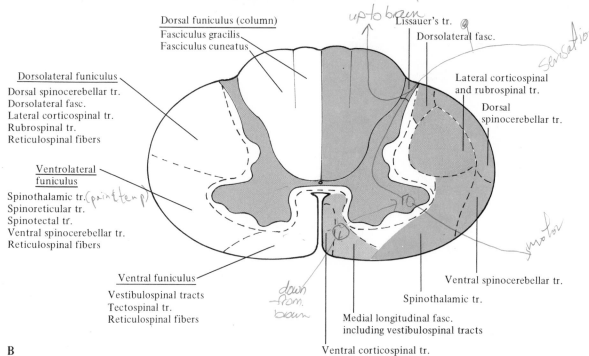

Dorsal funiculus (column)
Fasciculus gracilis
Fasciculus cuneatus

Dorsolateral funiculus
Dorsal spinocerebellar tr.
Dorsolateral fasc.
Lateral corticospinal tr.
Rubrospinal tr.
Reticulospinal fibers

Ventrolateral
funiculus
Spinothalamic tr.(point temp)
Spinoreticular tr.
Spinotectal tr.
Ventral spinocerebellar tr.
Reticulospinal fibers

Ventral funiculus
Vestibulospinal tracts
Tectospinal tr.
Reticulospinal fibers

up to brain
Lissauer's tr.
Dorsolateral fasc.

sensation

Lateral corticospinal
and rubrospinal tr.
Dorsal
spinocerebellar tr.

Ventral spinocerebellar tr.

motor

Spinothalamic tr.

down from brain

Medial longitudinal fasc.
including vestibulospinal tracts

Ventral corticospinal tr.

B

Fig. 99. White Matter of the Spinal Cord

A. Transverse myelin stained section of the spinal cord through the cervical enlargement. The ascending and descending pathways form the white matter of the spinal cord, which appears black in this myelin-stained preparation. (From Gluhbegovic, N. and T. H. Williams, 1980. The Human Brain and Spinal Cord. With permission of the authors and Harper and Row, Hagerstown.)

B. Since there is considerable overlap between different fiber tracts, it is difficult to illustrate all spinal cord tracts in a schematic drawing. Nevertheless, the position of some of the most important ascending (*blue*) and descending (*red*) pathways is indicated on the *right side*. The reticulospinal fibers, which serve many important somatomotor and autonomic functions, descend in all funiculi except the dorsal funiculus.

of the spinal cord, is to a large extent a propriospinal pathway.

The ascending somatosensory pathways, i.e., the dorsal column-medial lemniscus system and the spinocervicothalamic and the spinothalamic tracts, are described in more detail in Chapter 6, and the descending pathways in Chapter 7. The spinocerebellar pathways are discussed in relationship to the functional anatomy of cerebellum in Chapter 9.

CLINICAL NOTES

Segmental Signs and Symptoms in Diseases of the Spinal Nerves or the Nerve Roots

In contrast with a peripheral nerve disease, in which the signs and symptoms appear within the distribution of the affected nerve, diseases of the spinal nerves or the nerve roots are characterized by *segmental loss* of function. Lesions of the spinal cord may also give segmental symptoms, but such lesions are usually accompanied by involvement of long ascending or descending pathways as well.

Spinal nerve disorders cause both motor and sensory disturbances, whereas root disorders produce either motor or sensory symptoms depending on whether a ventral or dorsal root is affected. The stretch reflexes are affected in both dorsal and ventral root lesions.

Sensory Symptoms

Compression or inflammation of a root manifests itself as pain localized to the affected dermatome, i.e., *radicular* or *root pain*. Other types of abnormal sensation, or *paresthesias*, are tingling, prickling, burning, and itching. Increased sensitivity to various stimuli is called *hyperesthesia*. When the fibers lose their capacity to conduct sensory impulses, the corresponding symptoms are referred to as *hypesthesia* (diminished sensitivity) or *anesthesia* (loss of all forms of sensation).

When testing for sensory loss one should remember that there is a considerable overlap between neighbouring dermatomes. The upper half of dermatome T10, for instance, is innervated not only by fibers from T10, but also by fibers from T9, whereas the lower half of T10 receives additional innervation from T11 (Fig. 100). Therefore,

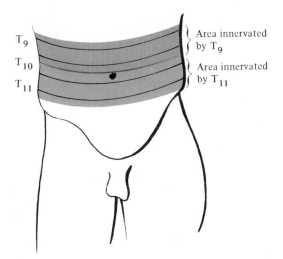

Fig. 100. Overlap of Dermatomes
There is considerable overlap between neighboring dermatomes, and the overlap is usually greater for touch than it is for pain. A small sensory deficit, therefore, is more easily detected by testing for pain rather than for touch.

interruption of one dorsal root may not be noticed. However, since the overlap is usually greater for touch than it is for pain, a small sensory deficit can be more easily detected by testing the sensibility for pain rather than for touch.

Motor Symptoms

A complete loss of motor function is referred to as *paralysis;* a lesser loss is called *paresis.* The motor deficits in spinal nerve or ventral root disorders are characterized by a flaccid (soft, flabby) paresis or paralysis of the affected muscles. There is also significant *atrophy* and reduced tonus, i.e., *hypotonus,* of the affected muscles, whose stretch reflexes are absent or weakened compared to the normal side. An affection of the peripheral motor neuron (lower motor neuron, see Fig. 114, Chapter 7), therefore, is characterized by flaccid paralysis, atrophy, hypotonus, and hyporeflexia.

Disc Prolapse

This is the major cause of backache (lumbago) and radicular pain in the leg corresponding to the distribution of the sciatic nerve (sciatica). It is often seen in middle-aged people, in whom degenerative changes in the anulus fibrosus and the posterior longitudinal ligament are common. The condition is often precipitated by a flexion injury that forces the disc (or prolapsing nucleus pulposus) in a posterolateral direction into the vertebral canal, where the disc compresses the nerve roots or the spinal nerve.

Flexion of the vertebral column mainly takes place in the lower lumbar region, and the discs between L4–L5 and L5–S1 are therefore most often affected. Intervertebral discs in the upper lumbar and lower thoracic regions are less commonly affected. Since the spinal cord ends at vertebral body L1, lumbar and sacral roots hang down below the cord at the cauda equina. Each set of roots proceeds obliquely toward its intervertebral foramen in such a manner that protrusion of an intervertebral disc may compress one or two existing roots, either right or left. For instance, protrusion of disc L4–L5 may compress either the 5th lumbar root or the 1st sacral root, or both (Fig. 101). The most common sites for disc protrusions in the cervical region are C5–6 and C6–7.

Compression of the 5th lumbar root usually produces radiating pain and sometimes corresponding sensory loss in the lateral calf, dorsal surface of the foot, and the first to third toes. Extension of the big toe and foot may be weakened.

Compression of the 1st sacral root produces radiating pain and sometimes corresponding sensory loss in the posterior surface of the leg and the outer plantar surface of the foot and fourth and fifth toes. The plantar flexors of the foot may be weakened and the achilles reflex is often diminished or absent.

Herpes Zoster

This disease is caused by a virus that is related to chicken pox virus. It causes inflammation of isolated posterior root ganglia, resulting in a skin lesion known as shingles. The symptoms are usually confined to one or two adjacent dermatomes, most often in the thoracic region. The initial symptom is radicular pain followed in a few days by reddening and the appearance of vesicles in a typical segmental distribution on one side of the body.

Spinal Cord Disorders

Spinal cord disorders are quite common and often produce distinctive syndroms, which can best be

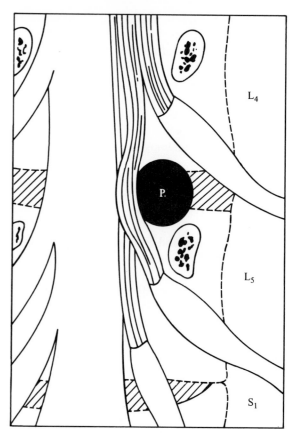

Fig. 101. Disc Prolapse
A protrusion (P) of the 4th intervertebral disc between L4 and L5 may compress either the 5th lumbar root or the 1st sacral root, or both. (Redrawn from Spurling and Grantham, 1940, Arch. of Surgery 40: 375–388. In: Brodal, A., 1981. Neurological Anatomy, Third Edition. With permission of Oxford University Press.)

understood following a discussion of the long ascending and descending pathways of the spinal cord (Chapters 6 and 7). Therefore, only a brief summary of the main diseases of the spinal cord is presented here.

Like all types of nervous diseases, the signs and symptoms of a spinal cord disorder are dependent on the extent of the damage and the level of the injury. For instance, a complete *transverse lesion* of the spinal cord, which is often traumatic in origin, results in loss of all voluntary movements and all sensations below the level of injury. A *degenerative disease,* on the other hand, is usually characterized by selective involvement of certain functional-anatomical systems, e.g., the motor neuronal cell groups in *amyotrophic lateral sclerosis,* or some of the long ascending and descending tracts in *Friedreich's ataxia* and other s.c. *spinocerebellar degenerations.* Another typical spinal cord disease is *syringomyelia,* a disease of unknown etiology, which is characterized by a pathologic cavitation of the central gray substance often in the cervical part of the spinal cord. The lesion produces a characteristic segmental loss of pain and temperature sense (Fig. 109 and Clinical Example in Chapter 6) by involving the second order neurones as they cross the midline.

Trauma

Automobile and diving accidents are two of the most common causes of severe *fracture-dislocations* of the spine and concommitant transverse lesions of the spinal cord. The most mobile parts of the vertebral columns, the lower cervical and the upper lumbar regions, are often damaged, and if the injury is severe enough, the patient will be suffering from a *paraplegia* (paralysis of both lower extremities) if the lower part of the spinal cord is damaged, or a *tetraplegia* (paralysis of all four extremities) if the lesion occurs in the cervical area (see Clinical Notes in Chapter 7).

Myelitis

An inflammatory disease of the spinal cord, i.e., a myelitis, is usually the result of a general infection of the nervous system. The cause of myelitis is often unknown; other times it is caused by a virus, e.g., *poliomyelitis, herpes zoster* (see above), or *rabies.*

Tabes dorsalis is a tertiary form of neurosyphilis, which is characterized primarily by degeneration of the dorsal roots and the dorsal columns, resulting, typically, in lighting pains and ataxia (loss of muscular coordination). Neurosyphilis, which usually develops 15–20 years following the initial infection with treponema pallidus, is today relatively uncommon because of successful therapy with penicillin.

Tumors

Since most of the tumors in the vertebral canal arise outside the spinal cord rather than within the substance of the cord, they can be removed surgically before they have produced irreversible damage, providing they are recognized at an early stage. Compression of a nerve root causes radicular pain and other sensory and motor disturbances,

and the segmental signs and symptoms usually indicate the location of the tumor. Further, compression of the long pathways may result in motor and sensory symptoms, which are often of an asymmetic distribution.

Vascular Lesions

Vascular disorders of the spinal cord are uncommon compared with cerebrovascular diseases. Nevertheless, infarctions and bleeding do occur, most often in the territory of the anterior spinal artery (see Clinical Examples in Chapter 21).

CLINICAL EXAMPLE

Disc Prolapse

A 38-year-old male manual laborer suffered acute onset of back pain while operating a pneumatic hammer. The pain radiated down the posterior aspect of his right leg and into the ventral surface of his foot. He noticed that coughing made the pain worse.

The neurologic examination was remarkable for percussion tenderness over his lower back with a sharp pain that radiated down the posterior aspect of his right leg. The right gastrocnemius muscle was weak and the Achilles reflex was absent on the right side. The motor deficits were matched by loss of pain and temperature sensitivity over the lateral surface of his right foot.

The man was treated with strict bed rest and his pain was alleviated with analgesics. However, his condition did not improve and a CT scan (Fig. B, next page) was obtained before he was transferred to a neurosurgical unit.

1. What do you think is the nature of his disease process?

2. What nerve root is most likely to be involved?

3. Into which large peripheral nerve does this nerve root contribute fibers?

4. Compare the CT scan from this patient with a normal CT scan taken from a higher level (Fig. A, next page). The arrow in the pathologic CT scan is pointing to disc material that should not be present in the vertebral canal. The herniated disk is pressing on an elliptically shaped area in the center of the picture. What does this area represent and what nervous structures are located there?

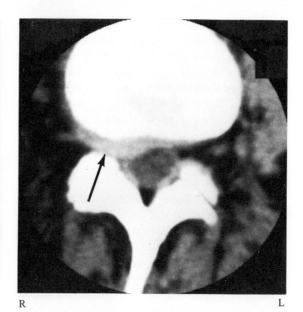

R   L

A. Normal

Fig. CE5A and B.
The CT scans were kindly provided by Dr. V. Haughton.

R   L

B. Disc Prolapse

Discussion

The patient's history is typical for a disc prolapse (herniated disc), and the radiation of pain down the posterior aspect of the leg into the foot indicates compression of the S1 nerve root (see Fig. 101). This root contributes fibers to the sciatic nerve and one of its branches, the tibial nerve, which innervates the medial and lateral heads of the gastrocnemius muscle. Selective loss of gastrocnemius power coupled with a reduced or absent Achilles reflex (mediated by the gastrocnemius muscle) is typical of an S1 root lesion. The sensory deficit is also consistent with such a lesion.

This type of herniation is referred to as a central–lateral disc herniation. The elliptically shaped structure against which the disc material is pressing is the dural sac, containing the cauda equina and leptomeninges. The ring of enhancement around the dural sac represents filling of the epidural venous plexus. Selective filling of this plexus with contrast dye (lumbar venogram) is also helpful in demonstrating herniated discs. Many patients with disc herniations improve with bed rest and analgesics, but some ultimately require surgery for removal of the extruded disc material.

SUGGESTED READING

1. Adams, R. D. and M. Victor, 1979. Principles of Neurology, 2nd ed. McGraw-Hill: New York, pp. 136–155.
2. Brown, A. G., 1981. Organization in the Spinal Cord. The Anatomy and Physiology of Identified Neurons. Springer-Verlag: Berlin.
3. DeMyer, W., 1981. Anatomy and Clinical Neurology of the Spinal Cord. In A. B. Baker and L. H. Baker (eds.): Clinical Neurology, Vol. 3. Harper and Row: Philadelphia, Chapter 31.
4. Henneman, E., 1980. Organization of the Spinal Cord and Its Reflexes. In V. B. Mountcastle (ed.): Medical Physiology, 14th ed., Vol. 1. C. V. Mosby: St. Louis, Missouri, pp. 762–786.
5. Patten, J., 1977. Neurological Differential Diagnosis. Springer-Verlag: New York, pp. 139–171.

6

Ascending Sensory Pathways

PATHWAYS FOR PAIN AND TEMPERATURE: THE
SPINOTHALAMIC TRACT
  Receptors and Peripheral Pathways
  Spinal Pathways
  Thalamocortical Projections and the
    Appreciation of Pain and Temperature
  Gate Control Hypothesis for Pain

PATHWAYS FOR TOUCH–PRESSURE, VIBRATION,
AND POSITION SENSE: THE DORSAL COLUMN–
MEDIAL LEMNISCUS SYSTEM AND THE
DORSOLATERAL FASCICULUS
  Receptors and Peripheral Pathways
  Spinal Pathways
  Thalamocortical Projections and the Primary
    Somatosensory Cortex

CLINICAL NOTES
  Peripheral Nerve Lesions
  Spinal Nerve and Nerve Root Lesions
  Spinal Cord Syndromes
  Lesions in the Postcentral Gyrus and Superior
    Parietal Lobule
  Pain: A Clinical Problem with Many
    Dimensions

CLINICAL EXAMPLES
  Syringomyelia
  Subacute Combined Degeneration

SUGGESTED READING

The classic view of two largely independent somatosensory channels, the dorsal column–medial
lemniscus system for tactile sensitivity and position
sense, and the spinothalamic system for pain and
temperature sensitivity, has been modified in recent years through the discovery of additional spinal pathways for transmission of sensory impulses
to the brain. This is highly significant, because
the sensory symptoms that appear in patients with
lesions in the CNS have sometimes been difficult
to explain by the traditional dual-processing theory. They can now be better appreciated on the
basis of a more dynamic view of the somatosensory
pathways.

Although sensory and motor neurons are closely
interconnected throughout the nervous system, the
ascending sensory pathways are to a large extent
separated from the structures and pathways that
control motor functions. Therefore, nervous system disorders can in large measure affect sensory
or motor functions independently.

The traditional view of the somatosensory pathways to the cerebral cortex is that the dorsal column–medial lemniscus pathway carries information necessary for discriminative touch, vibratory sensibility, and position sense, and that the spinothalamic pathway is mainly responsible for pain and temperature sensitivity. Although clinical findings could not always be explained on the basis of this dual-processing theory, the sensory deficits that appeared in patients with spinal cord disorders, nevertheless, seemed to be compatible with the presence of these two conduction routes. However, in recent years some additional ascending pathways have been discovered, and the classic view is gradually losing ground.

The changing view is related not so much to the pathway for pain and temperature but rather to the ascending systems that are responsible for tactile sensitivity and position sense. The picture that is about to emerge is rather complicated in the sense that there are several channels for both tactile and proprioceptive impulses. However, the different channels are not well segregated; there is considerable interaction between the different pathways.

The ascending sensory pathways can be divided into three groups:

1. Pathways for *pain and temperature*. The main pathway is the *spinothalamic tract,* which is accompanied in its course by fibers terminating in the reticular formation, the *spinoreticular tract,* and by fibers terminating in the mesencephalic tectum and central gray matter, the *spinotectal tract.* The spinothalamic, spinoreticular, and spinotectal tracts are sometimes included in the so-called anterolateral (AL) system.

The traditional subdivision of the spinothalamic tract into a lateral spinothalamic tract for pain and temperature and a ventral spinothalamic tract for tactile stimuli is of little value.

2. Pathways for *tactile information, vibration,* and *position sense* (static position sense and kinesthesia). Impulses related to these modalities are carried via several pathways, particularly in the *dorsal column* (funiculus) and in the *dorsolateral fasciculus,* which is located in the dorsal part of the lateral funiculus. Although some touch–pressure signals, and probably also proprioceptive impulses, can be mediated via the spinothalamic tract, the critical pathways for tactile information and position sense are located in the dorsal part of the spinal cord.

Lissauer's tract, which is a part of the propriospinal system, is sometimes referred to as the dorso-

lateral fasciculus. However, as indicated above, this term is also frequently used for the collection of ascending sensory fibers in the dorsal part of the lateral funiculus.

3. Pathways for *somatosensory impulses to the cerebellum* are described in Chapter 9.

PATHWAYS FOR PAIN AND TEMPERATURE: THE SPINOTHALAMIC TRACT (AL-SYSTEM)

The sense of pain has several submodalities. Intense stimulation of the skin results in *superficial pain,* which is well localized. *Deep (aching) pain,* which arises in skeletal muscles, tendons, and joints, is poorly localized. *Visceral pain,* like deep pain, has an aching character and is poorly localized. *Itch* is closely related to pain and the two modalities are transmitted by the same pathways.

Thermal sensation can be divided into two discrete modalities: *warm* and *cold.*

Receptors and Peripheral Pathways

Most, if not all, *nociceptors,*[1] (pain receptors) and *thermoreceptors* (cold and warm receptors) are represented by free nerve endings that are related to fine unmyelinated C fibers,[2] or thinly myelinated

---

1. Receptors can be subdivided in many ways, and there is no classification system that adequately incorporates either anatomic or physiologic characteristics. It is common to divide the receptors into *nociceptors* (pain receptors), *thermoreceptors,* and *mechanoreceptors.* Nociceptors and thermoreceptors are apparently represented by free nerve endings, whereas there are several varieties of mechanoreceptors responding to touch and pressure, or to movements and distentions in the joints, muscles, and viscera. If the receptors are located in the skin or the subcutaneous connective tissue, and respond to stimuli from the outside, they are referred to as *exteroceptors.* Those located in the visceral organs are called *interoceptors* (viscero-ceptors). *Proprioceptors* are located in muscles, tendons, and joints.

2. The classification of nerve fibers is somewhat confusing. In one classification the fibers are divided into A, B, and C fibers according to their diameter and physiologic properties. A fibers are somatic myelinated fibers, and they fall into four partly overlapping groups, α, β, γ, and δ, with decreasing diameter. B fibers are lightly myelinated preganglionic fibers in the autonomic nervous system, and C fibers include all unmyelinated fibers of both the somatic and autonomic (postganglionic fibers) system. Sensory fibers are either A$\alpha\beta$ fibers (conduction rate 120–30 m/sec), Aδ fibers (conduction rate 4–30 m/sec), or C fibers (conduction rate less than 2.5 m/sec).

Another classification that pertains to the afferent fibers in a muscle nerve recognizes four groups, I, II, III, and IV. Groups I and II correspond to A$\alpha\beta$, group III to Aδ, and group IV to C fibers.

A-delta (Aδ) fibers. The cell bodies of the fibers lie in the dorsal root ganglion, and the central axonal processes proceed through the dorsal root to terminate in the dorsal horn, primarily in the posteromarginal nucleus (lamina I), the substantia gelatinosa (laminae II and III), and the nucleus proprius (lamina V).

Many of the fibers that transmit pain and temperature impulses take part in reflexes of various types, e.g., autonomic responses and the flexion withdrawal response (Chapter 5). Other afferent fibers establish synaptic contacts with cells whose axons form the ascending spinal pathway for pain and temperature.

Spinal Pathways (Fig. 102)

Spinothalamic Tract

The spinothalamic tract is the main spinal cord pathway for transmission of pain and temperature impulses. Its cells of origin are located primarily in the *posteromarginal nucleus* (lamina I of Rexed) and the *nucleus proprius* (laminae IV and V). The majority of the axons cross in the white commissure in the same or adjacent segment and ascend in the anterolateral funiculus on the opposite side of the cord.

Since crossing fibers are added to the inner aspect of the tract, fibers from successively more rostral levels will occupy increasingly deeper parts of the tract. This provides for a *rough somatotopic organization* in the sense that the lower parts of the body are represented laterally and the upper parts medially.

The spinothalamic tract ascends in the anterolateral white matter toward the brain stem, where it is located on the dorsolateral aspect of the inferior olivary nucleus in the medulla oblongata. Higher in the brain stem, it is situated dorsal to the medial lemniscus, which gradually moves laterally through its ascent in the brain stem. The spinothalamic fibers terminate primarily in the *ventral posterolateral nucleus (VPL)* and in the nearby *posterior nuclei* of the thalamus. The *intralaminar thalamic nuclei* (Chapter 18) also receive significant contributions from the spinothalamic tract.

Spinoreticular and Spinotectal Tracts

The spinothalamic fibers are accompanied by fibers that terminate in the medial parts of the brain stem *reticular formation,* i.e., the spinoreticular tract, and in the *tectum* and *periaqueductal gray* of the midbrain, the spinotectal tract. The spinoreticular fibers, which are both crossed and uncrossed, are involved in various reflex adjustments. Further, the spinoreticular tract represents the first link in a spinoreticulothalamic pathway to the intralaminar and midline thalamic nuclei, which in turn seem to be able to activate widespread areas of the cerebral cortex (Chapter 10). The spinotectal tract establishes important synaptic relationships with a "pain inhibiting system," which apparently is located in the periaqueductal gray and midbrain raphe nuclei (see Clinical Notes).

Pathways for Pain and Temperature from the Face

Pain and temperature impulses from the face travel along fibers in the different components of the trigeminal nerve and reach the *nucleus of the spinal trigeminal tract.* Small fiber components of the facial, glossopharyngeal, and vagus nerves (from the external ear, auditory canal, and middle ear, as well as from the back of the tongue, pharynx, larynx, and esophagus) also terminate in the nucleus of the spinal tract.

Many of the fibers from the nucleus of the spinal tract cross to the opposite side of the medulla, join the medial lemniscus, and reach the *ventral posteromedial nucleus* (*VPM*) and intralaminar nuclei of the thalamus. Fibers also terminate in the reticular formation, and many fibers reach the ipsilateral VPM.

Thalamocortical Projections and the Appreciation of Pain and Temperature

The thalamus is apparently of great significance for the appreciation of pain and temperature, but how it is involved is not known. It should be reemphasized, however, that pain stimuli do reach several thalamic regions, including the intralaminar nuclei, which are important in behavioral arousal and EEG activation.

To what extent the perception of pain and temperature requires the cerebral cortex is not clear.

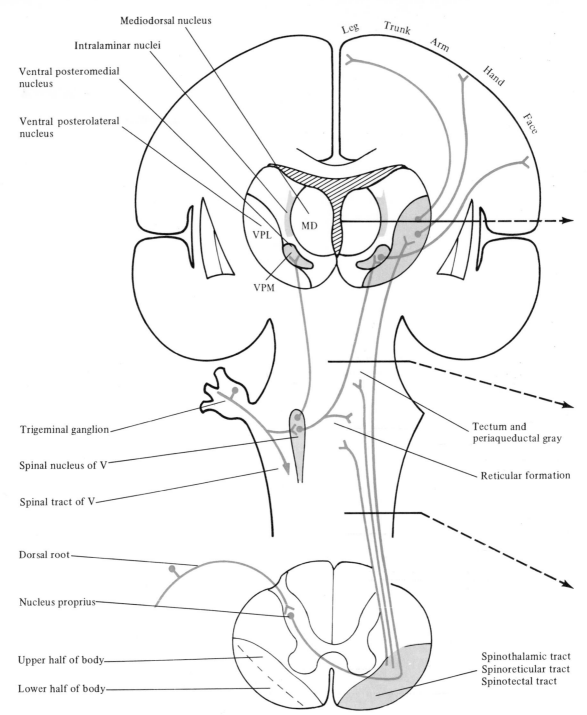

Fig. 102. Pathways for Pain and Temperature
Diagram illustrating the course and termination of the main pathways for pain and temperature, i.e., the spino-thalamic and trigeminothalamic tracts. Many of the ascending fibers in the anterolateral system of the spinal cord as well as from the trigeminal system terminate in the reticular formation, periaqueductal gray, and tectum. The ascending pathways for pain and temperature are colored *blue* in the cross-sections through medulla oblongata **(A)**, mesencephalon **(B)**, and internal capsule **(C)**.

Although clinical studies of patients with cortical lesions indicate that the cerebral cortex is not essential for conscious appreciation of pain, it is probably a mistake to think that the cortex is of no importance in pain mechanisms. Accurate localization is dependent on the cerebral cortex, and there are significant pathways both from the VPL–VPM and the posterior thalamic nuclei to the cerebral cortex. Fibers from the VPL and VPM project through the posterior limb of the internal capsule to the *first somatosensory area, SI,* in the postcentral gyrus (Broadmann's areas 3, 1 and 2) and the *second somatosensory area, SII,* in the superior lip of the lateral fissure (Fig. 108). Further, pathways descending from the cerebral cortex to the thalamus and different levels of the brain stem and spinal cord are likely to modify the transmission of pain impulses.

Gate Control Hypothesis for Pain

According to this theory the substantia gelatinosa acts as a gating mechanism for the control of afferent input to the spinothalamic neurons (blue in Fig. 103). The activity in small C fibers (pain) keeps the gate open, and activation of large myelinated A fibers closes the gate. To accomplish a closing of the gate, small substantia gelatinosa cells (Fig. 103, in black), which project to spinothalamic neurons in the nucleus proprius would have to be excited by large afferents. This would produce presynaptic inhibition of the afferent input to the spinothalamic neurons, and the pain impulses, which travel along the small fibers, would not be able to reach the brain.

The gating principle seemed to provide an elegant explanation for some well known phenomena, e.g., the tendency to rub a sore spot for relief from pain (the rubbing would activate the large fibers, thereby closing the gate). However, new scientific discoveries have made the theory less attractive, and it will probably not survive in its present form, at least not as a model for the substantia gelatinosa. Nevertheless, it provides a striking example of how an imaginative hypothesis can stimulate scientific inquiry and sometimes even bring about a change in therapy (see Clinical Notes).

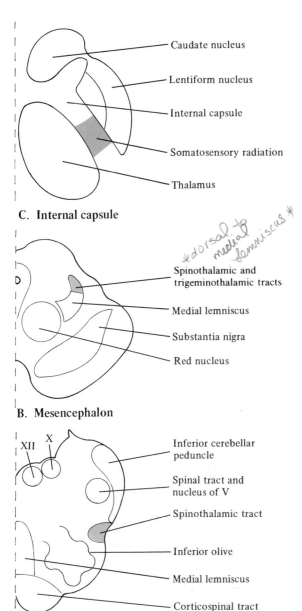

Caudate nucleus

Lentiform nucleus

Internal capsule

Somatosensory radiation

Thalamus

C. Internal capsule

dorsal to medial lemniscus

Spinothalamic and trigeminothalamic tracts

Medial lemniscus

Substantia nigra

Red nucleus

B. Mesencephalon

XII   X

Inferior cerebellar peduncle

Spinal tract and nucleus of V

Spinothalamic tract

Inferior olive

Medial lemniscus

Corticospinal tract

A. Medulla oblongata

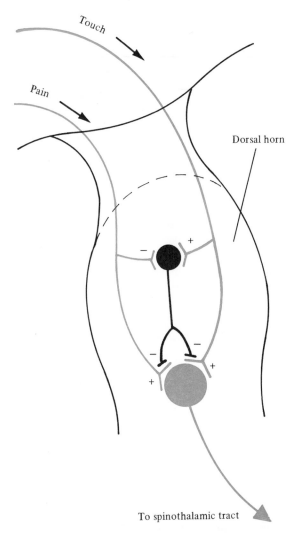

Touch

Pain

Dorsal horn

To spinothalamic tract

Fig. 103. The Gate Control Theory for Pain
Diagram explaining how activity in small C-fibers (pain) would keep the gate open, whereas impulses reaching the dorsal horn through large A-fibers in the medial portion of the dorsal root would close the gate. Although the gate control hypothesis has been severely criticized in recent years, it has stimulated much research and the development of therapeutic devices for pain control. *Black* neuron, Inhibitory interneuron. *Blue,* primary afferent fibers and spinal projection neuron. (Modified after Melzack R. and P. D. Wall, 1965. Pain mechanisms: A new theory. Science 150: 971–979.)

PATHWAYS FOR TOUCH–PRESSURE, VIBRATION, AND POSITION SENSE: THE DORSAL COLUMN–MEDIAL LEMNISCUS SYSTEM AND THE DORSOLATERAL FASCICULUS

Touch is the experience of light stimulation of the skin, whereas activation of receptors deeper in the skin arouses the sensation of pressure. Touch and pressure, however, can be thought of as representing a continuum of stimulus intensity, *touch–pressure.*

Vibration is aroused by an oscillating stimulus, applied by the aid of a tuning fork, that activates receptors deep to the skin.

Position sense is composed of two submodalities: *static position sense* and *kinesthesia.* Static position sense (postural sense) signals the position of a limb in space, whereas kinesthesia reveals the movement of a limb.

Receptors and Peripheral Pathways

In contrast with the pain and temperature receptors, which are represented by free nerve endings (Fig. 104A), the receptors related to touch–pressure, vibration, and position sense are more or less specialized and often encapsulated (Fig. 104).

The tactile receptors signaling information about touch–pressure are represented by specialized epithelial cells of Merkel, by *encapsulated nerve endings* (e.g., Ruffini's and Meissner's corpuscles), and by hair follicle[3] receptors.

Vibration is mediated by highly specialized encapsulated nerve endings, the *Pacinian corpuscles.*

Position sense is apparently dependent on various *proprioceptive receptors* in joints and tendons and probably also in the muscles.

The cell bodies of the fibers related to these various receptors are located in the dorsal root ganglion, and their central processes, many of which are large and myelinated, proceed through the dorsal root to the spinal cord, where they divide in an ascending and a descending branch, both of which contain many collaterals that establish synaptic contacts with various cell groups in

---

3. Although the specialists refer to the sensation generated by many of the hair follicle receptors (velocity receptors) as flutter, they are activated when the physician tests the sense of "touch" with a wisp of cotton, and for the sake of convenience they will be considered as touch receptors.

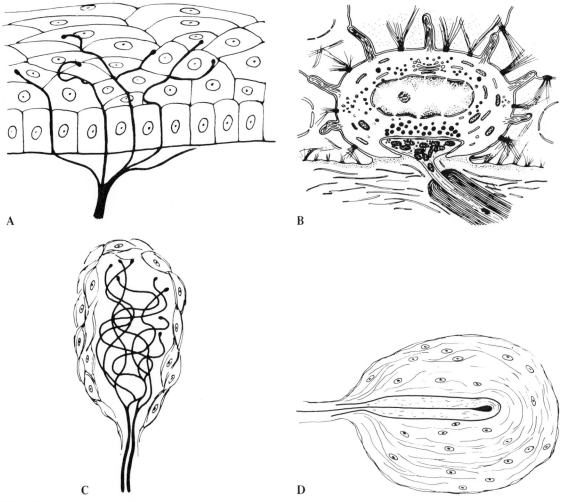

Fig. 104. Sensory Receptors
A. Free nerve endings. **B.** Merkel's specialized cell. **C.** Meissner's corpuscle. **D.** Pacinian corpuscle (**A, C** and **D** from Geneser, 1981. Histologi. With permission of the author and Munksgaard, Copenhagen, Denmark. **B** from Bannister, L. H., 1976. Sensory Terminals of Peripheral Nerves. In D. N. Landon (Ed.), The Peripheral Nerve. With permission of Chapman and Hall Ltd.).

the spinal cord. Many of the ascending collaterals enter the dorsal column and some of them reach the medulla oblongata, where they terminate in an orderly somatotopic fashion in the dorsal column nuclei, also called the gracile and cuneate nuclei.

Spinal Pathways (Figs. 105, 106, and 107)

Tactile Sensitivity

There are at least two major ascending systems, the *dorsal column–medial lemniscus pathway* and

the *spinocervicothalamic pathway,* for transmission of tactile impulses. The *spinothalamic tract* seems to provide a third alternative.

The Dorsal Column–Medial Lemniscus Pathway. Many of the fibers that enter the dorsal columns directly from the dorsal roots terminate at different levels in the spinal cord and only about 25% of the fibers reach the dorsal column nuclei, the *gracile* and *cuneate nuclei* in the medulla oblongata, where they establish synaptic contacts with cells, whose axons cross over to the other side of the medulla and form the *medial lemniscus.* The crossing fibers, the internal arcuate fibers,

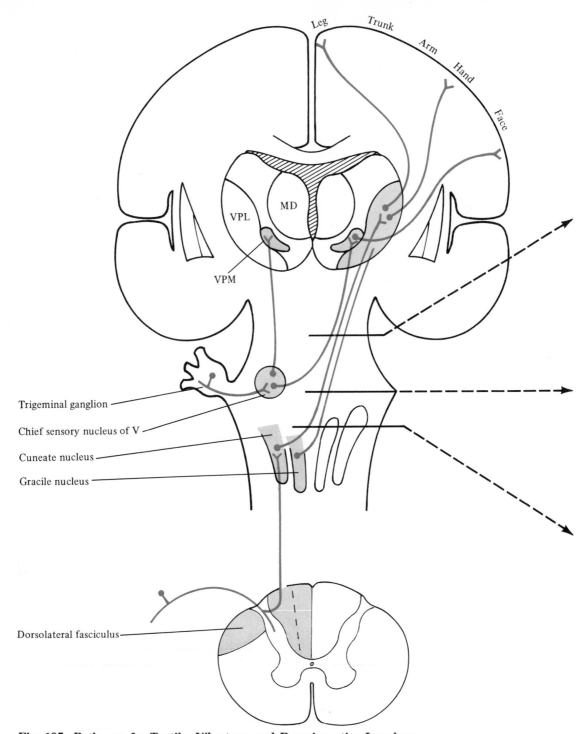

Leg

Trunk

Arm

Hand

Face

MD

VPL

VPM

Trigeminal ganglion

Chief sensory nucleus of V

Cuneate nucleus

Gracile nucleus

Dorsolateral fasciculus

Fig. 105. Pathways for Tactile, Vibratory, and Proprioceptive Impulses
Diagram illustrating the dorsal column–medial lemniscal system mediating proprioception and stereognosis. Proprioceptive impulses and impulses for tactile discrimination are also being transmitted in the dorsolateral fasciculus (see Figs. 106 and 107). **A–C.** Cross-sections showing the decussation of the medial lemniscus (**A**), and the position of the medial lemniscus in the medulla oblongata (**B**) and mesencephalon (**C**).

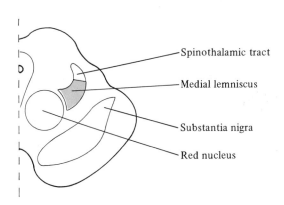

Spinothalamic tract

Medial lemniscus

Substantia nigra

Red nucleus

C. Mesencephalon

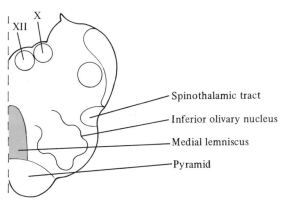

Spinothalamic tract

Inferior olivary nucleus

Medial lemniscus

Pyramid

B. Medulla oblongata

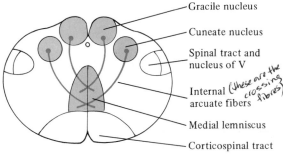

Gracile nucleus

Cuneate nucleus

Spinal tract and nucleus of V

Internal *(these are the crossing fibres)* arcuate fibers

Medial lemniscus

Corticospinal tract

A. Decussation of the medial lemniscus

form the *decussation of the medial lemniscus,* which is located in the lower part of the medulla (MEDIAL) (Fig. 105A) just rostral to the pyramidal decussation. The medial lemniscus is located medially in the medulla, but it gradually moves laterally through its ascent in the brain stem to reach the *ventral posterolateral nucleus (VPL)* in the thalamus. Some of the fibers in the dorsal column–medial lemniscus system also terminate in the posterior thalamic nucleus. 2/0 *not accord to R.M. S.P.R.M.*

The Spinocervicothalamic Pathway.   The other major spinal pathway for touch–pressure, the *dorsolateral fasciculus* (Fig. 106), originates primarily in the nucleus proprius (laminae IV–V) and ascends on the same side to the *lateral cervical nucleus,* which is located on the lateral aspect of the posterior horn in the uppermost part of the cervical cord. The axons from cells in the lateral cervical nucleus cross the midline in the white commissure, and ascend in the brain stem in close relation to the spinothalamic tract, to reach the VPL.

The Spinothalamic Tract.   Although the critical pathways for touch–pressure seem to be the two dorsal pathways just mentioned, there is evidence both from animal experiments and clinical studies that touch–pressure information can reach the brain also through the spinothalamic tracts on both sides. In other words, the transmission for impulses related to touch–pressure is quite complicated; the spinal pathways ascend in several parts of the spinal cord white matter (Fig. 107A) and the tactile sense involves both the medial lemniscal system and the spinothalamic tract.

Vibration

The vibratory impulses are conveyed through the *dorsal column–medial lemniscus system* to the VPL.

Position Sense

The traditional view is that the dorsal column–medial lemniscus system alone is responsible for the proprioceptive information. This concept, however, has been difficult to reconcile with the clinical experience that dorsal column lesions at

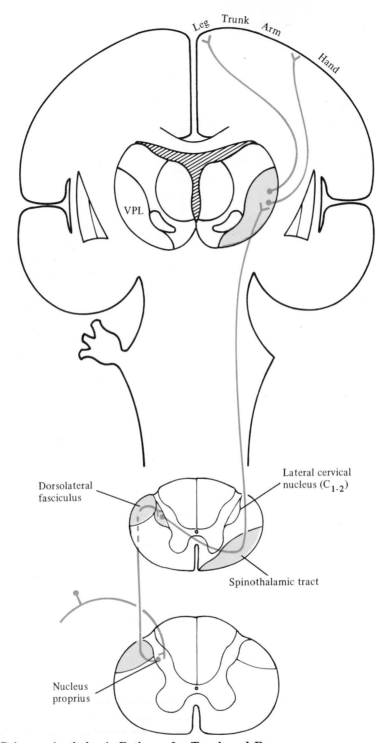

Fig. 106. The Spinocervicothalamic Pathway for Touch and Pressure
Diagram illustrating the second major pathway mediating impulses for tactile discrimination. Following a relay in the nucleus proprius, the impulses ascend in the dorsolateral fasciculus to the lateral cervical nucleus, which is located in the upper cervical region. Axons from the lateral cervical nucleus cross over to the other side and ascend in close relationship to the spinothalamic tract.

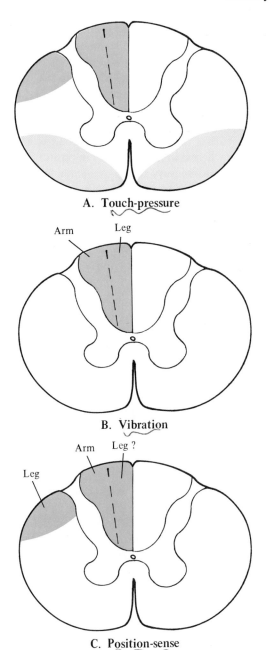

A. Touch-pressure

B. Vibration

C. Position-sense

Fig. 107. Somatosensory Pathways in the Spinal Cord

lateral fasciculus (Fig. 107). The fibers related to position sense in the dorsolateral fasciculus project to a cell group that is closely related to the dorsal column nuclei in the medulla oblongata. Axons from this cell group cross to the other side of the medulla and join the medial lemniscus in regular fashion.

Pathways from the Face

Fibers carrying tactile stimuli from the face reach the brain stem through the various components of the trigeminal nerve. The cell bodies of the fibers are located in the trigeminal (semilunar) ganglion, and the central processes terminate in the *chief sensory nucleus* of the trigeminal nerve (Fig. 105). Most of the axons from cells in this nucleus cross over to the other side and form part of the *trigeminothalamic tract,* which terminates in *VPM.* Some of the fibers from the trigeminal nucleus reach the ipsilateral VPM.

The fibers responsible for position sense are unique in that their perikarya are located within the CNS, specifically in the mesencephalic nucleus of the fifth cranial nerve. The central processes from these cells establish synaptic relationships with reticular formation cells, which in turn project to the VPM.

Thalamocortical Projections and the Primary Somatosensory Cortex

The medial lemniscus fibers and the trigeminothalamic fibers terminate in a somatotopic fashion in the VPL and the VPM, and this place specificity is maintained also in the thalamocortical projections, which proceed through the *posterior limb of the internal capsule* (Fig. 102C) to the primary somatosensory cortex, SI, in the postcentral gyrus and the secondary somatosensory cortex, SII, in the superior lip of the lateral fissure (Fig. 108A).

Within the primary *somatosensory cortex* the different parts of the body are represented in regions that are related to that part's importance in somatic sensation rather than to its actual size (Fig. 108B). In other words, the areas serving the lips, the tongue, and the hand are much larger than the regions related to other parts of the body.

The organization in the somatosensory cortex is characterized not only by a high degree of *space specificity* (somatotopic organization), but also by

the thoracic or lumbar levels may produce a reduction in vibratory sensitivity but not in the position sense of the leg. Recent discoveries seem to have settled this apparent contradiction.

In brief, the situation seems to be as follows. Whereas the cuneate fasciculus serves position sense in the arm, the spinal pathway for position sense in the leg is primarily located in the dorso-

First somatosensory cortex, SI

Central sulcus

Second somatosensory cortex, SII

A. Somatosensory cortices

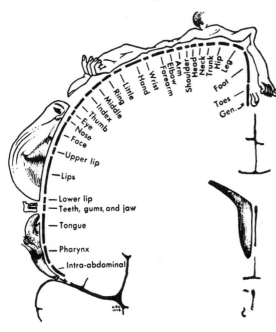

B. Sensory homunculus

Fig. 108. Somatosensory Cortices and the Sensory Homunculus

A. Primary somatosensory cortex, SI, is located in the postcentral gyrus and in the depth of the central sulcus. It corresponds to Brodmann's areas 3, 1, and 2 (see Fig. 176, Chapter 19). Another secondary sensory area is located in the upper lip of the lateral fissure. It was discovered more recently and is, therefore, *referred* to as the secondary somatosensory cortex, SII.

B. Within the primary somatosensory cortex various parts of the body are represented in regions that are related to that part's importance in somatic sensation rather than to its size. Note the large areas devoted to lips, thumb, and fingers. (From Penfield, N. and T. Rasmusson, 1955. The Cerebral Cortex of Man. With permission of MacMillan, New York.)

① space specificity (site of stimulus)
② stimulus specificity (character of stimulus)
stimulus specificity. Therefore, the cortex receives information concerning both the site of the stimulus and the character of the stimulus. The stimulus specificity is to some extent reflected in the cytoarchitectural subdivision of the somatosensory area, which is divided into three longitudinal zones, Brodmann's areas 3, 1, and 2 (Fig. 176, Chapter 19). Neurons in area 3 mainly respond to tactile stimuli, whereas area 2 is related to position sense.

The somatosensory cortex is essential for *sensory discrimination,* and patients with cortical lesions are tested specifically for loss of discriminative functions (see below). Lobulus parietalis superior (Brodmann's areas 5 and 7), which is closely related to somatosensory cortex, is also of importance for various discriminative functions.

CLINICAL NOTES

The examination of patients with sensory disorders is difficult because the test procedures are rather crude and the responses are dependent on the patient's cooperation. Although the results obtained in a sensory examination may appear perplexing, they may reflect accurately complicated mechanisms of sensory transmission that are still not fully understood.

The symptoms following lesions of the sensory pathways are to a certain extent dependent on the location of the lesion. Lesions of the *spinal nerves* or the *nerve roots,* for instance, result in characteristic segmental syndromes.

Spinal cord lesions often give rise to sensory deficits of a dissociated character. For instance, a lesion in the anterior part of the spinal cord may abolish the sensitivity for pain and temperature, but it may not interfere substantially with transmission of tactile and propioceptive impulses, e.g., anterior spinal artery syndrome (see below). A lesion in the *brain stem* is often characterized by involvement of one or several of the cranial nerve nuclei. *Parietal lobe* lesions, finally, are mainly characterized by disturbances in discriminative sensory functions.

Peripheral Nerve Lesions

The symptoms following interruption of a peripheral nerve will vary depending on whether a motor, a sensory, or a mixed nerve is affected. In regard to sensory symptoms, it is important to be familiar

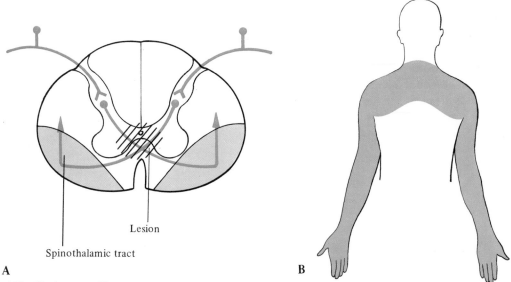

Fig. 109. Syringomyelia
A. Centrally located syringomyelic cavity in the spinal cord. The lesion interrupts the spinothalamic fibers as they cross the midline in the anterior white commissure. The sensory deficit following this type of lesion in lower cervical and upper thoracic region is shown in **B.**
B. Cape-like distribution of pain and temperature deficit caused by a syringomyelic cavity in the lower cervical and upper thoracic region. The lesion (A) and concommitant sensory deficits are usually not as symmetric as the ones indicated here (see Clinical Examples). *(one or both arms)*

with the cutaneous distribution of the more important peripheral nerves (see Appendix) to differentiate between a peripheral nerve lesion and a lesion of the nerve roots or the CNS. Since there is a considerable overlap between neighbouring nerves, the area of sensory loss following interruption of a cutaneous nerve is always smaller than its anatomic distribution.

Spinal Nerve and Nerve Root Lesions

Although the manifestations of spinal nerve and root lesions are similar to those accompanying peripheral nerve lesions, the distribution of various symptoms is different. Spinal nerve and root lesions have a typical segmental character.

Spinal Cord Syndromes

Segmental Symptoms with Lesions of the Spinal Cord

A segmental distribution of sensory symptoms is generally caused by diseases that affect the spinal nerves or the spinal roots, but can also occur in disorders that affect the center of the spinal cord. A typical example is the segmental sensory disturbances seen in patients with syringomyelia (syringomyelic syndrome).

Syringomyelia is a degenerative disease causing a pathologic cavity involving the central region of the gray matter (Fig. 109A), often with destruction of the decussating fibers in the anterior white commissure that carry impulses for pain and temperature. This results in a segmental anesthesia (loss of sensation) of dissociated type, i.e., loss of pain and temperature sense with preservation of tactile sensitivity. Since the cavity is often located in the lower cervical and upper thoracic region of the cord, one or both arms are usually involved (Fig. 109B). If the lesion extends to one or both ventral horns, there is also a segmental denervation of muscles supplying one or both arms. Symptoms from involvement of long pathways may appear in later stages of the disease.

Anterior Spinal Artery Syndrome

A thrombotic lesion in the anterior spinal artery may be secondary to atherosclerosis, an inflammatory disease, or to compression of the vessel by a tumor. Since the artery supplies the anterior two-thirds of the spinal cord, there is a bilateral loss of pain and temperature sensation (spinothalamic tract) below the level of the lesion. Further, involvement of the corticospinal tract and the ventral horns results in disturbances of motor functions (see also Clinical Example, Chapter 21). However, the ascending pathways in the dorsal part of the spinal cord are usually spared and there is accordingly little or no interference with touch, vibration, and position sense.

Dorsal Column Syndrome

Dorsal column lesions are characterized by deficits in vibration and joint-position sense. The impairment of proprioceptive sensibility results in disturbances in coordination, i.e., sensory ataxia.[4] If the lower extremities are affected, the patient has difficulty maintaining balance, especially when the eyes are closed (Romberg's sign). Interruption of the pathway for proprioceptive and tactile impulses also interferes with discriminative functions, such as the ability to recognize the shape and the form of an object by palpation.

There are several degenerative disorders that affect the dorsal columns, e.g., tabes dorsalis (a tertiary form of syphilis), Friedreich's ataxia (a heredo-familial spinocerebellar disease), and subacute combined degeneration (vitamin B_{12} deficiency). These disorders, however, invariably involve either the dorsal roots or other ascending pathways in addition to the dorsal columns, and it has therefore been extremely difficult to appraise the sensory deficits in lesions restricted to the dorsal columns.

Brown–Séquard Syndrome

This is the well known, although rarely seen, syndrome caused by hemisection of the spinal cord. It is characterized by a contralateral loss of pain and temperature sensations that begins one or two segments below the level of the lesion (Fig. 110).

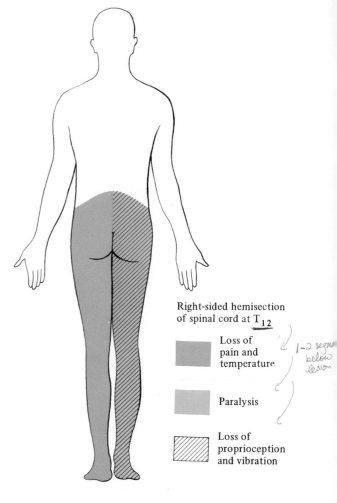

Right-sided hemisection of spinal cord at T_{12}

■ Loss of pain and temperature

▨ Paralysis

▩ Loss of proprioception and vibration

Fig. 110. Brown-Sequard Syndrome
Diagram illustrating the deficits following a hemisection of the right side of the spinal cord at the level of T12. A spinal cord lesion is hardly ever as precisely located to one half of the spinal cord as shown here, but the figure has been included for didactic purposes.

There is also ipsilateral loss of proprioceptive sensation and ipsilateral motor paralysis below the level of transection. The sense of touch is usually preserved, since tactile impulses from one side ascend on both sides of the spinal cord (Fig. 107).

Lesions in the Postcentral Gyrus and Superior Parietal Lobule

Because the somatosensory pathways to the cerebral cortex are crossed, a circumscribed lesion of the postcentral gyrus results in sensory loss in a part of the body on the opposite side. The primary

---

4. Although sensory ataxia is most often seen in dorsal column disorders, it can occur whenever the pathways for proprioceptive and tactile impulses are interrupted, e.g., as a result of a generalized lesion in the peripheral nerves (polyneuropathy) or following a lesion of the ascending lemniscal pathways in the brain.

modalities of pain, temperature, and touch may not be significantly impaired but the patient usually has difficulties localizing pain and touch stimuli. There is *loss of several discriminative sensory functions,* collectively called the cortical sensations.

One cortical sensation is two-point discrimination, the ability to separate two blunt points from one another. Normally, a double stimulus with a distance of about 5 mm can be recognized as two separate points on the fingertips, whereas the distance for two-point discrimination on the body surface varies between 4 and 8 cm.

Astereognosis is another well known symptom of a cortical sensory syndrome. This means that the patient cannot recognize an object by palpation in spite of the fact that primary sensory modalities, e.g., touch and vibration, are intact. It should be noted, however, that the ability to recognize the texture, shape, and size of an object by palpation is dependent on proprioceptive as well as exteroceptive input. Therefore, loss of position sense, which often is a prominent feature of a cortical sensory syndrome, contributes to astereognosia. *Agraphesthesia,* inability to recognize letters or numbers drawn on the hand, is another cortical sensory dysfunction.

As indicated above, inability to recognize the shape and form of an object can also be the result of a spinal cord or brain stem lesion that destroys the ascending pathways for tactile sensibility and position sense. In this case, the sensory deficit is called *stereoanesthesia.*

Pain: A Clinical Problem with Many Dimensions

Pain can be either a simple matter or a complex problem with many dimensions, including psychologic. It is always a warning that something is wrong, and the physician must be familiar with the functional anatomy of the pathways for pain, if for no other reason than that patients suffering from pain are a daily experience in most doctors' waiting rooms.

The character of a pain and its distribution is sometimes quite typical with little doubt about the underlying disease and its location in the body (see Disc Prolapse, Clinical Notes, Chapter 5, and Referred Pain, Clinical Notes, Chapter 16). Other "pain cases," e.g., the unfortunate patients suffer-

ing from chronic or intractable pain such as that caused by metastases from cancer, may require the attention of the most experienced and skillful medical team available.

Although removal of the disease causing the pain is usually the most effective way to deal with the pain problem, many diseases cannot be cured, and effective pain control becomes a matter of great importance. *Neurosurgical procedures* such as sectioning dorsal roots (rhizotomy), transection of the spinothalamic tract in the spinal cord (tractotomy or cordotomy), the cingulum bundle (cingulotomy) can be used in some cases. Exciting prospects for the future are based on recent studies of the gating mechanism and the discovery of an endogenous pain control mechanism (see below).

Stimulators

One method of pain amelioration is based on the theory of a gate control mechanism in the substantia gelatinosa. Stimulating electrodes may be pasted to the skin overlying the spinal cord (transcutaneous stimulator) or implanted directly against the spinal cord (dorsal column stimulator). The electrical stimulation, according to the "gate control theory," activates fibers capable of closing the hypothetical gate, thereby preventing pain stimuli from reaching the brain. Regardless of whether the "gate control theory" is right or wrong, stimulators have been used in many cases, and the therapy is not harmful.

Endogenous Pain Control

That sensory impulses are being subjected to central control at different relays in the afferent fiber systems is now clearly established, and many of the centrifugal pathways controlling various sensory inputs have been identified.

Important descending control systems for the impulses conveyed by the spinothalamic tract originate in the brain stem, and much interest has focused on a possible *"pain-inhibiting system"* located primarily in the region of the periaqueductal gray matter and in the serotonin-producing brain stem raphe nuclei. Electrical stimulation of these regions increases the threshold for pain, probably by releasing *enkephalin,* or *endorphin* ("the morphine within"), i.e., an endogenous substance with opiate-like activity. Implantation of stimulating electrodes at some point in the "pain-inhibiting system" has already been tried, and it is possible that such procedures, called stimulation-produced analgesia (SPA), will emerge as an attractive alternative for pain relief in difficult cases. The pain inhibiting system can also be activated by somatosensory impulses reaching it from the periphery, and it has been suggested that the *acupuncture* needle might generate such impulses in large muscle afferent fibers.

Although the details of the endogenous pain control mechanisms are still poorly understood, much interest has recently focused on the dorsal horn, where the pain fibers establish their first synaptic contact after having entered the CNS (Fig. 111). A pharmacologically active polypeptide, *substance P,* apparently acts as a neurotransmitter in the pain fiber system. It is believed that enkephalinergic inhibitory interneurons establish synaptic contact with the substance P-containing terminals in the dorsal horn. Activation of the enkephalinergic interneurons, for instance by the descending "pain-inhibiting system," would release enkephalin, which in turn inhibits the release of substance P from the pain fibers, thereby suppressing the transmission of pain impulses to the brain. Unoccupied enkephalin receptors on the terminals of the pain fibers could conceivably be occupied by *morphine,* as well, which would mimic the pain-inhibiting effect of enkephalin.

CLINICAL EXAMPLES

Syringomyelia

A 28-year-old woman complained of numbness in her right arm. Over the preceding 5 years she had gradually lost sensation in her right arm and hand, and over the last few months she had occasionally burned her right fingertips while cooking but had not been aware of the injuries at the time they occurred.

On examination, a Horner syndrome was evident on her right side. She also had mild atrophy of her right shoulder muscles and marked atrophy of the intrinsic hand muscles and thenar and hypothenar muscles on the right side. Several poorly healing burn scars were noticed on her right fingers. Muscle tone was reduced, and the stretch

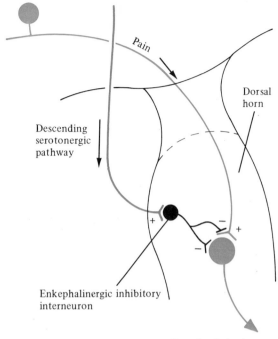

Fig. 111. Descending Control of Pain Transmission

Modulation of pain transmission is believed to occur at the level of the dorsal horn by a descending serotonergic pathway (*red*) originating in the brain stem raphé system. The pathway would activate enkephalinergic interneurons, which may exert postsynaptic and maybe even presynaptic inhibitory control over incoming fibers transmitting pain impulses (*blue*).

reflexes were absent in the right arm. The left arm and both legs were normal.

Sensory examination revealed loss of pain and temperature sensation in the right arm and shoulder in a cape-like distribution, but position and vibratory sensations were normal. i.e. dorsolat. columns o.k.

An EMG study of the left arm showed pronounced fibrillations of all muscle groups innervated by spinal cord segments C5–T1.

1. Where is the lesion located?
2. Why do fibrillations occur in the muscles of her left arm and hand?
3. Why are the sensory deficits related only to one arm?
4. Why does the patient have a Horner's syndrome?

Discussion

Denervation of muscles and sensory loss in a limb can arise from a variety of pathologic processes

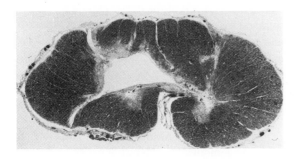

Fig. CE6A. Syringomyelia
Syringomyelic cavity in the spinal cord. (From Escourolle and Poirier, 1978. Manual of Basic Neuropathology, 2nd ed. Translated by L. J. Rubinstein. W. B. Saunders: Philadelphia. With permission of Masson et Cie, Paris.)

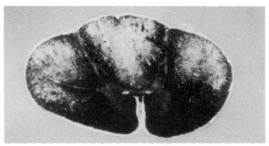

Fig. CE6B. Subacute Combined Degeneration
Myelin-stained section through the thoracal part of the spinal cord from a patient with subacute combined degeneration. (From Escourolle and Poirier, 1978. Manual of Basic Neuropathology, 2nd ed. Translated by L. J. Rubinstein. W. B. Saunders: Philadelphia. With permission of Masson et Cie, Paris.)

involving the spinal cord, nerve roots, nerve plexuses, or peripheral nerves. In this case, preservation of position and vibratory sensation in the right arm militates against peripheral nerve, plexus, or root disease.

The symptoms and signs presented by this patient are typical of syringomyelia of the cervical spinal cord, in this case on the right side. This patient probably has a cervical syrinx similar to the one shown in Fig. 6A above from another patient, who died of an unrelated disease.

Extension of the syrinx cavity into the anterior gray matter results in progressive loss of anterior horn cells and denervation/atrophy of the corresponding muscles with concomitant fibrillations.

Ipsilateral spinothalamic fibers are disrupted as they approach the anterior white commissure (Fig. 109), resulting in a "suspended" sensory level typically in a cape distribution involving an arm and part of the shoulder.

If the descending sympathetic fibers or the ciliospinal center in T1–T2 are involved in the lesion, an ipsilateral Horner's syndrome appears as in this case. If the cavity continues to enlarge, posterior column fibers or corticospinal tract fibers may also be damaged.

Subacute Combined Degeneration

A 60-year-old woman had noticed a progressive weakness and unsteadiness when walking for the last couple of months. Six months earlier she noted tingling in her toes. Her vision had also deteriorated during the last month, and she had become irritable and somewhat disoriented.

Examination showed that she was suffering from mild dementia. She had bilateral optic atrophy, and a marked reduction of position and vibratory sensations in her hands and feet. However, superficial sensations, including pain and temperature, were normal. Her stretch reflexes were increased and she had bilateral Babinski's signs. She was also ataxic in her limbs and gait, and the Romberg test was positive.

Laboratory studies revealed anemia with increased size of red cells (macrocytosis) and a very low vitamin B_{12} level in the serum. She was given large doses of intramuscular vitamin B_{12} and made a slow but steady recovery.

The patient has pernicious anemia, which most likely is related to an inability to absorb a sufficient amount of vitamin B_{12} from the diet. The most dramatic effects of pernicious anemia occur on the nervous system and include optic atrophy and dementia, sometimes with psychosis, peripheral neuropathy, and myelopathy.

Figure 6B (above) shows a myelin-stained spinal cord section from a patient who suffered from subacute combined degeneration. The primary lesion in this disorder appears to be swelling and degeneration of myelin sheaths in certain fiber tracts, primarily in the spinal cord.

1. Which fiber tracts appear to be demyelinated?
2. Are the deficits of sensation and motor function con-

sistent with the areas of demyelination?

3. Why was the patient ataxic?

4. Why was sensation to pain and temperature preserved?

Discussion

The spinal cord section demonstrates demyelination of the dorsal columns (fasciculus cuneatus and gracilis), dorsolateral fasciculi, lateral corticospinal tracts, and spinocerebellar tracts (see also Fig. 99B). The reason for the predilection for this pattern of demyelination is unknown.

The involvement of the dorsal columns and dorsolateral fasciculi causes disturbances in vibration and position sense, whereas weakness, spasticity, and Babinski's signs are due to damage of the corticospinal tracts.

Ataxia may arise because of damage to cerebellum or cerebellar pathways (cerebellar ataxia) or to the dorsal columns with subsequent disturbance of proprioceptive sensibility (sensory ataxia). In subacute combined degeneration patients are commonly ataxic for both these reasons.

The spinothalamic tracts, which transmit impulses for pain and temperature, seem to be relatively well preserved.

SUGGESTED READING

1. Boivie, J. J. G. and E. R. Perl, 1975. Neural substrates of somatic sensation. In C. C. Hunt (ed.): MTP International Review of Science. Physiology Series One, Vol. 3. Butterworths: London, pp. 303–411.

2. Brodal, A., 1981. Neurological Anatomy in Relation to Clinical Medicine, 3rd ed. Oxford University Press: New York, Oxford, pp. 46–148.

3. DeJong, R., 1979. The Neurologic Examination, 4th ed. Harper and Row: Hagerstown, Maryland, pp. 40–80.

4. Fields, H. L. and A. J. Basbaum, 1978. Brainstem control of spinal pain-transmission neurons. Annu. Rev. Physiol. 40: 217–248.

5. Mountcastle, V. B., 1980. Central Nervous Mechanisms in Sensation. In V. B. Mountcastle (ed.): Medical Physiology, 14th ed., Vol. 1. C. V. Mosby, St. Louis, Missouri, pp. 327–427.

6. Wall, P. D., 1980. The substantia gelatinosa, a gate control mechanism set across a sensory pathway. Trends in Neurosciences. 3: 221–224.

7. Willis, W. D. and R. E. Coggeshall, 1978. Sensory Mechanism of the Spinal Cord. Plenum Press: New York.

7

The Lower Motor Neuron and the Descending Supraspinal Pathways

LOWER MOTOR NEURONS AND MUSCLE RECEPTORS
  Motor Neurons
  The Motor Unit and the Motor End-Plate
  Muscle Receptors
  Functional Considerations

DESCENDING SUPRASPINAL PATHWAYS
  The Corticospinal Tract
  The Rubrospinal Tract
  The Vestibulospinal Tracts
  The Reticulospinal Tracts
  Functional Considerations

CLINICAL NOTES
  Lower Motor Neuron Paralysis
  Electromyography, Fibrillations, and Fasciculations
  Upper Motor Neuron Paralysis
  Comparison between LMN and UMN Lesions
  Monoplegia, Paraplegia, and Tetraplegia

CLINICAL EXAMPLES
  Subdural Hematoma
  Capsular Infarct

SUGGESTED READING

The motor neurons in the spinal cord and the cranial nerve nuclei, the lower motor neurons (LMNs), represent the "final common path" for all the impulses that are transmitted to the striated muscles. All movements are brought about by influences that ultimately converge on these neurons from many sources, including both peripheral sensory receptors and structures in the CNS, e.g., cerebral cortex, basal ganglia, brain stem, and cerebellum. These latter structures exert their influence through the descending supraspinal pathways.

One of the main functions of the CNS is to produce purposeful movements, and since many parts of the brain and spinal cord are concerned with motor functions, disorders of motility following lesions in the nervous system are extremely common. The type of motor disturbance that occurs in a patient is largely dependent on the location of the lesion, and it is therefore important to have a good understanding of the various components of the motor system.

Coordinated movements result from a harmonious interaction between a variety of different structures throughout the nervous system, and it is customary to refer to all these structures and their related pathways as the motor system. However, practically all parts of the nervous system, including the sensory pathways, are to some extent concerned with movements, and the motor system, therefore, cannot be strictly delimited from the rest of the nervous system.

Any subdivision of the motor system into different functional–anatomic units will of necessity be somewhat arbitrary. Nevertheless, to appreciate the organization of the motor system and to recognize the main clinical syndromes resulting from lesions of its various parts, it is necessary to subdivide the subject into a few major topics. It is convenient to deal first with the LMNs and the descending pathways [upper motor neurons (UMNs)][1] that more or less directly influence their activity. It is through these descending pathways that the motor cortex, basal ganglia, and cerebellum, ultimately influence the activity in the LMNs. The basal ganglia and the cerebellum will be discussed in subsequent chapters.

LOWER MOTOR NEURONS AND MUSCLE RECEPTORS

The motor neurons, whose axons project to the striated muscles, are often referred to as the primary or *lower motor neurons*. These neurons are located in the ventral horns of the spinal cord and in some of the cranial nerve nuclei, and they represent the "final common path" for all impulses coursing to the striated muscles.

Motor Neurons

It is customary to distinguish between two types of motor neurons, α (alpha) and γ (gamma) motor neurons. The large α motor neurons are responsible for the contraction of a muscle, whereas the smaller γ motor neurons innervate specialized muscle receptors, the muscle spindles (see below).

---

1. Although many clinicians seem to use the term upper motor neuron in reference to the corticospinal tract only, it is more appropriate to refer to the neurons of all descending pathways as upper motor neurons.

Topographic Arrangement

The spinal motor neuronal cell groups, which together form Rexed's lamina IX (Fig. 97), are located according to a general somatotopic pattern. The neurons that supply the axial musculature are located medially, whereas the neurons that innervate the musculature of the limbs are located in the lateral part of the ventral horn (Fig. 96). Further, the motor neurons related to the distal musculature are located in the more caudal segments of the enlargements, and also more dorsally than the neurons that innervate the proximal part of the limbs. The somatotopic localization of the motor neurons is important for understanding the relationship between the descending pathways and various motor neuron pools (see below). It also explains why a localized lesion in the ventral horn may result in a segmentally distributed paralysis.

Interneurons and Their Relationship to the Motor Neurons

Interneurons play an essential role in any type of motor performance. Most of the boutons that impinge on the motor neurons belong to interneurons, many of which are located in the intermediate gray matter in the same or neighbouring segments of the spinal cord. Indeed, most of the afferent input through the dorsal roots, as well as the motor commands, that reach the motor neurons through the descending pathways are being mediated by interneurons. The importance of the interneuronal system, therefore, can hardly be overestimated. The variability in motor performance and the flexibility that the motor system shows in response to various stimuli are made possible largely by the interneuronal system.

The Motor Unit and the Motor End-Plate

The axon of a motor neuron arborizes extensively to supply many muscle fibers. The motor neuron, together with the muscle fibers it supplies, is called a *motor unit*. Muscles used for delicate movements, e.g., hand muscles and extrinsic eye muscles, have small motor units in the sense that one motor neuron may supply less than 10 muscle fibers. In some of the other muscles in the body, the motor unit may contain many hundred muscle fibers.

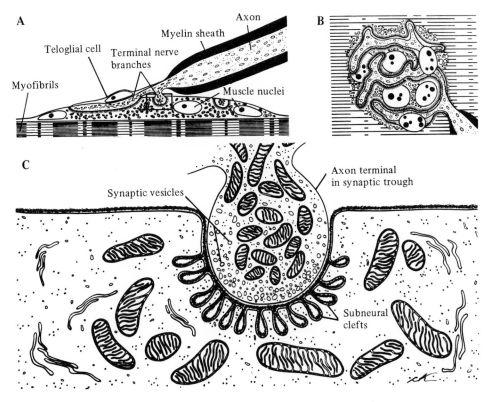

Fig. 112. Motor End-Plates

Motor end-plates are specialized synapses between the motor nerve and the muscle fibers **(A)**. They form slightly elevated plaques on the surface of the muscle fibers, where the axons form terminal arborizations among clusters of muscle nuclei **(B)**. **C.** The axonal part of the end-plate contains swellings that occupy synaptic troughs. The troughs, in turn, contain a number of folds, which greatly increase the postsynaptic surface. (The drawings, which are modified after R. Couteaux, are reprinted from Bloom, W. and D. W. Fawcett, 1975. A textbook of Histology, Tenth Edition. With permission of W. B. Saunders Company, Philadelphia.)

The junction between the terminal branches of the axon and the muscle fiber, i.e., the neuromuscular junction, is known as the *motor end-plate* (Fig. 112). The axonal part of the end-plate contains a number of swellings that resemble the boutons in the CNS. These swellings, which contain synaptic vesicles and mitrochondria, dip into grooves or troughs on the surface of the muscle cell. The trough, in turn, contains a number of junctional folds, which greatly enlarges the surface area of the muscle membrane. When the action potential reaches the end-plate, the neurotransmitter acetylcholine is released into the synaptic cleft. The transmitter binds to specific receptors on the muscle cell membrane, thereby altering its ionic permeability. When the end-plate potential in the muscle fiber has reached a certain value, an action potential is propagated along the muscle fiber, which results in a contraction of its myofibrils. The muscle fiber action potential is recorded in the examination known as electromyography (EMG).

Muscle Receptors

Muscle Spindle

Intrafusal Muscle Fibers. The muscle spindle is an intricate sense organ, consisting of an encapsulated bundle of specialized muscle fibers, the intrafusal fibers. The intrafusal fibers attach to the extremities of the capsule, which ultimately attach to the tendon like the extrafusal muscle fibers. The intrafusal fibers, therefore, are arranged in parallel with the extrafusal fibers. This means that the tension in the intrafusal muscle fibers increases if the muscle is stretched and decreases when the muscle contracts. The muscle spindles, therefore, can be referred to as "length recorders" since they record

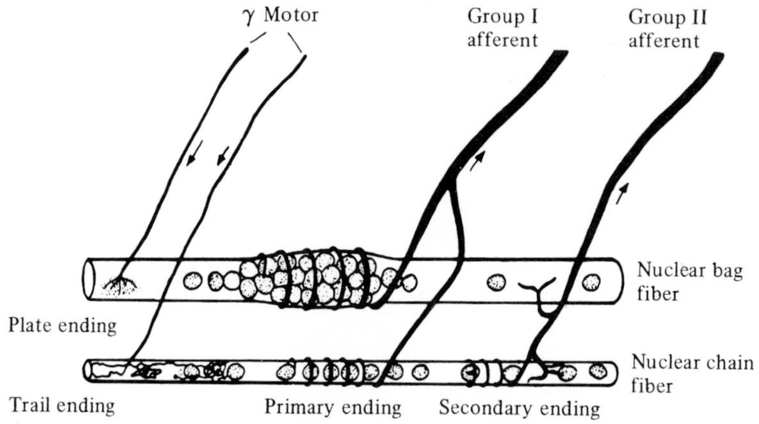

Fig. 113. The Muscle Spindle
Simplified diagram of the central region of a muscle spindle showing the two types of intrafusal muscle fibers and their sensory and motor innervation. (From Brodal, A. 1981. Neurological Anatomy. Third edition. With permission of the author and Oxford University Press.)

the length of the muscle. This is known as the static response. The muscle spindle can also mediate a dynamic response, which provides information about the speed of stretching. The static response is mainly related to thin, intrafusal fibers called nuclear chain fibers, whereas the dynamic response originates in thicker intrafusal fibers, i.e., nuclear bag fibers (Fig. 113).

Primary and Secondary Endings. There are two types of sensory terminals in the muscle spindles, referred to as primary and secondary endings. All intrafusal fibers contain primary endings, whereas secondary endings are related primarily to the nuclear chain fibers. The impulses from the endings, which are located in the central parts of the intrafusal fibers, are transmitted to the CNS either by large, fast-conducting group Ia afferent fibers (from primary endings) or by thinner and more slowly conducting group II fibers (from secondary endings).

Fusimotor Fibers. The contractile polar parts of the intrafusal fibers are innervated by fusimotor fibers, i.e., the axons of the γ motor neurons, which are intermingled with the α motor neurons of the same muscle. The spindle, in other words, has its own motor innervation and its sensitivity is subjected to central control. It is important to recognize this fact, because it means that the sensory part of the spindle can be kept under tension and continue to send information about the length of the muscle during the full range of a contraction. If the intrafusal fibers could not be contracted,

the spindle would quickly be unloaded or silenced at the very beginning of the muscle contraction.

The Golgi Tendon Organ

This is another important muscle receptor, which is innervated by a large group 1b afferent fiber. It consists of a small capsule, which surrounds a number of collagen fiber bundles, and it is located in the tendon, or more precisely, at the junction between the tendon and the muscle fibers. The tendon organs, therefore, are arranged in series with the extrafusal muscle fibers, and they are stimulated regardless of whether the muscle contracts or is stretched. They are "tension recorders" rather than "length recorders," and they are generally considered to safeguard the muscle from excessive contraction. Apart from that, little is known regarding their functions, but there is evidence that the tendon organs, as well as the joint receptors, i.e., specialized mechanoreceptors in the joint capsules, serve important functions in the general control of movements.

Functional Considerations

The Stretch Reflex and Muscle Tone

The contraction of a muscle in response to stretching, e.g., by a tap on its tendon, is known as the myotatic or *stretch reflex.* The most famous stretch reflex is the patellar reflex (Fig. 98), which is tested routinely by the physician. A tap on the patellar tendon stretches not only the extrafusal muscle fibers but also the muscle spindles, thereby stimulating the sensory endings of the intrafusal fibers. This leads to an increased activity in the afferent input to the motor neuron pool of the quadriceps muscle, and the large group la afferent fibers stimulate directly the α motor neurons, which are responsible for the contraction of the quadriceps. Since there are only two neurons, or one synapse, involved in the stretch reflex, it is referred to as a *monosynaptic reflex.* A list of the most commonly tested stretch reflexes and their spinal reflex centers are presented in Chapter 5.

The majority of the spinal reflexes are disynaptic or polysynaptic, i.e., they involve more than one synapse. An example of a disynaptic reflex is the reflex that provides for an inhibitory influence on the knee flexors from group la afferent fibers when the patellar tendon is tapped (Fig. 98). Reciprocal inhibition of the antagonist is a prerequisite for the execution of a stretch reflex. Stretch reflexes can be provoked in all muscles and they, like other spinal reflexes, are modified by the descending supraspinal pathways.

The normal tension in a muscle is referred to as *muscle tone.* It is in large part a reflex phenomenon dependent on the activity in the muscle spindles, and it is tested by palpation or passive movement. Experience tells the clinician when the muscle tone is abnormal.

α–γ Linkage

The descending supraspinal pathways apparently activate the α and γ motor neurons simultaneously. This coactivation of the α and γ motor neurons is referred to as α–γ *linkage,* and this linkage is probably an important feature in many motor acts. However, it is not a rigid linkage. The contractions needed for complicated movements call for a high degree of flexibility in the α–γ linkage, and for the possibility to activate the α and γ systems independently.

DESCENDING SUPRASPINAL PATHWAYS

Many fiber tracts descend to the spinal cord from supraspinal structures including the cerebral cortex. Although these tracts are often referred to as motor tracts, it is important to remember that they also have other important functions besides influencing movements, namely to control the activity in the sensory pathways and in spinal reflexes. The most important descending fiber tracts are the following (Fig. 114):

1. The corticospinal (pyramidal) tract
2. The rubrospinal tract
3. The reticulospinal tracts
4. The vestibulospinal tracts

There are several other descending tracts, with less well known functions. These include the tectospinal and interstitiospinal tracts, as well as descending noradrenergic and serotonergic fiber tracts.

The corticospinal and rubrospinal tracts, which descend in the dorsal part of the lateral funiculus, are sometimes referred to as the *lateral group,* whereas the vestibulospinal tracts and the medial (pontine) reticulospinal fibers are components of the *ventromedial group.* This distinction between a lateral and a ventromedial descending system, however, is no doubt an oversimplification. Nevertheless, the fibers in the lateral system terminate to a large extent on laterally placed interneurons in the intermediate gray matter, and these interneurons are related primarily to the dorsolateral part of the ventral horn, whose motor neurons innervate the limb muscles, i.e., those muscles that are especially important for skilled movements. The ventromedial system is more closely related to medially placed interneurons and motor neurons concerned not only with limb muscles but also with the axial musculature, which is of special importance for postural activities and gross aspects of movements.

The Corticospinal Tract

Origin of the Corticospinal Tract

Each corticospinal tract contains about 1 million fibers, more than half of which originate in pyramidal cells[2] in the *motor cortex* (Brodmann's area

---

2. Since there are about 20–30,000 giant pyramidal cells of Betz in the motor cortex, only 2–3% of the pyramidal fibers come from giant cells. The pyramidal tract has received its name from the fact that its fibers form the pyramid of the medulla oblongata, and not because its fibers originate in pyramidal cells in the cerebral cortex.

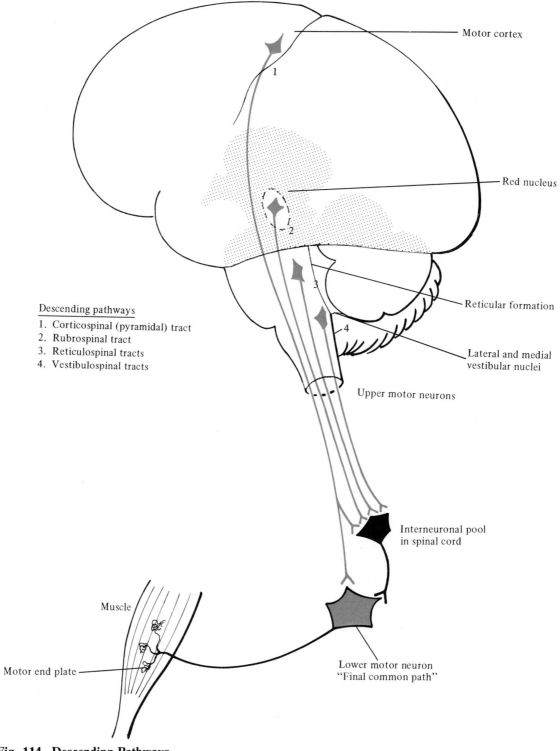

Descending pathways
1. Corticospinal (pyramidal) tract
2. Rubrospinal tract
3. Reticulospinal tracts
4. Vestibulospinal tracts

Motor cortex

Red nucleus

Reticular formation

Lateral and medial
vestibular nuclei

Upper motor neurons

Interneuronal pool
in spinal cord

Muscle

Motor end plate

Lower motor neuron
"Final common path"

Fig. 114. Descending Pathways
Most of the descending pathways (upper motor neurons) influence the peripheral motor neuron (lower motor neuron) via interneurons in the spinal cord.

4) in precentral gyrus (Fig. 115A). Additional corticospinal tract fibers come from *premotor cortex* (areas 6 and 8), including the *supplementary motor area* on the medial side of the hemisphere in front of the paracentral lobule. It is worth emphasizing that the *primary somatosensory cortex* (areas 3, 1, and 2) and the *superior parietal lobule* (area 5) also contribute fibers to the corticospinal tract.

The motor cortex in precentral gyrus forms a band that stretches from the lateral fissure upward and around the dorsal border of the hemisphere to its medial side including the rostral part of the paracentral lobule. Characteristically, discrete movements can be obtained on the opposite side of the body by the application of weak electrical stimulation of the motor cortex. The different parts of the body are represented by cortical areas of varying size dependent on the functional importance of the body parts; i.e., those parts that are capable of the most delicate movements have the largest representation. This representation can be illustrated by a so-called motor homunculus (Fig. 115B).

Course and Termination of the Corticospinal Tract

The corticospinal tract fibers converge toward the posterior limb of the internal capsule, where they occupy a rather small area (Fig. 116). As the tract descends through the capsule, it shifts position from the genu to the posterior part of the posterior limb in order to accommodate the large amount of descending frontal lobe fibers, which are also heading for the base of the cerebral peduncle. It is important to remember that the corticospinal fibers are intermingled with other fiber systems in the internal capsule. Therefore, a capsular lesion that affects the corticospinal tract of necessity will influence also other fiber systems, including corticorubral, corticoreticular, and corticopontine fibers.

After having passed through the middle part of the base of the cerebral peduncle (Fig. 116B), the pyramidal fibers break up into several bundles in the basilar part of pons before they come together again to form the pyramid of the medulla oblongata (Fig. 116C). At the lower level of the medulla, most of the fibers cross to the opposite side in the *pyramidal decussation,* and proceed through the lateral funiculus as the *lateral cortico-*

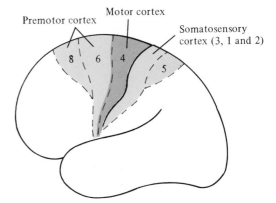

A. Origin of corticospinal tract

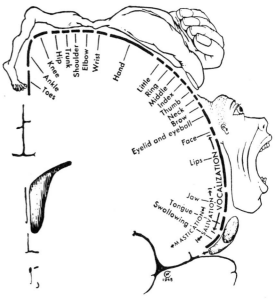

B. Motor homunculus

Fig. 115. Origin of Corticospinal Tract
A. The corticospinal fibers originate primarily in the area of the precentral gyrus (area 4) and to a lesser extent in nearby regions of the frontal and parietal lobes.
B. Diagram showing the motor representation of the various part of the body in the motor cortex. Note the large areas devoted to the fingers, thumb, and face. (From Penfield, W. and Rasmussen, T. 1955. The Cerebral Cortex of Man. With permission of Macmillan, New York.)

spinal tract to all levels of the spinal cord. Although most of the corticospinal fibers terminate on interneurons in the lateral aspect of the intermediate gray matter (laminae IV–VII of Rexed), some of the fibers synapse direct on α and γ motor neurons. Less than 10% of the corticospinal fibers

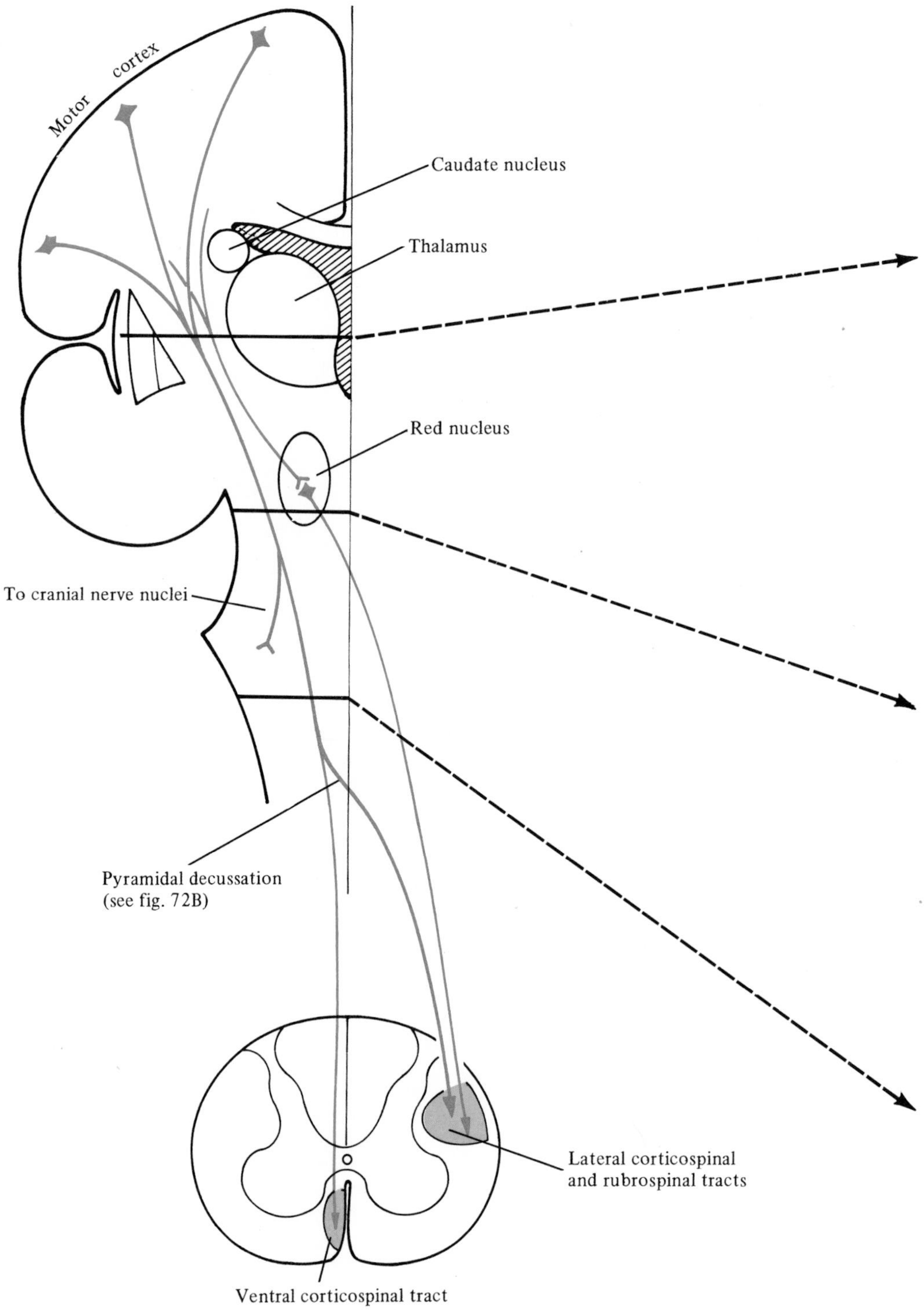

Fig. 116. Corticospinal Tract
Diagram of the corticospinal pathway which descends in the spinal cord in close relationship to the rubrospinal tract. The corticofugal fibers to the cranial nerve nuclei are referred to as the corticobulbar tract. Although there are some indications of a topographic localization in the corticospinal tract, it is not of great clinical relevance.

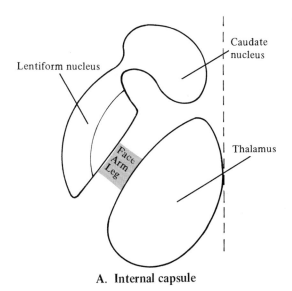

A. Internal capsule

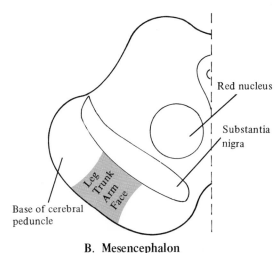

B. Mesencephalon

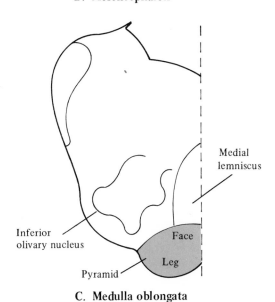

C. Medulla oblongata

descend uncrossed in the ventral funiculus to the midthoracic level as the *ventral corticospinal tract.*

The Corticobulbar Tract

Although gross dissections may give the impression that the corticospinal tract represents a well confined bundle that proceeds in relative isolation from the cerebral cortex to the spinal cord, this is far from the case. The striatum, the red nucleus, the reticular formation, and many of the cranial nerve nuclei receive direct terminal fibers from the cerebral cortex. It is possible that some of these structures also receive collaterals from corticospinal fibers. The corticofugal fibers that end in the cranial nerve nuclei are collectively referred to as the *corticobulbar tract,* and since the function of the corticobulbar fibers is similar to the function of the rest of the pyramidal tract fibers, the corticobulbar tract is usually conceived of as an integral part of the pyramidal tract.

The Rubrospinal Tract

This tract is closely related to the corticospinal tract, both anatomically and physiologically. It descends through the spinal cord together with the corticospinal tract, and the two tracts terminate in approximately the same region. Further, like the corticospinal fibers, the rubrospinal fibers mediate primarily a facilitatory effect on the flexor motor neurons. To complete the comparison, it should also be noted that the red nucleus serves as a relay station in an indirect corticorubrospinal pathway, which, like the corticospinal system, originates primarily in the motor cortex. Another even more important input to the red nucleus comes from the cerebellum (Chapter 9).

The Vestibulospinal Tracts

The most important vestibulospinal fibers come from the lateral vestibular nucleus, and they form the *lateral vestibulospinal tract* in the ventral funiculus. The fibers terminate primarily in the medial parts of the ventral horn where they establish synaptic contacts with interneurons and motor neurons related to both trunk muscles and limb muscles. Since one of the most significant inputs to the lateral vestibular nucleus comes from the cerebellum, the vestibulospinal tract is an important mediator of cerebellar influence on the lower motor neuron.

The less well known *medial vestibulospinal tract* originates in the medial vestibular nucleus and terminates in approximately the same region as the lateral vestibulospinal tract in the upper half of the spinal cord. The medial vestibular nucleus receives input from the cerebellum.

The Reticulospinal Tracts

The reticulospinal fibers are sometimes divided in a lateral and a medial reticulospinal tract on anatomic grounds. It is questionable, however, if such a subdivision is useful. Reticulospinal fibers originate in several cell groups in the medial reticular formation (Chapter 10) and they descend both in the ventrolateral and dorsolateral funiculi (Fig. 99). The reticulospinal fibersystems are involved in many functions related to both somatomotor and visceromotor functions including the control of cardiovascular and respiratory mechanisms (Chapter 16).

Although little is known regarding the effects of reticulospinal activity on movements, it is important to realize that the reticular formation receives input from many brain regions, including *cerebral cortex, tectum,* and the *fastigial nucleus.* These structures, therefore, can use the reticulospinal pathways in their control of movements.

The term *bulbospinal tract* is sometimes used for the reticulospinal fibers originating in the medulla oblongata as opposed to those with cells of origin in the pons, i.e., the *pontospinal tract.* Physiologists tend to use the term *bulbospinal* when they are unable to distinguish between reticulospinal and vestibulospinal effects.

Functional Considerations

The Corticospinal and Rubrospinal Tracts

The corticospinal and rubrospinal fibers terminate in the ventrolateral part of the dorsal horn and the intermediate zone (laminae V–VII), adjacent to interneurons that influence spinal reflexes and motor neurons in the more lateral parts of the ventral horn. The pathways, therefore, are in a position to regulate the activities in the distal and proximal limb musculature. Some of the fibers in the corticospinal tract end directly on α and γ motor neurons.

It is generally believed that the corticospinal tract can control all types of movements but that it is of special importance for skilled and precise finger movements, and it seems that the activity in the tract is of special importance for the timing of muscle contractions. Correct timing is a requirement for the high degree of precision that characterizes fine manipulative finger movements. There is apparently a high degree of integrated activity already on the spinal cord level, and it seems that the function of the descending systems, including the corticospinal system, is primarily to modulate spinal reflexes and spinal patterns of movements.

Motor Cortex as a "Distribution Center." The fact that the corticospinal system is of special importance for independent finger movements does not mean that "skilled movements" are represented in motor cortex. Electrical stimulation of the primary motor cortex does not give rise to coordinated purposeful movements on the contralateral side, but to simple flexion or extension of one or more joints.

Considering the functions of the motor cortex and the corticospinal system, one should also take note of the fact that the motor cortex and premotor cortex receive input from many sources including some of the thalamic nuclei, e.g., the VA–VL (ventralis anterior and lateralis) complex, as well as from various cortical areas, especially the somatosensory cortex. For instance, the VA–VL complex is a formidable gateway for basal ganglia and cerebellar input to the motor-premotor cortex. Whatever role the motor cortex has in motor performance, it is clear that its functional attributes are to a large extent determined by the information that reaches it from other cortical areas as well as from the basal ganglia and the cerebellum by way of the thalamus.

The *supplementary motor cortex* on the dorsal and medial side of the hemisphere seems to be of special importance for the planning or "programming" of movements.

The Vestibulo- and Reticulospinal Tracts

These descending tracts exert their influence on motor neurons related to both axial musculature and limb muscles. The vestibulospinal tract, which is closely associated with the vestibular apparatus and the vestibular and spinal parts of the cerebellum (Chapter 9), is of special importance for postural reflexes.

The functions of the reticulospinal tracts are not well known, but it is generally believed that the reticulospinal tracts cooperate with the vestibulospinal tracts in the control of postural reflexes and movements.

Supraspinal Control of Afferent Input and Reflex Transmission

As already indicated, the descending supraspinal pathways not only have motor functions; they also control the afferent input to the spinal cord, the cerebellum, and the forebrain, and they influence reflex transmission. These functions are reflected in the termination of corticospinal tract axons in laminae IV and V of the dorsal horn where they are in a position to control incoming impulses from muscles, joints, and skin. Corticobulbar fibers to the sensory cranial nerve nuclei and to the dorsal column nuclei, similarly, control the transmission of sensory impulses in these relay nuclei.

CLINICAL NOTES

Lower Motor Neuron Paralysis

A lesion that destroys the peripheral motor neurons in the ventral horn or interrupts their axons produces a loss of voluntary movements in the affected muscles. All reflexes, including the stretch reflex, are abolished, and the muscles, therefore, lose their normal tonus. This produces a *flaccid paralysis,* which together with a *pronounced atrophy* constitutes a characteristic LMN paralysis. This form of paralysis is typical for poliomyelitis, a viral infection of the LMNs.

If only part of the motor innervation to a muscle is lost, there will be a partial paralysis, known as *paresis,* and the stretch reflex will be weakened, rather than abolished. The atrophy, likewise, will be less pronounced.

Electromyography, Fibrillations, and Fasciculations

The electrical activities in a muscle can be tested by inserting needle electrodes into the muscle. The electrodes pick up the electrical activity of the muscle fibers as they contract. The potentials are transmitted, amplified, and displayed on a cathode ray oscilloscope. The technique, which is referred to as electromyography (EMG), is a valuable aid in the diagnosis of LMN disorders and in primary muscle disorders. It is of little use in UMN disorders.

There should be no electrical activity in a relaxed muscle. Spontaneous activity is abnormal. The spontaneous discharge of a single muscle fiber is known as *fibrillation,* which is characterized by small potentials of short duration. Although fibrillation usually appears in denervated muscles, it can also occur in primary diseases of the muscle. A fibrillation cannot be seen through the intact skin, since the contraction of a single muscle fiber is too small. Fibrillation is an EMG observation.

The spontaneous contraction of the muscle fibers comprising a motor unit or a group of motor units is known as *fasciculation,* and it may be noticed as a twitching under the skin. Fasciculation is a sign of irritation rather than denervation, and it is a common phenomenon in chronic affections of the motor neurons, such as amyotrophic lateral sclerosis. It is important to remember, however, that fasciculations do occasionally occur in healthy persons.

Upper Motor Neuron Paralysis

The descending supraspinal pathways can be interrupted by lesions at many levels from the cerebral cortex to the spinal cord, and the distribution of an UMN paralysis is to some extent dependent on the location of the lesion. A lesion involving the motor cortex gives rise to circumscribed weakness or paralysis of a limb (monoplegia) or part of a limb, whereas a lesion in the internal capsule (capsular lesion) or the brain stem usually involves both the arm and the leg on one side of the body (hemiplegia).

Spasticity, the "Clasp-Knife Phenomenon" and Clonus

A chronic UMN paralysis is characterized by *spastic paralysis,*[3] i.e., the stretch reflexes are exaggerated and there is no significant atrophy of the affected muscles. As a result of the increased reactivity to stretch stimuli, a "clasp-knife phenomenon" may be elicited. That is, if an affected muscle is stretched rapidly it increases muscular resistance to a certain point; then all of a sudden, the resistance melts away, which is due to inhibitory effects from muscle receptors. *Clonus* is another sign of spasticity worthy of attention. It is a series of rhythmic contractions elicited by a sudden stretch of a muscle.

Spastic Hemiplegia

The most common form of paralysis in a human is a spastic hemiplegia. A patient suffering from a spastic hemiplegia secondary to a cerebral lesion presents the following signs and symptoms: (1) weakness or paralysis in arm, leg, and often lower half of face contralateral to the cerebral lesion, (2) hyperreflexia, i.e., exaggerated stretch reflexes, and (3) Babinski sign (dorsiflexion of the great toe instead of the normal plantar flexion to plantar stimulation by stroking the sole of the foot with a blunt point).

An UMN paralysis primarily affects limb muscles. It seldom involves all the muscles on one entire side of the body. Although most cranial motor and spinal motor neurons innervating neck and axial musculature receive corticofugal innervation from both hemispheres, the part of the facial nucleus that innervates the lower half of the face receives only crossed innervation. The lower half of the face, therefore, is usually affected in a hemiparesis, but there is sparing of muscles in the upper part of the face, because their cranial motor neurons receive bilateral innervation from the motor cortex. The hypoglossal nucleus and the nucleus of the accessory nerve are two other motor nuclei that receive only crossed innervation from the ce-

rebral cortex. Extraocular nuclei, however, receive bilateral corticobulbar innervation.

It must be emphasized that a hemiplegic patient is often suffering from other symptoms as well, and the site of the lesion can often be determined on the basis of the additional signs and symptoms. The most common cause of hemiplegia is a vascular lesion in the internal capsule and a capsular lesion is likely to involve sensory and visual fibers with impairment of postural sensibility and homonymous hemianopia in addition to the hemiplegia. An extensive lesion in the cerebral cortex and the subcortical white matter, especially in the left hemisphere (see Clinical Examples, Chapter 21) may result in speech defects (aphasia) in addition to the hemiplegia. A brain stem lesion can also cause a spastic hemiplegia. Depending on the level of the damage, one or several of the cranial nerve nuclei are usually involved. Typically, the hemiplegia is contralateral to the lesion, whereas the cranial nerve disorder appears on the side of the lesion. This is referred to as a "crossed (alternating) syndrome" (e.g., Wallenberg's syndrome, see Clinical Examples, Chapter 11).

The "Pyramidal Syndrome"

Although the motor symptoms that characterize an UMN paralysis following a capsular lesion has traditionally been referred to as a "pyramidal tract syndrome," or "corticospinal tract syndrome," it must be emphasized that such a lesion involves more than the corticospinal tract. Even if a lesion is restricted to the posterior limb of the internal capsule, it always involves other fiber systems besides the corticospinal tract. Corticostriatal, corticothalamic, corticopontine, and corticoreticular fibers, as well as ascending fiber systems from the thalamus, are also likely to be involved to some extent. The use of the term "pyramidal tract syndrome" for a spastic hemiplegia, therefore, is not correct and should be discontinued. The only place where the corticospinal tract can be damaged selectively is in the pyramids of the medulla, and such pathologic processes are extremely rare. If it occurs, the patient loses the ability to perform coordinated finger movements, but there is no spasticity.

---

3. Often the acute paralysis following an intracerebral catastrophe such as intracranial bleeding (cerebral stroke) is flaccid (shock stage). The stretch reflexes subsequently slowly reappear and the paralysis becomes increasingly more spastic as the patient recovers.

Comparison between LMN and UMN Lesions

LMN lesion	*UMN lesion*
Flaccid paralysis	Spastic paralysis
Pronounced atrophy	No significant atrophy
Hyporeflexia	Hyperreflexia; clonus
No Babinski sign	Babinski sign usually present
Fibrillations and fasciculations	No fibrillations or fasciculations

Monoplegia, Paraplegia, and Tetraplegia

Paralysis of one limb is often the result of a LMN disorder, in which case there might be a significant degree of muscle atrophy as well as fasciculations and fibrillations. Monoplegia without muscular atrophy may be seen in UMN disorders. A lesion in the paracentral lobulus, for instance, may cause a spastic paralysis of the leg and foot.

Paralysis of the two lower or upper limbs, *paraplegia,* or of all four limbs, *tetraplegia,* occurs especially in spinal cord disorders. A lesion confined to the thoracic or lumbar part of the spinal cord results in a spastic paraplegia, whereas a lesion in the cervical part of the spinal cord may give rise to a spastic tetraplegia.

CLINICAL EXAMPLES

Subdural Hematoma

A 45-year-old man suffering from chronic alcoholism was brought to the Emergency Room after having been found lying on the street in a daze. He had been hospitalized 2 months earlier, when, in a drunken condition, he had fallen against a lamp post. At that time he was observed for a couple of days, his sensorium cleared without any neurologic deficits, and he was released.

The man was stuporous when he was brought to the hospital, but he could be aroused to answer simple questions. His speech was slow but not noticeably slurred. The only abnormality in regard to his cranial nerves was some difficulty with conjugate lateral gaze to the right. Motor examination showed a mild right hemiparesis, with increased reflexes and a Babinski sign on the right side. His serum alcohol level was not significantly raised.

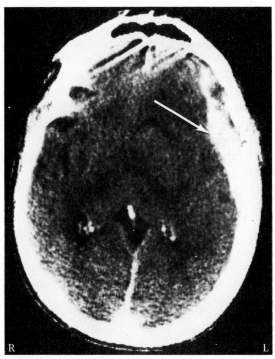

Fig. CE7A. Subdural Hematoma
The CT scan was kindly provided by Dr. V. Haughton.

In view of the focal neurologic signs, a CT scan was obtained (see the above figure).

1. Where is the abnormality located?
2. Why does he have a right hemiparesis?
3. Why does he have difficulty with conjugate lateral gaze to the right side?
4. What is the elliptically shaped white structure near the midline, and why is the space around this structure dark?

Discussion

The CT scan demonstrates a crescent-shaped dense area that overlies the left frontal and parietal lobes, and is causing compression of the left hemisphere with a shift of the midline brain structures from left to right. Slight movement artefact is present in the picture.

The clinical history and radiologic findings are typical for a subdural hematoma, which is particularly common in persons who drink large amounts of alcohol or other persons subjected to repeated head injury. They may also occur without a history of trauma in elderly individuals. The neurologic deficits are often appropriate to the side of the lesion, but this is not always the case.

Because the hematoma is pressing primarily on the left frontal lobe, it is reasonable to expect that the patient may have deficits referable to the motor areas in the left frontal lobe, i.e., right-sided hemiparesis. His difficulty with conjugate eye movements to the right is consistent with the fact that supranuclear control of conjugate lateral gaze originates in the frontal eye field (area 8) contralateral to the direction of intended gaze (signals to look rapidly to the right originate in the left frontal lobe).

The hematoma was evacuated and the patient recovered fully.

The structure near the midline is the pineal gland, which is calcified in about 50% of individuals over the age of 25. A calcified pineal gland is helpful in delineating the midline on plain skull X-rays. The space around the pineal gland, the superior cistern, is dark because it is filled with CSF, which has a low density compared with surrounding brain structures. The speckled structure on either side of the superior cistern corresponds to the choroid plexus, which is also commonly calcified.

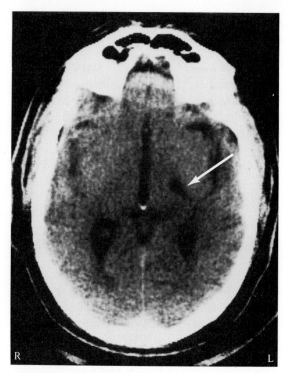

Fig. CE7B. Capsular Infarct
The CT scan was kindly provided by Dr. V. Haughton.

Capsular Infarct

A 70-year-old male was admitted for evaluation of acute onset of weakness and sensory loss. He had at least a 20-year history of hypertension. Erratic compliance with medication however, resulted in poor control of his hypertension. On the morning of admission, while having his breakfast as usual, he noticed a feeling of numbness in his right leg and arm. When he tried to leave the table he realized that his right leg was too weak to support him.

When seen in the emergency room 2 hours later, he was alert and oriented, and his blood pressure was 180/110. Neurologic examination revealed a mild weakness in the lower right side of the face but no other cranial nerve deficits. Muscle strength and tonus were significantly reduced in his right leg and arm. There was a moderate sensory deficit involving pain, temperature, vibration, and proprioception in his right leg and arm. The patient was admitted for observation, and a CT scan obtained shortly thereafter was normal. During the following days his blood pressure decreased slowly with medication. Whereas the somatosensory deficits became less and less pronounced, the weakness

in his arm and leg did not improve significantly. Muscle tone and stretch reflexes slowly increased in the right arm and leg associated with the development of a Babinski sign on that side. Two weeks after admission another CT scan was obtained. This time a lesion was clearly seen in the brain substance (see arrow in CT scan above).

1. Where is the lesion located?
2. Why does he have weakness in his right arm and leg but only in the lower half of the face on the right side?
3. Why did he initially have sensory loss?

Discussion

The lesion, an ischemic infarct, is located in the posterior limb of the left internal capsule. This type of lesion, involving the small penetrating branches of the cerebral arteries, is commonly found in persons with long-standing hypertension and atherosclerosis and is designated by the eponym of "lacunar infarct." When the softened tissue in the infarct has been removed it leaves a cavity, which can be as large as 1–1½ cm in diameter.

The lesion involves the posterior limb of the internal capsule, apparently including the corticospinal tract (see Fig. 116A). The corticospinal fibers innervating the face may be less involved because they are located at the rostral border of the infarct. Since the part of the facial nucleus that innervates the upper half of the face receives corticofugal fibers from both hemispheres, there is no weakness in the upper part of his face on the right side.

The transient hemisensory deficit was most likely due to some involvement of VPL or the very first part of the somatosensory radiation before its fibers start to diverge to different parts of the cerebral cortex. The optic radiation, which is located primarily in the retro- and sublenticular parts of the internal capsule, was not involved.

The lacunar infarct described above is somewhat unusual in the sense that it involves both motor and sensory pathways in the internal capsule. The lacunae are usually small enough and strategically located in the basal ganglia, thalamus, or internal capsule to produce either pure motor strokes when the lesion is located in the internal capsule or the base of the pons, or pure sensory strokes, especially if the lacune is located in VPL. The lacunar infarcts have become more rare after the introduction of effective antihypertensive therapy.

SUGGESTED READING

1. Adams, R. D. and M. Victor, 1981. Principles of Neurology, 2nd ed. McGraw-Hill: New York, pp. 33–47.
2. Brodal, A. L., 1981. Neurological anatomy in relation to Clinical Medicine, 3rd ed. Oxford University Press, New York, pp. 148–179.
3. Evarts, E. V., 1979. Brain Mechanisms of Movement. Scientific American 241(3): 146–156.
4. Kuypers, H. G. J. M., 1981. Anatomy of the descending pathways. In: Handbook of Physiology, Sec. 1, The Nervous System, Vol. 2: Motor Control Part 2. American Physiological Society, pp. 597–666.
5. Lundberg, A., 1975. Control of spinal mechanisms from the brain. In D. B. Tower (ed.): The Nervous System, Vol. 1: The Basic Neurosciences. Raven Press: New York, pp. 253–265.
6. Patten, J., 1977. Neurological Differential Diagnosis. Springer-Verlag: New York, pp. 172–193.

8

Basal Ganglia

COMPONENTS
   Striatum
   Globus Pallidus
   Substantia Innominata, Ventral Pallidum and
      Basal Nucleus of Meynert
   Substantia Nigra
   Subthalamic Nucleus

CONNECTIONS
   The Striatopallidothalamic Loop
   Important Side Loops

FUNCTIONAL CONSIDERATIONS

CLINICAL NOTES
   Parkinson's Disease (Paralysis Agitans)
   Huntington's Disease
   Extrapyramidal Syndromes and Antipsychotic
      Drugs
   Hemiballismus

SUGGESTED READING

The following structures are usually included in the designation basal ganglia: caudate nucleus, putamen, globus pallidus, substantia nigra, and subthalamic nucleus. The interrelationships between these various parts and their relationship to the rest of the CNS are extremely complicated and not yet fully known. Nor is it known how these nuclei ultimately affect the striated muscles. There is a growing awareness, however, that several components of the basal ganglia play an important role, not only in motor functions, but also in mood and behavior and in their relationships to movements.

Diseases of the basal ganglia produce characteristic symptoms, and our knowledge regarding the function of the basal ganglia is to a large extent based on the motor abnormalities produced by basal ganglia disorders. The classic syndromes of *akinesia–rigidity–tremor* seen in Parkinson's disease and the *chorea–athetosis* of Huntington's disease represent the two extremes in basal ganglia dysfunction.

There is no generally accepted definition of the term *basal ganglia*. Early anatomists included most of the subcortical gray matter in the forebrain, i.e., the caudate nucleus, the lentiform nucleus, the claustrum, the thalamus, and the amygdaloid body. However, clinicians often use the term basal ganglia in the context of the motor system, and since the amygdaloid body and a large part of the thalamus are conceived of as primarily nonmotor in function, these two structures are generally excluded. However, the substantia nigra and the subthalamic nucleus, both of which have important motor functions, are often included in the basal ganglia. The functions of the claustrum are unknown, and this structure is not considered in the following discussion.

COMPONENTS

The main components of the basal ganglia, the *caudate* and *lentiform nuclei,* i.e., the *corpus striatum,*

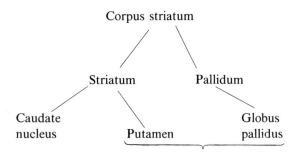

are large subcortical structures that can be recognized easily during dissections of the brain. The lentiform nucleus consists of two parts, the *putamen* and *globus pallidus* (pallidum), which are characterized by great differences in histologic structure and anatomic relationships. The putamen, which is the lateral part of the lentiform nucleus, is similar to the caudate nucleus, and the two structures are collectively called *striatum.*

Striatum

The *caudate nucleus* and *putamen* are derived from the telencephalon, and their development parallels that of the cerebral cortex, from which they receive a large part of their input. Although the caudate nucleus and putamen are partly separated by the fiber bundles of the internal capsule, bridges of cells connect the two parts in many places. Such striatal cell bridges, which are most clearly seen among the fiber bundles in the anterior portion of the internal capsule (Fig. 60 in dissection guide), indicate the common origin of the caudate and putamen.

The ventral parts of the striatum, including the caudatoputamenal junction area as well as the accumbens and the olfactory tubercle, can be referred to collectively as the *ventral striatum* (*VS*). Although the histologic characteristics and general pattern of connections of the ventral striatum are similar to those of the rest of the striatum, the ventral striatum is characterized foremost by its relationships to limbic cortical areas. The rest of the striatum is related, not only to limbic cortical regions, but especially to the sensorimotor and sensory association cortices (see Functional Aspects).

Globus Pallidus

Globus pallidus (GP) consists of an outer (lateral) and an inner (medial) division, the latter of which is continuous caudally with the substantia nigra. GP can easily be distinguished from the putamen in a freshly cut brain because of its pale color (Fig. 78 in dissection guide), which reflects the presence of a large number of myelinated fibers. The neurons in the GP are generally larger than those in the striatum, and they are less densely packed.

Substantia Innominata, Ventral Pallidum, and Basal Nucleus of Meynert (Fig. 117)

The *substantia innominata* (SI) is located between the anterior perforated space ventrally and the lentiform nucleus and the temporal limb of the anterior commissure dorsally. It interdigitates with the central nucleus of the amygdaloid body laterally and borders on the lateral hypothalamus medially.

The region, which is poorly defined and difficult to delineate from nearby basal forebrain regions, is characterized by a variety of different cell populations including both medium-sized striatal cell populations as well as collections of large neurons. Whereas the striatal-like cells in the SI most likely form part of the ventral striatum, many of the larger cells probably represent a ventral extension of the GP. Since this ventral extension of GP seems to be related to the ventral striatum in the same way as the main dorsal part of GP is related to the caudate–putamen, it has been referred to as the *ventral pallidum* (*VP*).

The basal nucleus of Meynert, which is sometimes called the nucleus of the substantia innominata, is composed of large cells that project to the cerebral cortex. As the name indicates, the nucleus is located primarily in the SI, but other cells of the same type are scattered throughout the basal forebrain. Some even extend up into the medullary laminae of the GP. It has long been known that the cells of the nucleus basalis undergo pronounced degeneration in old age, and recent studies have indicated that there is a selective destruction of the nucleus basalis in patients with Alzheimer's presenile dementia.[1] However, some caution may be appropriate. The basal nucleus is a very prominent structure in the human brain, and a depletion of its cells may well appear as one of the central pathological feature in Alzheimer's disease, even if many other parts of the brain are involved. To what extent, if any, these neurons are involved in the neuronal circuitry of the basal ganglia is not known.

Substantia Nigra

The substantia nigra can be easily recognized with the naked eye as a darkly colored band on each side of the midline in the cerebral peduncle (Fig. 69 in dissection guide). The dark color is the result of the presence of melanin pigment[2] in the cells of the *pars compacta,* i.e., the compact dorsal part of the substantia nigra. This part contains cells that project rostrally to the striatum and that synthesize and utilize dopamine as the neurotransmitter. The ventral reticular part of the substantia nigra, *pars reticularis,* is directly continuous with the GP through strands of gray matter between the fiber bundles of the internal capsule. Pars reticularis shares the same histologic characteristics as the GP including iron-containing glial cells, and the two structures may well be part of the same entity. The substantia nigra forms a tissue plate that extends throughout the mesencephalon from the rostral border of pons into the subthalamic area.

Ventral Tegmental Area (Tsai)

This area is located on the medial side of the substantia nigra in the midbrain tegmentum. It contains dopaminergic cells that project to the nucleus accumbens and the olfactory tubercle, i.e., the ventral striatum, as well as to the amygdaloid body, the entorhinal, orbitofrontal, and medial frontal cortices. This part of the ascending dopaminergic system has been called the *mesolimbic dopaminergic system.*

Subthalamic Nucleus

This is a lens-shaped nucleus located on the medial side of the internal capsule at the border between diencephalon and mesencephalon, and it is contiguous caudally with the substantia nigra. A destructive lesion in the subthalamic nucleus pro-

---

1. Growing old means different things to different people. For those who are fortunate enough and able to protect their health, the later years can be a gratifying experience. However, the process of growing old is inevitably characterized by a decrease in various functional abilities. Functional decline related to the nervous system is becoming increasingly more important as life expectancy increases. Old brains are regularly afflicted by degenerative changes. If these become severe, they often result in mental deterioration with failing memory and loss of intellectual functions, i.e., *senile dementia.*

Unfortunately, brain degeneration can occur before old age and result in *presenile dementia.* One of the most common forms of presenile dementia is Alzheimer's disease. The brains from patients who have died from Alzheimer's disease show widespread neuronal degeneration in the forebrain, and especially in the cerebral cortex and the basal nucleus of Meynert. Other important histopathological features include *senile plaques* (aggregates of amorphous argentophilic material) and Alzheimer's *neurofibrillary changes* (intracellular tangles of pathological neurotubules). Although senile dementia can be associated with several disorders (e.g., arteriosclerosis, tumors, endocrine abnormalities), the most common form is identical to the pathology of Alzheimer's disease. The etiology of the senile–presenile dementia of Alzheimer is unknown.

---

2. Melanin is a polymerized form of dopamine and norepinephrine metabolites. Melanin is also located in the cells of some other brain stem nuclei, including locus ceruleus.

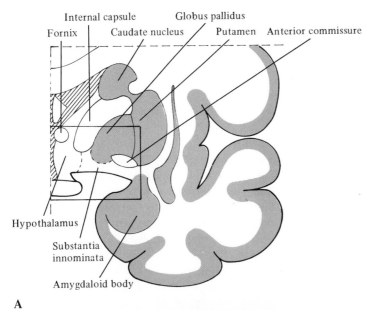

Internal capsule   Globus pallidus

Fornix   Caudate nucleus   Putamen   Anterior commissure

Hypothalamus

Substantia innominata

Amygdaloid body

A

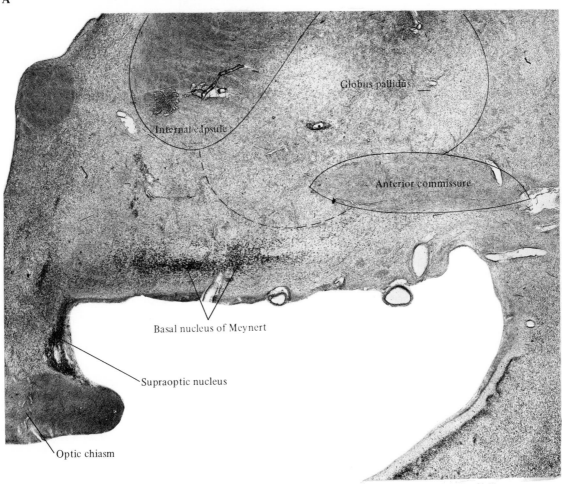

Globus pallidus

Internal capsule

Anterior commissure

Basal nucleus of Meynert

Supraoptic nucleus

Optic chiasm

B

◁ **Fig. 117. Substantia Innominata and Basal Nucleus of Meynert**
A. Schematic drawing to show general position of substantia innominata in the basal forebrain.
B. Nissl-stained frontal section through the hypothalamus and substantia innominata of the human brain corresponding to the area indicated by a rectangle in **A.** The most conspicuous structure in the substantia innominata is the basal nucleus of Meynert.

duces an unusual disorder called *hemiballismus* (see Clinical Notes).

CONNECTIONS

The connections of the basal ganglia are complicated and not yet fully known. However, the main connections discussed below are of great clinical relevance.

The Striatopallidothalamic Loop

The input side of the basal ganglia, the striatum, receives input from three main sources (Fig. 118A): the cerebral cortex, the intralaminar thalamic nuclei, and the dopaminergic cells in the substantia nigra–ventral tegmental area. The amygdaloid body also projects to most of the striatum. Striatum, in turn, projects to the GP, whose output is directed primarily to the premotor area (area 6) via the ventralis anterior–ventralis lateralis (VA–VL) nuclei of the thalamus (Fig. 118B). Cerebellum, incidentally, influences both the primary motor area (area 4) and premotor area (area 6) via the VA–VL complex. The distinction between motor and premotor area, however, loses some significance when one realizes that short association fibers tie the two regions closely together, and that corticospinal fibers originate in both regions. The distinction, therefore, is not of immediate concern to the neurologist, and both the premotor and the motor areas will be referred to as motor cortex, especially since both regions are directly concerned with the control of movements.

The above mentioned striatopallidothalamic loop, which is the major conduction route through the basal ganglia, provides a mechanism whereby information from many sources including various cortical regions can be successively processed and integrated in the basal ganglia and the thalamus before it reaches the motor cortex.

Ansa Lenticularis and Fasciculus Lenticularis

The output side of the basal ganglia, i.e., the GP, projects to the thalamus, and hence to the motor cortex, via two different pathways (Fig. 118B). Fibers from the dorsal part of the internal segment of GP traverse the internal capsule as the *fasciculus lenticularis*, whereas axons of more ventrally located cells in GP sweep around the medial edge of the internal capsule as the *ansa lenticularis*. After having either traversed or looped around the internal capsule, the fibers combine to form a massive fiber system (field H_2 of Forel), which courses medially and caudally to the prerubral area (field H of Forel) just rostral to the red nucleus. At this point, the fibers make a sharp U-turn and proceed to the VA–VL complex via the *thalamic fasciculus* (field H_1 of Forel).

Important Side Loops

The Striatonigrostriatal Loop

The striatum and substantia nigra are closely related through fibers projecting in both directions. The nigrostriatal projection system (Fig. 118A), which uses dopamine as transmitter, has received considerable attention following the discovery in the late 1950s that *Parkinson's disease* (see Clinical Notes) was related to a reduced amount of dopamine in the striatum. The dopamine-synthesizing cells are located not only in the pars compacta of the substantia nigra but also in the more medial ventral tegmental area. This widespread system of dopaminergic cells projects in a more or less topographic fashion to all parts of the striatum in the sense that the main dorsal part of striatum (caudate and putamen) receives input primarily from pars compacta of the substantia nigra whereas the ventral striatum, including the accumbens and the olfactory tubercle, receives input from the ventral tegmental area. The ascending dopa-

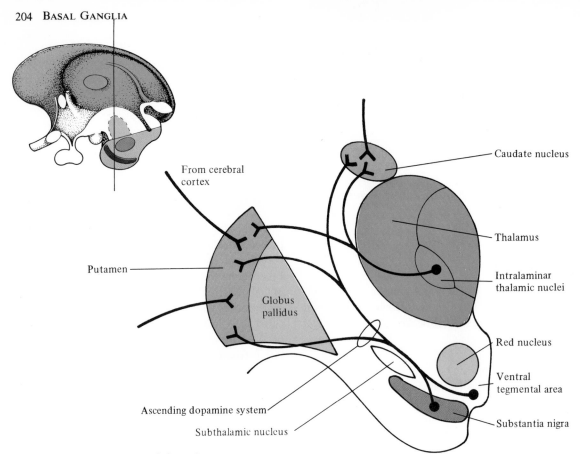

Caudate nucleus

From cerebral cortex

Thalamus

Putamen

Intralaminar thalamic nuclei

Globus pallidus

Red nucleus

Ventral tegmental area

Ascending dopamine system

Substantia nigra

Subthalamic nucleus

A. Afferent connections of the striatum

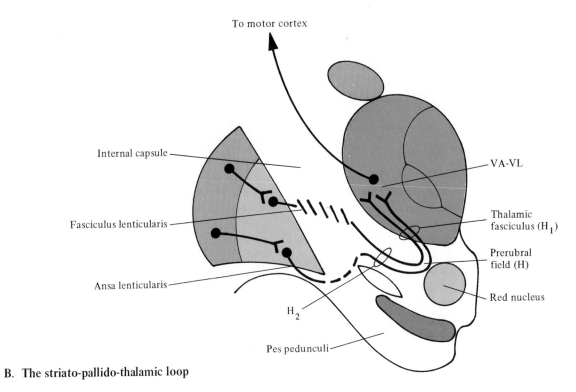

To motor cortex

Internal capsule

VA-VL

Fasciculus lenticularis

Thalamic fasciculus (H$_1$)

Prerubral field (H)

Ansa lenticularis

Red nucleus

H$_2$

Pes pedunculi

B. The striato-pallido-thalamic loop

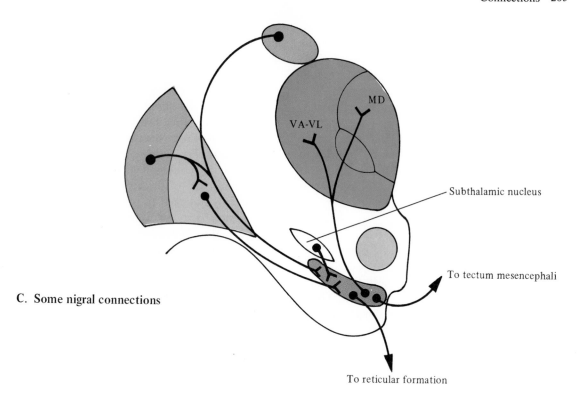

Subthalamic nucleus

To tectum mesencephali

C. Some nigral connections

To reticular formation

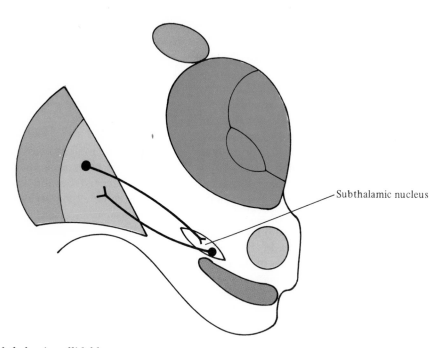

Subthalamic nucleus

D. The pallido-subthalamic-pallidal loop

Fig. 118. Connections of the Basal Ganglia
The diagrammatic key figure in the *upper left corner* (opposite page) illustrates the topographic relationships of some of the main components of the basal ganglia. The *vertical line* indicates the approximate level for the frontal sections shown in **A–D**. H, H$_1$ and H$_2$ = Tegmental fields of Forel.

minergic system from the ventral tegmental area to the ventral striatum is a prominent part of the *mesolimbic dopaminergic system.*

Although the relationships between the striatum and the substantia nigra–ventral tegmental area are especially close, it is important to realize that the striatonigrostriatal loop is not a closed circuit. Substantia nigra receives input from many other structures besides the striatum, and it projects to several nonstriatal structures, including the thalamus, the tectum mesencephali, and the brain stem reticular formation (Fig. 118C).

The Pallidosubthalamicpallidal Loop

The external segment of GP projects to the subthalamic nucleus, which in turn sends fibers back to the GP (Fig. 118D), thus establishing an important side loop whereby the subthalamic nucleus is brought in close relationship with the main striatopallidothalamic circuit.

FUNCTIONAL CONSIDERATIONS

The basal ganglia are best known for their motor functions, and clinicians have long been aware of the fact that basal ganglia disorders are characterized primarily by the appearance of *involuntary movements, difficulties in movement initiation or control,* and *changes in muscle tone.* Further, different basal ganglia syndromes can, at least to some extent, be correlated with lesion or dysfunction of specific parts or circuits of the basal ganglia. Typical examples are Parkinson's disease, hemiballismus, and Huntington's disease (see Clinical Notes).

Although dysfunction of the basal ganglia may give rise to striking abnormalities in movements, the precise role of the basal ganglia in the regulation of normal movements is still a matter of speculation. A look at the basal ganglia connections, however, does offer some suggestions. For instance, the major output from the basal ganglia is directed to the thalamus rather than the brain stem reticular formation, and the pallidothalamic pathway terminates in the VA–VL complex, which projects to the motor cortex (Fig. 119). The activity of the basal ganglia, therefore, primarily affects the descending corticoreticulospinal and corticospinal pathways, which regulate voluntary movements in the axial musculature as well as in the limb muscles, primarily on the opposite side of the body.

Although it is not known what type of instructions the motor cortex receives from the basal ganglia, it has often been suggested that the basal ganglia are concerned primarily with the planning and initiation of movements. The prominent input from all parts of the cerebral cortex to the striatum would certainly be consistent with this notion. The main dorsal part of the striatum (caudate–putamen) is closely linked to sensory association and sensorimotor cortices, whereas the ventral striatum (accumbens, olfactory tubercle, and caudate–putamenal junction area) is more strongly related to areas within the limbic system (Chapter 17), e.g., hippocampus, orbitofrontal and temporal association cortices, and the amygdaloid body. However, both the dorsal and the ventral striatopallidal systems apparently give rise to transthalamic projections that eventually affect the descending corticospinal systems. Therefore, it is reasonable to suggest that the dorsal striatopallidal system may play a preeminent role in the initiation of motor activities stemming from cognitive activities, whereas the ventral striatopallidal system, which is closely related to the limbic system, has a stronger role in planning and initiating movements in response to motivational or emotionally powerful stimuli.

CLINICAL NOTES

Clinicians often refer to basal ganglia and cerebellar disorders as extrapyramidal.[3] Such disorders are characterized by abnormal movements and change in muscle tone (rigidity) as opposed to upper motor neuron disorders (Chapter 7), which

---

3. Many clinicians use the term *extrapyramidal disorders* as a synonym for basal ganglia disorders only. Considering the origin of the term extrapyramidal, however, it seems more appropriate to include both basal ganglia and cerebellar disorders. In the past, the motor system was divided into pyramidal and extrapyramidal parts, which implied that every motor structure, except the pyramidal or corticospinal tract, belonged to the extrapyramidal system. This distinction, however, is highly artificial and of little use for several reasons. For instance, it is impossible to separate completely the corticospinal tract from other descending tracts; the cortical areas that give rise to the corticospinal fibers also give rise to other descending (extrapyramidal) fibers. Further, the two main components of the extrapyramidal system, i.e., the basal ganglia and cerebellum, use the corticospinal tract to a considerable extent to influence the lower motor neuron.

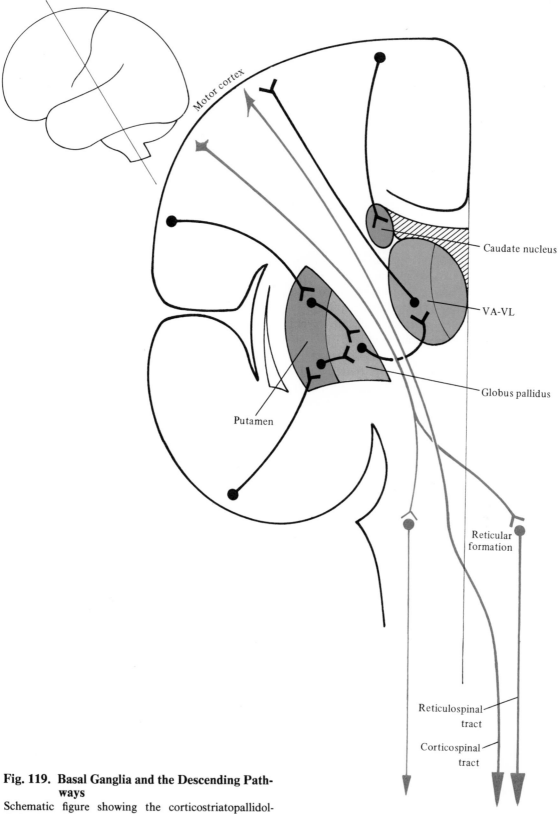

Fig. 119. Basal Ganglia and the Descending Pathways

Schematic figure showing the corticostriatopallidothalamic loop and its relationship to the descending corticospinal and corticoreticulospinal pathways.

Motor cortex

Caudate nucleus

VA-VL

Globus pallidus

Putamen

Reticular formation

Reticulospinal tract

Corticospinal tract

are characterized by a loss of voluntary movements and spasticity. This classification is useful because it makes a distinction between two major supraspinal motor syndromes, one characterized by alteration in the execution of voluntary movements, the other by paresis or paralysis. It should be kept in mind, however, that all motor activities of supraspinal origin are conveyed through the same descending pathways.

Parkinson's Disease (Paralysis Agitans)

Parkinson's disease is a common degenerative disorder of the brain. The causes are unknown. It begins insidiously in middle or old age and usually slowly progresses. The manifestations of Parkinsonism can be greatly ameliorated with proper therapy, providing patients with many more years of normal or useful life. The four cardinal manifestations are bradykinesia (slowness of movement), rigidity, tremor, and postural instability. The typical patient has decreased facial expressiveness as a result of muscular rigidity, a pill-rolling tremor at rest involving the hands more than other parts of the body, a stooped posture with a tendency to fall unexpectedly, and increased tone in the form of cogwheel rigidity. The patient, in addition, may develop a shuffling gait with short, increasingly rapid steps (festination), micrographia, and a low volume voice making him difficult to hear. Anticholinergic and dopaminergic medication, primarily in the form of levodopa (L-Dopa) with carbidopa, minimizes many of these manifestations and is particularly helpful in decreasing the degree of Parkinsonism's most crippling feature, bradykinesia.

The discovery, in the late 1950s, that Parkinson's disease was related to a selective reduction of dopamine content in the striatum indicated for the first time that a disorder in the CNS could be caused by a deficiency of a specific neurotransmitter. On the basis of our understanding of the basal ganglia, Parkinson's disease is believed to result from dysfunction of the nigrostriatal dopaminergic system caused by neuronal degeneration in the substantia nigra. Since the Parkinson's patient suffers from a reduction of dopamine in the striatum, a rational treatment might be to give the patient dopamine. Dopamine, however, does not cross the blood–brain barrier, and the patient is therefore treated with a precursor of dopamine, the amino acid L-Dopa, which is converted to dopamine, presumably by the remaining dopaminergic neurons in the substantia nigra.

Although L-Dopa therapy is helpful to many patients, it does not prevent or retard the degenerative process, and the search continues for more effective treatment. The pathophysiology of Parkinson's disease is probably more complex than indicated above. There is usually degeneration of other monoaminergic cells in the ventral tegmental area and the locus ceruleus. Further, other transmitters such as gamma-aminobutyric acid (GABA), are also related to nigral pathways, and they are likely to be involved in Parkinson's disease. *Surgical treatment* is sometimes tried as a last resort in Parkinson's disease, but is rarely used today because of improvements in medical therapy. Since the principal effect of the basal ganglia activity is channeled via GP and the VA–VL complex to the motor cortex, stereotaxic lesions have been performed either in the VA–VL nuclei (thalamotomy) or the medial portion of the GP (pallidotomy). Such lesions can lessen rigidity and involuntary movements (tremor) with little or no impairment of voluntary movements.

Huntington's Disease

Huntington's disease is a rare hereditary disorder caused by degeneration of neurons primarily in the striatum and the cerebral cortex. It is characterized by widespread and arrhythmic involuntary movements (choreiform movements) and progressive dementia.

In several respects, Huntington's disease represents the opposite of Parkinson's disease. In Parkinson's disease, the major (but certainly not only) alteration is progressive loss of dopaminergic neurons in the substantia nigra, which results in decreased dopamine content and function in the striatum. In Huntington's disease, on the other hand, the major basal ganglia deficits appear to be due to loss of acetylcholine and GABA-utilizing interneurons in the striatum and pallidum. The dopamine content in the brain is normal in Huntington's disease.

If Parkinson's disease is viewed as a case of functional dopamine deficiency, Huntington's disease is the result of dopamine overactivity in the striatum. The reason for the overactivity is not known, but the most plausible hypothesis is that the loss of GABA-utilizing inhibitory neurons in the striatum and pallidum, which in turn project to the dopaminergic substantia nigra cells, results in increased activity of the nigral cells and excessive dopamine release in the striatum. This somewhat simplified scheme is supported by postmortem studies of brains from patients with Huntington's disease. Such brains show a marked loss of biochemical markers for GABA neurons in the striatum and pallidum. The movement disorder (chorea) of Huntington's disease, further, is ameliorated by drugs that decrease dopamine transmission in the striatum. Lastly, small doses of L-Dopa, which would have no discernible effect in normal individuals, worsen the chorea in patients with Huntington's disease.

Extrapyramidal Syndromes and Antipsychotic Drugs

The discovery of the antipsychotic drugs in the 1950s revolutionized the treatment of psychotic patients, especially those suffering from schizophrenia, and helped stem the tide of psychosurgery (p. 82). Most antipsychotic drugs however, have undesirable side effects, including the appearance of Parkinsonian rigidity and bradykinesia. It is believed that these extrapyramidal symptoms appear because the antipsychotic drugs block dopamine transmission. A neurologic disorder called *tardive dyskinesia,* characterized by abnormal choreiform movements, commonly of the face, mouth, and tongue is associated with prolonged treatment with antipsychotic drugs. The reason for this tardive (late) disorder is not known, but one hypothesis is that the postsynaptic dopamine receptors have become hypersensitive as a result of the prolonged treatment.

Dopamine Hypothesis of Schizophrenia

On the basis of the hypothesis that the major clinically relevant action of antipsychotic drugs is to block dopamine transmission, it has been proposed that schizophrenia results from an excess of dopamine transmission. There is even some speculation that the major site of dysfunction is the mesolimbic dopamine system or its target areas in the ventral striatum or limbic cortical areas in the frontal lobe. However, there is little direct evidence for this proposed selective dysfunction of mesolimbic dopaminergic transmission.

Hemiballismus

This is a rare and very characteristic disorder, most often caused by a vascular lesion in the subthalamic nucleus. The symptoms usually develop suddenly, and they are dominated by violent flinging movements of the extremities on the side contralateral to the lesion.

SUGGESTED READING

1. Adams, R. D. and M. Victor, 1981. Principles of Neurology, 2nd ed. McGraw-Hill: New York, pp. 48–86.
2. Carpenter, M. B., 1981. Anatomy of the corpus striatum and brainstem integrating systems. In: Handbook of Physiology, Sec. 1, The Nervous System, Vol. 2: Motor Control. Part 2. American Physiological Society, pp. 947–995.
3. DeLong, M. R. and A. P. Georgopoulos, 1981. Motor functions of the basal ganglia. In: Handbook of Physiology, Sec. 1, The Nervous System, Vol. 2: Motor Control. Part 2. American Physiological Society, pp. 1017–1261.
4. Graybiel, A. M. and C. Ragsdale, 1979. Fiber connections of the basal ganglia. In M. Cuenod, G. W. Kreutzberg, and F. E. Bloom (eds.): Development and Chemical Specificity of Neurons. Progress in Brain Research, Vol. 51, pp. 239–282.
5. Mehler, W. R., 1982. The basal ganglia—circa 1982. A review and commentary. In A. L. Gildenberg (ed.): Applied Neurophysiology. Karger: Basel, pp. 261–290.

9

Cerebellum

CEREBELLAR CORTEX
  Cortical Layers
  Intrinsic Circuitry
  Functional Anatomic Organization

AFFERENT CEREBELLAR CONNECTIONS
  Spinocerebellar Tracts
  Vestibulocerebellar Fibers
  Reticulocerebellar Fibers
  Pontocerebellar Fibers
  Olivocerebellar Fibers; Sagittal Zonal
    Organization
  Aminergic Fibers from Raphe Nuclei and Locus
    Ceruleus

INTRACEREBELLAR NUCLEI
  Corticonuclear Relations

EFFERENT CEREBELLAR CONNECTIONS
  Cerebellovestibular Fibers
  Cerebelloreticular Fibers
  Cerebellorubral and Cerebellothalamic Fibers

CEREBELLAR FUNCTIONS
  Cerebellum and the Motor System
  Relationships between the Cerebellum, the
    Vestibular System and the Oculomotor
    Centers

CLINICAL NOTES
  Cerebellar Ataxia
  Localization of Cerebellar Disease

CLINICAL EXAMPLE
  Metastatic Cerebellar Hemisphere Lesion

SUGGESTED READING

The overall structure of the cerebellum is similar to that of the cerebrum in the sense that superficial cellular layers form a cortex, which covers several deep nuclei embedded in the white substance. The cerebellar cortex is heavily folded, but its histologic structure is stereotype and relatively simple compared with that of the cerebral cortex.

By observing patients with cerebellar disease, it becomes evident that the cerebellum is an important center for coordination of movements and postural adjustments. To regulate these functions, the cerebellum receives information from all parts of the body: proprioceptive and interoceptive impulses from muscles and joints and from visceral organs; messages from the skin and from the visual, the auditory, and the vestibular systems; as well as a variety of impulses from motor centers of the CNS.

CEREBELLAR CORTEX

Cortical Layers

One of the most characteristic features in the cerebellum is the stereotyped histology of its cortex. The cerebellar cortex is in this respect different from the cerebral cortex, in which various regions can be identified on the basis of their histologic characteristics. Although the cerebellar cortex contains several billions of neurons, most of them granule cells, its design is nevertheless relatively simple compared with that of the cerebral cortex. The five major cell types of the cerebellar cortex, *granular cells, Golgi cells, Purkinje cells, basket cells,* and *stellate cells* are arranged in a trilaminar pattern. From within, moving outward, these layers are the granular layer, the Purkinje layer, and the molecular layer (Fig. 120).

1. *The granular layer* contains an abundance of small relay neurons, the granular cells (red in Fig. 120), as well as a more limited number of larger interneurons, the Golgi cells (in yellow), whose large dendritic tree extends in all directions in the molecular layer.

2. *The Purkinje cell layer* is formed by a sheet of large Purkinje cells, whose richly branching, characteristically flattened dendritic tree extends throughout the thickness of the molecular layer in a plane perpendicular to the longitudinal axis of the folium.

3. *The molecular layer* contains two types of interneurons, the stellate cells and the basket cells (in black), in addition to the dendritic arborizations of Purkinje and Golgi cells. It is also characterized by an abundance of tightly packed granular cell axons, i.e., parallel fibers, which run parallel to the direction of the folia.

Intrinsic Circuitry

Familiarity with the intrinsic neuron circuits in the cerebellar cortex will not be of immediate relevance for the practicing physician. However, the geometric patterns formed by the neuronal components, and the remarkable regularity with which the different types of cells are interrelated, has made the cerebellar cortex a favorite research object for correlative anatomic–physiologic studies. Therefore, even if the physiologic significance of the neuron circuitry is not fully understood, an illustration of the different components of the cerebellar cortex is of great interest to anyone studying the brain. The stereotyped wiring diagram (Fig. 121) exemplifies beautifully some of the neuronal mechanisms related to important regulatory functions of the CNS.

Three different categories of afferent nerve fibers conduct nerve impulses to cerebellum. Two types, the *climbing fibers* (CF) and the *mossy fibers* (MF), have been known for a long time, whereas the third fiber system, the *aminergic fibers* (AF), has been discovered only recently with the aid of histofluorescence methods. The activity in these fiber systems ultimately affects the Purkinje cells. Most of the Purkinje cell axons, in turn, project to the intracerebellar nuclei, where the majority of the efferent cerebellar fibers originate. The arrangement through which the climbing and the mossy fibers influence the Purkinje cells are very different.

A climbing fiber, which typically originates in the inferior olive, makes multiple and powerful contacts directly with proximal dendritic branches of a limited number of Purkinje cells. Each one of the more numerous mossy fibers, on the other hand, which may come from a variety of different sources, influences a large number of Purkinje cells in an indirect fashion. To accomplish this, the mossy fiber branches extensively both in the white matter and in the granular layer, and establishes synaptic contacts with the dendrites of several granule cells in complex synapses called *glomeruli.*[1] The glomeruli contain a central mossy fiber terminal and boutons of the Golgi cell axons, both of which synapse with the granule cell dendrites (inset in Fig. 120) The axons of the granule cells, in turn, project upward to the molecular layer, where they bifurcate in a typical T-shaped manner to form the *parallel fibers,* each of which runs for several millimeters along the longitudinal extent of a folium. In other words, the parallel fiber passes perpendicular to the flattened dendritic tree of the Purkinje cell and it establishes synaptic contacts with spiny distal dendritic branchlets of many hundreds of Purkinje cells. Therefore, whereas the climbing fiber provides a powerful input to a few specific Purkinje cells, the mossy fiber input is greatly dispersed to a large number

---

1. The name glomerulus derives from the similarity this formation shows with the classic glomerulus in the olfactory bulb.

Cerebellar cortex

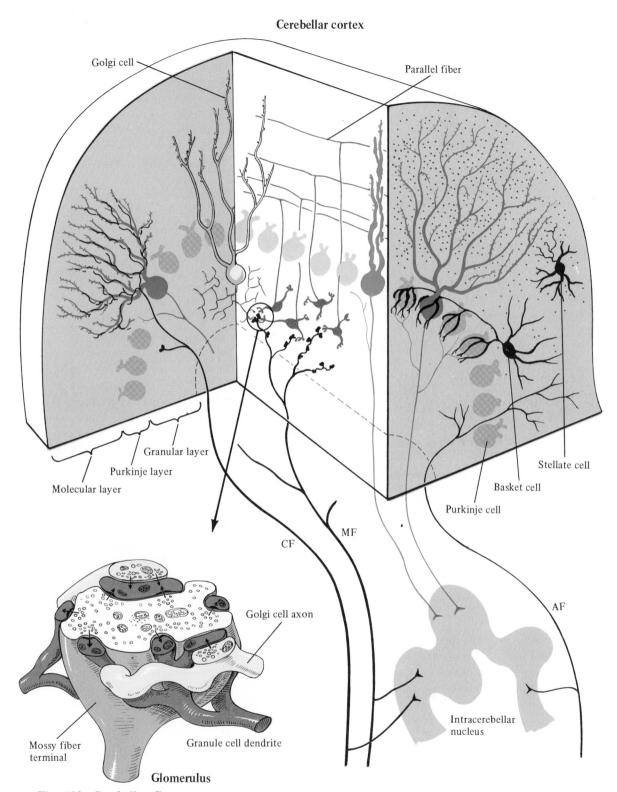

Fig. 120. Cerebellar Cortex

A single cerebellar folium has been sectioned vertically, both in longitudinal and transverse planes to illustrate the general organization of the cerebellar cortex. Purkinje cells, *blue;* granule cells, *red;* Golgi cell, *yellow;* basket and stellate cells, *black.* CF, climbing fiber; MF, mossy fiber; AF, aminergic fiber. The stereodiagram in the *lower left hand corner* illustrates the structure of a cerebellar glomerulus.

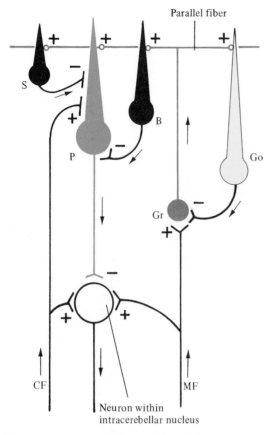

Parallel fiber

Fig. 121. Basic Circuitry in Cerebellum
Diagram of the most significant connections in the cerebellum. B, Basket cell; CF, climbing fiber; Go, Golgi cell; Gr, granular cell; MF, mossy Fiber; P, Purkinje cell; S, stellate cell. (Modified after Eccles, T. C. 1966. Functional organization of the cerebellum in relation to its role in motor control. In: Muscular afferents and motor control. First Nobel Symposium (R. Granit, ed.) Almquist and Wiksell, Stockholm.)

of Purkinje cells through glomerular relays in the granular layer.

Afferent axons in the third category, the aminergic fibers (AF), are characterized by their content of biogenic amines and by their widespread distribution in the cerebellar cortex. The aminergic fibers are of two different types, serotonin axons originating in the raphe nuclei of the brain stem, and norepinephrine-containing axons originating in the locus ceruleus.

The relatively simple input–output system described above is modified by a number of intrinsic neuron circuits formed with the aid of the three types of inhibitory interneurons, the Golgi cells (yellow in Figs. 120 and 121), and the basket and stellate cells (black). These interneurons, which are being contacted either directly or indirectly

by extrinsic afferent fibers of all categories, seem to serve as modulators of Purkinje cell activity. A remarkable feature of the cerebellar cortex is that its only output neurons, the Purkinje cells, have an inhibitory effect on the intracerebellar nuclei and the lateral vestibular nucleus. Indeed, four of the five major cell types in the cerebellar cortex are inhibitory, and immunocytochemical studies indicate that they all use γ-aminobutyric acid (GABA) as their neurotransmitter. The best available marker for GABA-ergic neurons is glutamic acid decarboxylase (GAD), the biosynthetic enzyme for GABA, and this enzyme has been localized by the aid of immunohistochemical methods both in Purkinje, basket, stellate, and Golgi cells (Fig. 122A), as well as in synaptic terminals of these cells (Fig. 122B).

Functional Anatomic Organization

The nervous elements of the cerebellar cortex and their afferent and efferent connections are organized in two perpendicularly oriented planes (Fig. 123). The Purkinje cells and their axons, which constitute the only efferent system of the cortex, are oriented in the parasagittal plane. Purkinje cells, whose axons terminate in a certain central cerebellar nucleus, constitute narrow sagittal zones, which are distributed across the cerebellar cortex, parallel to the median line. These longitudinal zones cut across the transversely organized cerebellar fissures. With the exception of the border between vermis and hemisphere, the borders between these zones are not visible at gross inspection. A similar longitudinal zonal organization is present in the afferent system of climbing fibers that originates in the inferior olive and terminates directly on the Purkinje cell dendrites.

The mossy fiber–parallel fiber system exhibits a mainly transverse orientation. Functionally different mossy fiber systems tend to terminate in different cerebellar lobules. In this way the cerebellum can be subdivided in a somewhat imprecise manner into three different parts that receive mossy fibers from the vestibular apparatus, the spinal cord, and the cerebral cortex.

Vestibulocerebellum

Vestibulocerebellum (archicerebellum: obsolete term), consists primarily of the flocculonodular

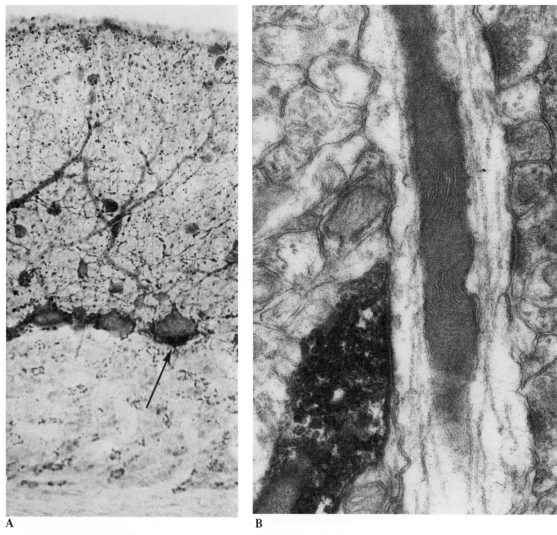

A   B

Fig. 122. Inhibitory GABAergic Neurons in Cerebellar Cortex
A. Lightmicrograph of an histologic section of the cerebellar cortex stained with an immunohistochemical technique for the localization of glutamic acid decarboxylase (GAD). Three large and moderately stained Purkinje cells are surrounded by heavily stained fibers and terminals. Note the heavy stain around the initial axon segment of one of the Purkinje cells (*arrow*). This is the place where basket fibers and terminals are known to congregate. Purkinje cell dendrites as well as many smaller neurons (basket and stellate cells) are stained in the molecular layer (*upper half of figure*). Most of the black granules in the molecular layer probably represent GABAergic inhibitory boutons.
B. Electron micrograph from the molecular layer showing a heavily stained terminal forming a symmetric synapse with a dendrite. The two boutons forming asymmetric contacts on the right side of the dendrite are unstained. (A and B, Micrograph courtesy of Dr. Enrico Mugnaini.)

lobe. Apart from vestibulocerebellar mossy fibers it receives pontocerebellar fibers concerned with the oculomotor system. Purkinje cell axons from the vestibulocerebellum terminate mainly in the vestibular nuclei.

Spinocerebellum

Spinocerebellum (palaeocerebellum: obsolete term), i.e., the anterior lobe and the region immediately caudal to the primary fissure as well as the pyramis and uvula. Apart from the direct and indirect mossy fiber pathways from the spinal cord and secordary trigeminocerebellar connections,

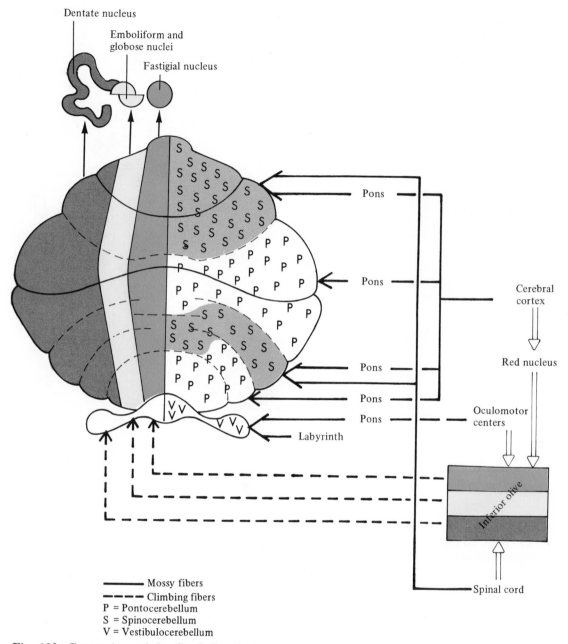

Fig. 123. Connections of the Cerebellar Cortex

Summary diagram of the afferent and efferent connections of the cerebellar cortex. The *left half of the figure* illustrates the climbing fiber input from the inferior olive to the Purkinje cells as well as the projections from the Purkinje cells to the intracerebellar nuclei. Both systems show a longitudinal zonal organization. The *right half of the figure* illustrates the mossy fiber systems from the spinal cord, vestibular apparatus, and cerebral cortex (via pons), all of which exhibit a mainly transverse orientation. Compare with Fig. 64, which illustrates the main subdivisions of cerebellum. P, Pontocerebellum; S, spinocerebellum; V, vestibulocerebellum. (Based on an original drawing by J. Voogd.)

the spinocerebellum receives a corticopontocerebellar projection from the sensorimotor cortex.

Pontocerebellum

Pontocerebellum (neocerebellum: obsolete term) consists of the portions of the vermis and hemispheres between the two spinal and the vestibular region of the cerebellum. The pontocerebellum therefore consists of two largely separate regions (Fig. 123). The pontocerebellum receives mossy fibers belonging to corticopontocerebellar projections from visual, acoustic, and association areas of the cerebral cortex. It comprises the major part of the cerebellar hemipshere, and its development parallels that of the cerebral cortex. Pontocerebellum is apparently involved in the coordination of skilled movement and speech.

AFFERENT CEREBELLAR CONNECTIONS

The fiber tracts, which carry information to the cerebellum from different sources in the spinal cord, the brain stem, and the cerebral cortex, converge primarily on the inferior and the middle cerebellar peduncles (Fig. 124). The major afferent systems can be subdivided as follows:

Mossy fibers:
1. From spinal cord
2. From vestibular system
3. From reticular formation
4. From pontine nuclei

Climbing fibers:
5. From inferior olive

Aminergic fibers:
6. From raphe nuclei and locus ceruleus

Some of the fibers arising from the spinal cord and the vestibular system are ipsilateral, whereas others have a bilateral distribution. The fibers originating in the inferior olive and the pontine nuclei cross the midline to terminate on the opposite side of cerebellum. The reticulocerebellar fibers, as well as the aminergic fibers, i.e., serotonin and norepinephrine fibers from the raphe nuclei and the locus ceruleus, are both crossed and uncrossed. Many of the afferent fibers send collateral

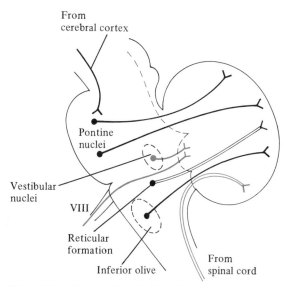

Fig. 124. Afferent Cerebellar Connections

projections to one of the cerebellar nuclei along the path to the cerebellar cortex.

Spinocerebellar Tracts

Through the spinocerebellar tracts (Fig. 99B) the cerebellum receives information from both the periphery and motor reflex centers in the spinal cord. According to the incoming information cerebellum can then elicit the appropriate regulatory response. The cerebellar response is transmitted to the motor cortex and to different brain stem centers for further delivery to motor centers in the spinal cord. All spinocerebellar pathways, except the ventral spinocerebellar tract, which enters through the superior cerebellar peduncle, reach cerebellum through the inferior cerebellar peduncle.

Dorsal Spinocerebellar Tract

Dorsal spinocerebellar tract (DSCT) and *cuneocerebellar tract* (CCT) transmit highly specific and discriminating proprioceptive and exteroceptive impulses from lower and upper parts of the body, respectively. DSCT originates in the *nucleus dorsalis of Clarke* (T1–L2), whereas the CCT originates in the *external* (accessory) *cuneate nucleus* (proprioceptive impulses) and in the *internal cuneate* and *gracile nuclei* (exteroceptive impulses).

The cells in Clarke's column receive dorsal root afferents from the lower part of the body (up to about midthoracic level) and the cells in the external cuneate nucleus from the upper part of the body.

Ventral Spinocerebellar Tract

Ventral spinocerebellar tract (VSCT) seems to transmit information about activity in motor reflex centers in the spinal cord. It originates in cell bodies located in the intermediate and ventral gray matter in the lower half of the spinal cord, as well as in cell bodies in the ventral horn of the cervical enlargement. VSCT enters the cerebellum through the superior cerebellar peduncle. Most of its axons cross twice, both in the spinal cord and in the cerebellar white matter.

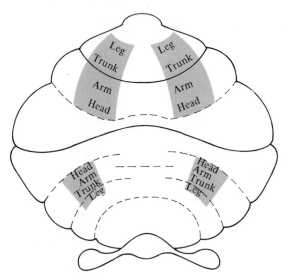

Fig. 125. Somatotopic Organization in Cerebellar Cortex

Trigeminocerebellar Fibers

Trigeminocerebellar fibers in the inferior cerebellar peduncle transmit properioceptive and exteroceptive impulses from areas of the face to the cerebellum.

Somatotopic Organization in the Cerebellar Cortex. The spinocerebellar fibers terminate in the "spinocerebellum," represented by the anterior lobe, pyramis, and uvula, as well as in adjoining parts of the hemisphere in the posterior lobe. The fibers terminate in a somatotopic fashion, in the sense that different regions of the body are represented separately in the anterior lobe and in the posterior lobe (Fig. 125). There are, in other words, two sets of topographically organized spinocerebellar receiving areas in the cerebellar cortex.

Vestibulocerebellar Fibers

The vestibular impulses, which arrive through the inferior cerebellar peduncle, provide the necessary information for proper reflex control of posture and eye position during head movements and changes in position of the head.

Primary Fibers

Primary fibers, with cell bodies located in the vestibular ganglion, carry information directly from the labyrinth receptors primarily to the ipsilateral cerebellum.

Secondary Fibers

Secondary fibers arise from cell bodies in the vestibular nuclei and have a symmetric, bilateral distribution.

"Vestibulocerebellum." The vestibulocerebellar fibers terminate primarily in the flocculonodular lobe, which therefore is referred to as "vestibulocerebellum."

Reticulocerebellar Fibers

Fibers from the reticular formation arise from several nuclear groups and project primarily through the inferior cerebellar peduncle to both the ipsilateral and the contralateral halves of the cerebellum. The reticular nuclear groups, like inferior olive, serve as relay and integration centers through which information from spinal cord as well as other parts of the CNS can reach the cerebellum.

Pontocerebellar Fibers

The pontocerebellar fibers, which convey impulses from the cerebral cortex to the cerebellum, form the massive middle cerebellar peduncles. The first link in this important cerebrocerebellar projection system (Fig. 126A) is represented by the cortico-pontine fibers, which converge toward the internal capsule from all cerebral lobes and proceed through the cerebral peduncle to the base of the pons, where they terminate in the *pontine nuclei.* The axonal projections of the pontine nuclei, the pontocerebellar fibers, enter the cerebellum through the middle cerebellar peduncles. Although it is generally believed that the pontocere-bellar fibers cross over in pons before they enter the cerebellum, recent studies indicate that a significant number do not cross. The large number of pontocerebellar fibers reflects the importance of close cooperation between the cerebral cortex and the cerebellum in the regulation of movements. Although the majority of the pontocerebellar fibers terminate in the s.c. "pontocerebellum" in the cerebellar hemispheres, there are a significant number of pontocerebellar projection fibers also to the more medial "spinocerebellar" parts of the cerebellar cortex, as well as to the "vestibulocerebellum" (Fig. 123).

Olivocerebellar Fibers; Sagittal Zonal Organization

The *inferior olive* is the only known source of the climbing fibers. It constitutes an important relay and integration center, through which information from many different sources in the spinal cord as well as in the brain stem and the forebrain, including cerebral cortex, is processed in parallel with the corresponding mossy fiber systems. The fibers from the inferior olive cross the midline before they enter the cerebellum to terminate in the intracerebellar nuclei and, as climbing fibers, directly on the Purkinje cells throughout the cerebellar cortex.

Prominent among the projection areas to the inferior olive are the spinal cord, the dorsal column nuclei, oculomotor centers in the midbrain, including the superior colliculus, and the parvocellular part of the red nucleus, which mediates the projections from the cerebral cortex, including a somatotopically arranged projection from the senso-

rimotor cortex. Direct corticoolivary fibers are probably few in number. The axons from different groups of neurons in the inferior olive project to narrow sagittal zones, which may extend over the entire rostrocaudal length of the cerebellum, and which contain the Purkinje cells projecting to a certain central cerebellar nucleus. These longitudinal zones cut through the transverse, spinal, vestibular, and pontine subdivisions of the cerebellum. This means that the information from vestibular, spinal, and cortical levels, which reaches the inferior olive, becomes fragmented over a number of longitudinal zones. Each of these zones contains the appropriate vestibular, spinal, and cortical information in its portion corresponding to the particular transverse subdivision of the cerebellum.

The input to the cerebellar cortex therefore shows a high degree of convergence of different pathways carrying information of the same modality. Spinocerebellar and corticopontocerebellar mossy fiber pathways and the different longitudinally organized olivocerebellar paths, which receive somatotopically organized information from the spinal cord and the sensorimotor cortex through the red nucleus, converge on the appropriate portions of the spinocerebellum. Similar examples can be cited for the afferent connections of the "vestibulocerebellum" and the pontocerebellum.

Aminergic Fibers from Raphe Nuclei and Locus Ceruleus

Serotonin-containing fibers from the raphe nuclei and norepinephrine-containing fibers from locus ceruleus reach the intracerebellar nuclei and cerebellar cortex through the superior and inferior cerebellar peduncles. The functional significance of biogenic amine-containing fibers is not clear. Their anatomic arrangement suggests a modulating effect on neuronal activities in general. The norepinephrine input from the locus ceruleus may be of special importance for cerebellar mechanisms related to the regulation of autonomic responses.

INTRACEREBELLAR NUCLEI

The intracerebellar nuclei within the white matter are from lateral to medial (Fig. 67B in dissection guide):

1. *Dentate nucleus*
2. *Emboliform nucleus*
3. *Globose nuclei*
4. *Fastigial nucleus*

The activity generated in the cerebellar cortex is ultimately channeled to the intracerebellar nuclei, as well as to the vestibular nuclei, via the Purkinje cells, which have an inhibitory effect on the cells with which they establish synaptic contact. The intracerebellar nuclei, however, do receive significant excitatory input through collateral projections of the afferent cerebellar fibers that pass by en route to cerebellar cortex. The activity generated in the intracerebellar nuclei, finally, is transmitted to other parts of the CNS through the efferent cerebellar pathways.

Corticonuclear Relationships

The projections from the cerebellar cortex to the intracerebellar nuclei tend to be organized in a longitudinal or sagittal fashion, in the sense that the axons of the Purkinje cells extend to the nearby deep nucleus (Fig. 123). In other words, a medial zone represented by vermis is primarily related to the fastigial nucleus and Deiters' nucleus, an intermediate zone consisting of the medial parts of the cerebellar hemisphere is related to the emboliform and globose nuclei, and a lateral zone including the rest of the hemisphere is related to the dentate nucleus. Although this subdivision of the cerebellum into three longitudinal zones is an oversimplification, the terms medial, intermediate, and lateral zones, which reflect the anatomic relationships between the cerebellar cortex, the intracerebellar nuclei, and the inferior olive, have a certain physiologic and clinical significance (see below).

EFFERENT CEREBELLAR CONNECTIONS

The distribution patterns of the cerebellofugal projections are very complicated and only the main features are summarized below. The efferent fibers, which leave the cerebellum in the inferior or superior cerebellar peduncle, terminate in brain stem and forebrain regions, many of which are directly or indirectly related to descending spinal pathways. These regions include the vestibular nuclei, the reticular formation, oculomotor centers in the brain stem, the red nucleus, and the ventrolateral thalamus.

Cerebellovestibular Fibers

The fibers to the vestibular nuclei project through the inferior cerebellar peduncle. Since many of the fibers arise directly from the cerebellar cortex, the vestibular nuclei can to some extent be compared with the intracerebellar nuclei. The two major contingents of cerebellovestibular fibers are: (1) fibers from flocculonodular lobe ("vestibulocerebellum") and fastigial nucleus to all four vestibular nuclei; and (2) fibers from anterior vermis ("spinocerebellum") to lateral vestibular nucleus of Deiters.

Cerebelloreticular Fibers

A considerable portion of the cerebelloreticular fibers originate in the fastigial nucleus and pass through the inferior cerebellar peduncle to the reticular formation in pons and medulla oblongata.

Cerebellorubral and Cerebellothalamic Fibers

Ascending cerebellar projections, which originate in dentate, emboliform, and globose nuclei, leave cerebellum in the superior cerebellar peduncle and cross the midline in the decussation of the superior cerebellar peduncles. Important areas of termination include the red nucleus and the oculomotor centers in the midbrain and the ventral lateral (VL) and ventral anterior (VA) nuclei of the thalamus.

The projection to the VL–VA complex, which in turn projects to the motor cortex, establishes a cerebellocerebral projection system, which reciprocates the corticopontocerebellar projection system. However, there is an important difference between the two systems. Whereas the cerebellum receives information from extensive regions of the cerebral cortex through the corticopontocerebellar system, the cerebellar activity mediated through the cerebellothalamocortical pathway affects primarily the motor cortex.

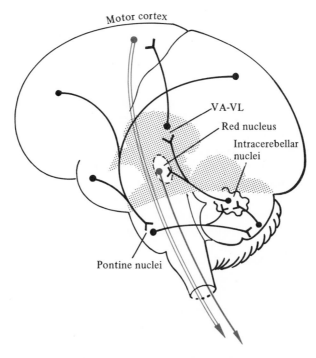

A. Cerebellar input to the corticospinal and rubrospinal tracts

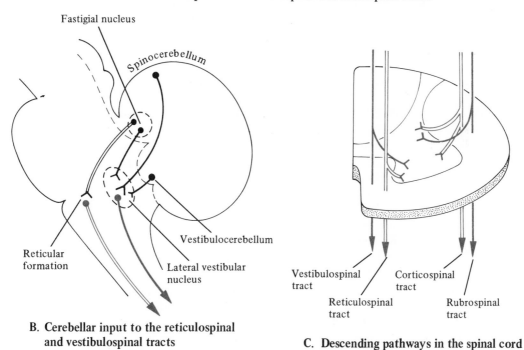

**B. Cerebellar input to the reticulospinal
and vestibulospinal tracts**

C. Descending pathways in the spinal cord

Fig. 126. Cerebellum and the Motor System
A. Highly schematic drawing of the corticopontocerebellar projection system and the efferent cerebellar projections to the red nucleus and the VA–VL complex of the thalamus. The VA–VL complex in turn, projects to the motor cortex, which provide access to the lateral descending system in the spinal cord.
B. Efferent cerebellar connections to the lateral vestibular nucleus and the reticular formation provide access to vestibulospinal and reticulospinal pathways.
C. Descending pathways in the spinal cord.

CEREBELLAR FUNCTIONS

A review of cerebellar anatomy reveals some striking features. Quite characteristic, for instance, is the stereotyped cortical histology. However, different parts of cerebellum are related to different regions of the nervous system. Therefore, although the intrinsic neuronal mechanisms seem to be similar throughout the cerebellum, the regulatory activities in different parts of the cerebellum are apparently related to different functions or to different parts of the body. Another striking feature is the large number of pathways carrying information to cerebellum from a variety of different sources. In other words, cerebellum must be concerned with the regulation of bodily functions in response to a variety of different stimuli.

A survey of the efferent cerebellar pathways indicates that a large part of the cerebellar output ultimately affects the motor system. How cerebellum is related functionally to the rest of the motor system is not altogether clear. What is obvious, however, is that the most striking symptom in a patient with cerebellar disease is loss of muscle coordination (see Clinical Notes).

Cerebellum and the Motor System

The efferent cerebellar pathways project primarily to motor nuclei in the brain stem, or to forebrain structures that serve as origin for major descending pathways, a fact that clearly reflects the importance of the cerebellum in motor functions (Fig. 126).

Fibers from emboliform and globose nuclei and from dentate nucleus project to the red nucleus, and via VL and VA of thalamus, to the motor cortex. Through these connections the intermediate and lateral parts of cerebellum have direct access to the lateral descending system in the spinal cord (see Chapter 7), i.e., the rubrospinal and the corticospinal tracts (Fig. 126A and C). These pathways are primarily related to limb musculature and fine manipulative movements, and there are indications that the cerebellum is important both for the initiation and coordination of limb movements.

The fastigial nucleus and the vermis represent major areas of origin for fibers to the reticular formation and the vestibular nuclei. The lateral vestibular nucleus of Deiters is influenced primarily by the vermis in the anterior lobe. The reticular formation and the vestibular nuclei give rise the reticulospinal and vestibulospinal tracts that control both postural activity and limb movements (Figs. 126 B and C).

Relationships between the Cerebellum and the Vestibular System and Oculomotor Centers

The vestibular system and cerebellum cooperate closely in motor functions related to the maintenance of equilibrium. They are also closely related to various oculomotor centers in the brain stem and the "vestibulocerebellum" plays an important regulating role in the so-called "vestibulo-ocular" reflex, i.e., adjustment of eye position in response to head movement. The importance of cerebellar control of vestibular and vestibulo-ocular reflexes is reflected in the massive reciprocal connections between the vestibular system and the cerebellum. Cerebellar relationships with the oculomotor centers are established via the inferior olive and its projections to the cerebellum, as well as by efferent cerebellar connections to the oculomotor centers. Impulses between the vestibular system and eye movement centers are mediated by the medial longitudinal fasciculus (Fig. 142).

Through its relationships to both the vestibular system and the oculomotor centers, as well as its projections to the red nucleus and the motor cortex, the cerebellum emerges as a crucial component in the neuron circuitry responsible for the coordination of voluntary eye, head, and hand movements that characterize most human activities.

CLINICAL NOTES

Cerebellar Ataxia

Ataxia, loss of muscular coordination, is most strikingly seen in cerebellar disease. It is best detected in the patient's gait and complicated limb movements. The gait is broad-based, irregular, and staggering, like that of an intoxicated person. When the patient is asked to put his finger on the nose (finger-to-nose test), the finger starts on its course normally but gradually begins to oscillate more and more violently as it approaches the nose. These tremulous movements are referred to as "cerebellar tremor" or "intention tremor." Cerebellar ataxia is often evident also in conjugate eye movements, which become jerky, and in speech, which has a tendency to become irregular and explosive with a slurring of words (cerebellar speech).

Although a cerebellar lesion is a common cause of ataxia, incoordination of movements can also be caused by loss of afferent proprioceptive input, e.g., by a lesion in the somatosensory pathways, in which case it is referred to as *sensory ataxia*.

Localization of Cerebellar Disease

Although there seems to be some validity in the functional subdivisions of cerebellum into "vestibulocerebellum," "spinocerebellum," and "pontocerebellum," considerable overlap exists among the three parts, and it is often difficult to determine the position of a focal cerebellar lesion, e.g., a tumor, on the basis of the patient's symptoms. The situation is further complicated by the fact that there is little room for expansion in the infratentorial part of the cranial cavity. A space-occupying lesion in the posterior fossa, therefore, may cause symptoms from pressure on surrounding brain stem and cerebellar structures.

Of importance, however, is the fact that each cerebellar hemisphere exerts its influence primarily on the ipsilateral half of the body. In other words, if cerebellar ataxia is evident in limb movements on only one side of the body, the lesion is likely to be present in the ipsilateral cerebellar hemisphere or its extrinsic pathways. The explanation for this is quite simple. Most of the cerebellofugal fibers from the hemisphere depart through the superior cerebellar peduncle and cross in its decussation before terminating in the red nucleus and the motor cortex (via the VL–VA thalamic complex) on the opposite side. The red nucleus and the motor cortex in turn give rise to descending pathways, which primarily affect the motor centers in the contralateral half of the spinal cord, i.e., that same side from which the cerebellofugal part of the circuit originated.

Whereas cerebellar hemisphere lesions primarily cause ipsilateral incoordination (ataxia and tremor), midline or vermis cerebellar disease may be manifest by impairment of equilibrium. Such deficits in upright posture cause titubation (a staggering and stumbling gait with shaking of the trunk and head), wide-based stance, and Romberg's sign (difficulty in standing erect with feet approximated and eyes closed).

In summary, one may say that the most common objective signs of a cerebellar tumor are disturbances of gait and posture, regardless of whether the tumor is located in the area of the vermis or in the hemisphere. Although ataxic limb movements can be seen in patients with both lateral and medial disease, unilateral limb movement disturbances indicate the presence of a lesion in the ipsilateral cerebellar hemisphere. It is important to remember, however, that a space-occupying lesion in the posterior fossa quickly produces increased intracranial pressure. Therefore, subjective symptoms, such as headache and vomiting with or without disturbances in balance, may be the first symptoms of a cerebellar tumor.

CLINICAL EXAMPLE

Metastatic Cerebellar Hemisphere Lesion

A 65-year-old male with a long history of cigarette smoking was found on routine chest X-ray to have a lesion in the upper lobe of his right lung, and bronchoscopy and biopsies revealed a lung cancer (bronchogenic squamous cell carcinoma). Examination of his scalene lymph nodes showed evidence of metastatic tumor, and he was treated with palliative radiotherapy.

Three months later, the man developed progressive gait difficulties. Examination at that time showed that he was alert and oriented, his cranial nerves were normal, but he had decreased muscle tone in his left arm and leg. The stretch reflexes were reduced on the left side compared with the right. He also had "intention tremor" in his left arm and leg while performing the finger-to-nose test or when trying to put his left heel on his right knee when lying in bed (heel-to-shin test). Although his balance was relatively good, he did have difficulty with heel-to-toe walking, and tended to veer toward the left side.

A CT scan (Fig. CE9) was obtained after infusion of intravenous contrast.

1. Where is the lesion in the CNS?
2. Given the clinical history, what do you think the lesion most likely represents?
3. The lesion is on the left side of his brain. Why then are his deficits also on the left side?
4. If the lesion were to expand, what adjacent brain structure would be compressed?

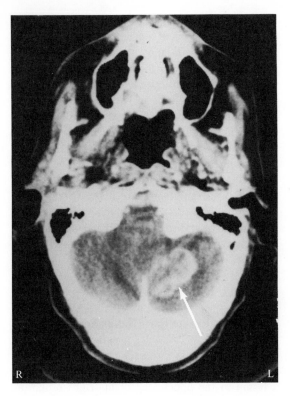

Discussion

The CT scan, which is taken through the posterior fossa, shows an elliptically shaped lesion in the left cerebellar hemisphere. With a history of lung cancer that had already spread to regional lymph

Fig. CE9. Metastatic Cerebellar Hemisphere Lesion

The CT scan was kindly provided by Dr. V. Haughton.

nodes, the most likely etiology is further metastatic spread of the lung tumor. Brain metastasis can involve virtually any part of the brain, but typically occurs at the junction of gray and white matter.

The patient's symptoms and signs are typical for a hemispheric cerebellar lesion in the sense that the cerebellar deficits (decreased muscle tone, hyporeflexia, and ataxia) involve the arm and the leg on the same side of the body as the lesion. This reflects the fact that the cerebellar hemisphere is involved primarily in the control of the ipsilateral limbs. Spinocerebellar pathways to the cerebellar hemispheres are mainly uncrossed and the cerebellofugal pathways from the cerebellar hemispheres via the motor cortex to the spinal cord are "doubly crossed" (see Fig. 126A).

If the lesion were to expand, the adjacent brain stem would gradually be compressed. In addition, the fourth ventricle would probably become obliterated thereby causing an acute obstructive hydrocephalus. Because of their accessibility in the posterior fossa, cerebellar metastases are commonly removed surgically if they are the only metastasis found in the brain. An alternative mode of therapy would be radiation treatments to the posterior fossa.

SUGGESTED READING

1. Adams, R. D. and M. Victor, 1981. Principles of Neurology, 2nd ed. McGraw-Hill: New York, pp. 60–68.
2. Brodal, A., 1981. Neurological Anatomy in Relation to Clinical Medicine, 3rd ed. Oxford University Press: New York, pp. 294–393.
3. Gilman, S., J. R. Bloedel, and R. Lechtenberg, 1981.

Disorders of the Cerebellum, F. A. Davis: Philadelphia.
4. Llinas, R. R., 1975. The Cortex of Cerebellum. Scientific American 232 (1): 56–71.
5. Palay, S. L. and V. Chan-Palay, 1974. Cerebellar Cortex: Cytology and Organization. Springer-Verlag: Heidelberg.

10

Brain Stem, Reticular Formation, and Monoaminergic Pathways

CROSS-SECTIONS THROUGH THE BRAIN STEM
  Medulla Oblongata
  Pons
  Mesencephalon

RETICULAR FORMATION
  Anatomic Organization
  Influences on the Spinal Cord
  The Ascending Activating System: Sleep and Wakefulness

MONOAMINERGIC PATHWAYS
  Serotonergic Pathways
  Noradrenergic Pathways
  Dopaminergic Pathways

CLINICAL NOTES
  Disorders of Consciousness

SUGGESTED READING

The brain stem is densely packed with many vital structures such as long ascending and descending pathways and specific nuclear groups including the nuclei of the cranial nerves. The central core of the brain stem is occupied by the reticular formation, i.e., diffuse aggregations of cells surrounded by a wealth of interlacing fibers. It is an extremely complicated but highly organized area of crucial importance for a variety of functions, including motor activities, respiration, cardiovascular functions, and mechanisms related to sleep and consciousness.

Although the monoamine neurotransmitters (dopamine, noradrenaline, and serotonin) are widely distributed in the CNS, the cell groups from which the monoaminergic pathways arise are almost without exception located within the brain stem. The monoaminergic systems participate in the regulation of sleep–wake cycles, feeding behaviors, motor and neuroendocrine regulation, reward mechanisms, and probably many other functions.

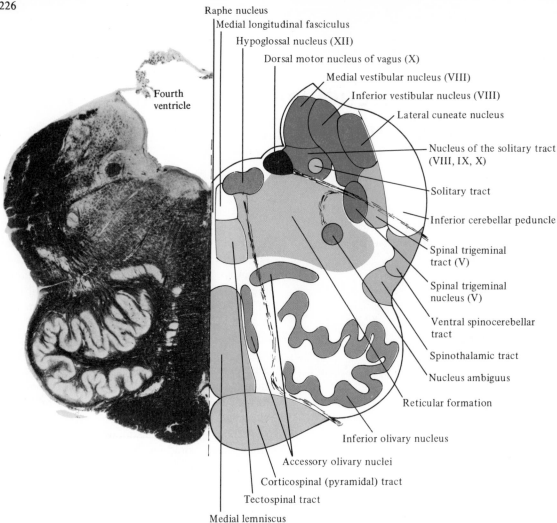

Raphe nucleus
Medial longitudinal fasciculus
Hypoglossal nucleus (XII)
Dorsal motor nucleus of vagus (X)
Medial vestibular nucleus (VIII)
Inferior vestibular nucleus (VIII)
Lateral cuneate nucleus
Fourth ventricle
Nucleus of the solitary tract (VIII, IX, X)
Solitary tract
Inferior cerebellar peduncle
Spinal trigeminal tract (V)
Spinal trigeminal nucleus (V)
Ventral spinocerebellar tract
Spinothalamic tract
Nucleus ambiguus
Reticular formation
Inferior olivary nucleus
Accessory olivary nuclei
Corticospinal (pyramidal) tract
Tectospinal tract
Medial lemniscus

Fig. 127. Cross-Section of Rostral Medulla Oblongata
Motor nuclei and pathways are colored *red,* sensory nuclei and pathways *blue,* and parasympathetic nuclei *black.* (The myelin stained left half of the brain stem is reprinted from DeArmond, S. J., M. M. Fusco, and M. M. Dewey, 1976. Structure of the Human Brain, 2nd ed. With permission of Oxford University Press.)

CROSS-SECTIONS THROUGH THE BRAIN STEM

Medulla Oblongata

The transition between the spinal cord and the medulla oblongata is characterized by a gradual change of gross anatomic features and internal structure. The central canal is gradually displaced in a dorsal direction through the appearance of the pyramidal and lemniscal decussations, until it finally opens up into the fourth ventricle.

Pyramidal Decussation

The majority of the fibers in each pyramid cross over the midline and continue as the *lateral corticospinal tract* on the opposite side of the spinal cord (Fig. 72B).

Lemniscal Decussation

Immediately above the pyramidal decussation the *internal arcuate fibers* cross the midline in front of the central canal (Fig. 72A). The fibers originate in the dorsal column nuclei and continue as the *medial lemniscus.*

The typical spinal cord section with a centrally located gray matter surrounded by white matter

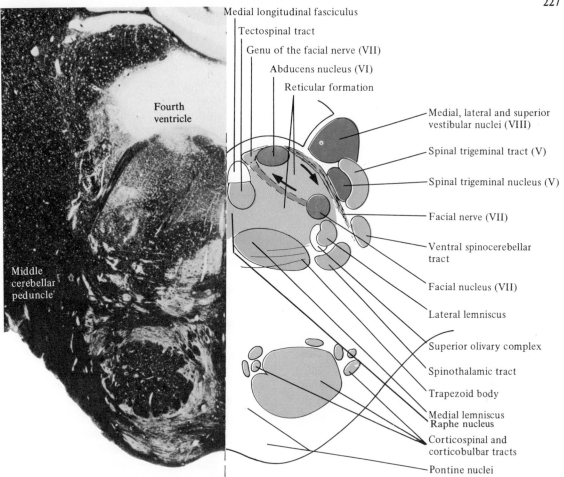

Medial longitudinal fasciculus
Tectospinal tract
Genu of the facial nerve (VII)
Abducens nucleus (VI)
Reticular formation

Fourth ventricle

Middle cerebellar peduncle

Medial, lateral and superior vestibular nuclei (VIII)
Spinal trigeminal tract (V)
Spinal trigeminal nucleus (V)
Facial nerve (VII)
Ventral spinocerebellar tract
Facial nucleus (VII)
Lateral lemniscus
Superior olivary complex
Spinothalamic tract
Trapezoid body
Medial lemniscus
Raphe nucleus
Corticospinal and corticobulbar tracts
Pontine nuclei

Fig. 128. Cross-Section of Caudal Pons. (The myelin stained left half of the brain stem is reprinted from DeArmond, S. J., M. M. Fusco, and M. M. Dewey, 1976. Structure of the Human Brain, 2nd ed. With permission of Oxford University Press).

can no longer be recognized at the level of the lemniscal decussation; instead, the dorsal column nuclei, i.e., the *nucleus gracilis* and *cuneatus,* as well as the *spinal trigeminal nucleus,* form well-circumscribed areas of gray matter.

A cross-section through the rostral part of the medulla oblongata is shown in Fig. 127. The gray matter underneath the floor of the fourth ventricle is represented by a number of specific nuclei and diffuse aggregations of cells. The *hypoglossal nucleus* (XII), *dorsal motor nucleus of vagus* (X), and *nucleus of the solitary tract* (VII, IX, and X) are located immediately below the fourth ventricle, whereas the *nucleus ambiguus* (IX, X) is embedded in the ventral part of the reticular formation. Specific nuclei in the more lateral part of the medulla include the *spinal trigeminal nucleus* (V) and part of the *vestibular complex* (VIII). The most conspicuous nucleus, however, is the *inferior olivary nucleus.*

The *medial lemniscus, tectospinal tract,* and *me-dial longitudinal fasciculus* (MLF) are located close to the midline, whereas the *spinothalamic tract* and *ventral* and *dorsal spinocerebellar tracts* are situated close to the lateral surface. A characteristic feature of the rostral medulla is the *inferior cerebellar peduncle,* a large part of which is represented by *olivocerebellar fibers,* which originate in the inferior olivary nucleus on the opposite side. The dorsal spinocerebellar tract also reaches the cerebellum through the inferior cerebellar peduncle. The ventral spinocerebellar tract traverses the superior cerebellar peduncle.

Pons

A cross-section through the caudal pons (Fig. 128) features the *superior vestibular nucleus* (VIII), *spinal trigeminal nucleus* (V), and *facial nucleus* (VII). The *facial nerve* makes a dorsally directed detour toward the floor of the fourth ventricle, where it bends over the *abducens nucleus* (VI) and then passes in a ventrolateral direction to its point of exit between pons and medulla oblongata in the cerebellopontine angle. The loop of the facial nerve over the abducens nucleus is referred to as the *genu of the facial nerve.* The area overlying the genu and the abducens nucleus is indicated by a slight elevation, the *facial colliculus,* in the rhomboid fossa (Fig. 68 in dissection guide).

The *trigeminal motor nucleus* (V) and the *main sensory nucleus of the trigeminus* (V) are located in the rostral pons.

The *medial lemniscus,* which is situated close to the midline in the ventral part of the tegmentum, is being penetrated by the *trapezoid body* containing crossing secondary auditory fibers. The trapezoid body continues in a rostral direction as the *lateral lemniscus.*

The massive basal part of pons contains a large number of transversely oriented fibers, which originate in the *pontine nuclei* and enter the cerebellum via the *middle cerebellar peduncle.* These pontocerebellar fibers form the second link in an important pathway between the cerebral cortex and the cerebellum. The first link is represented by longitudinally oriented fiber bundles, the *corticopontine tracts.* Other components of the longitudinally oriented fiber bundles in the basal pons are the *corticobulbar* and *corticospinal tracts.*

Mesencephalon (Fig. 129)

Tectum contains important reflex centers for visual and auditory impulses in the *superior* and *inferior colliculi,* respectively. The inferior colliculus, further, constitutes a relay center in the auditory pathway from the coclear nuclei to the medial geniculate body (Chapter 12). The *brachium of the inferior colliculus,* which connects the inferior colliculus with the medial geniculate body, forms a circumscribed bundle underneath the superior colliculus. The *oculomotor* (III) and *trochlear* (IV) *nuclei,* which are located in the ventral part of the central gray matter underneath the superior and inferior colliculi, respectively, are closely related to the MLF. This complicated bundle, which connects the oculomotor centers with the vestibular nuclei and motor centers in the cervical cord, is essential for the coordination of eye and head movements.

The somatosensory pathways, the *medial lemniscus* and *spinothalamic tract,* are located dorso-

lateral to the red nucleus as they ascend toward the ventrobasal complex of the thalamus. The red nucleus gives rise to an important descending pathway, the *rubrospinal tract,* which is closely related to the corticospinal tract (Chapter 7). The crossing of the rubrospinal and rubroreticular fibers in the ventral tegmentum is referred to as the *ventral tegmental decussation.* Tectospinal fibers cross the midline in the *dorsal tegmental decussation.*

The ventral portion of the cerebral peduncle, the *basis pedunculi,* is composed of a cellular part, the *substantia nigra,* and white matter, the *pes pedunculi,* which contains the *corticopontine, corticospinal,* and *corticobulbar tracts.*

RETICULAR FORMATION

Anatomic Organization

Intrinsic Structure

The reticular formation is located in the central parts of the brain stem (Figs. 127, 128 and 129). It is characterized by "diffuse aggregations of cells of different types and sizes, separated by a wealth of fibers travelling in all directions" (Brodal, in Suggested Reading). The reticular, or "net-like" appearance is easily appreciated in histologic sections, where the reticular formation can be distinguished from specific cell groups such as the red nucleus and the cranial nerve nuclei. The reticular formation, however, is not a diffuse, undifferentiated structure. On the contrary, cytoarchitectonic differences exist between different parts of the reticular formation, and the different cell groups are characterized by specific connections.

In general, large cells are restricted to the medial two-thirds of the reticular formation. This is the *magnocellular zone,* which gives rise to long ascending and descending pathways (see below), and which can be referred to as the "effector" region of the reticular formation. The lateral *parvocellular zone* contains primarily small cells. These two zones can be easily distinguished only in the pons and the rostral part of medulla oblongata (Fig. 130).

The magnocellular zone is characterized by a specific type of neuron with long radiating dendrites that are usually spread out in a plane perpendicular to the long axis of the brain stem. The dendrites of different neurons overlap extensively, and the neurons seem to be eminently suited to

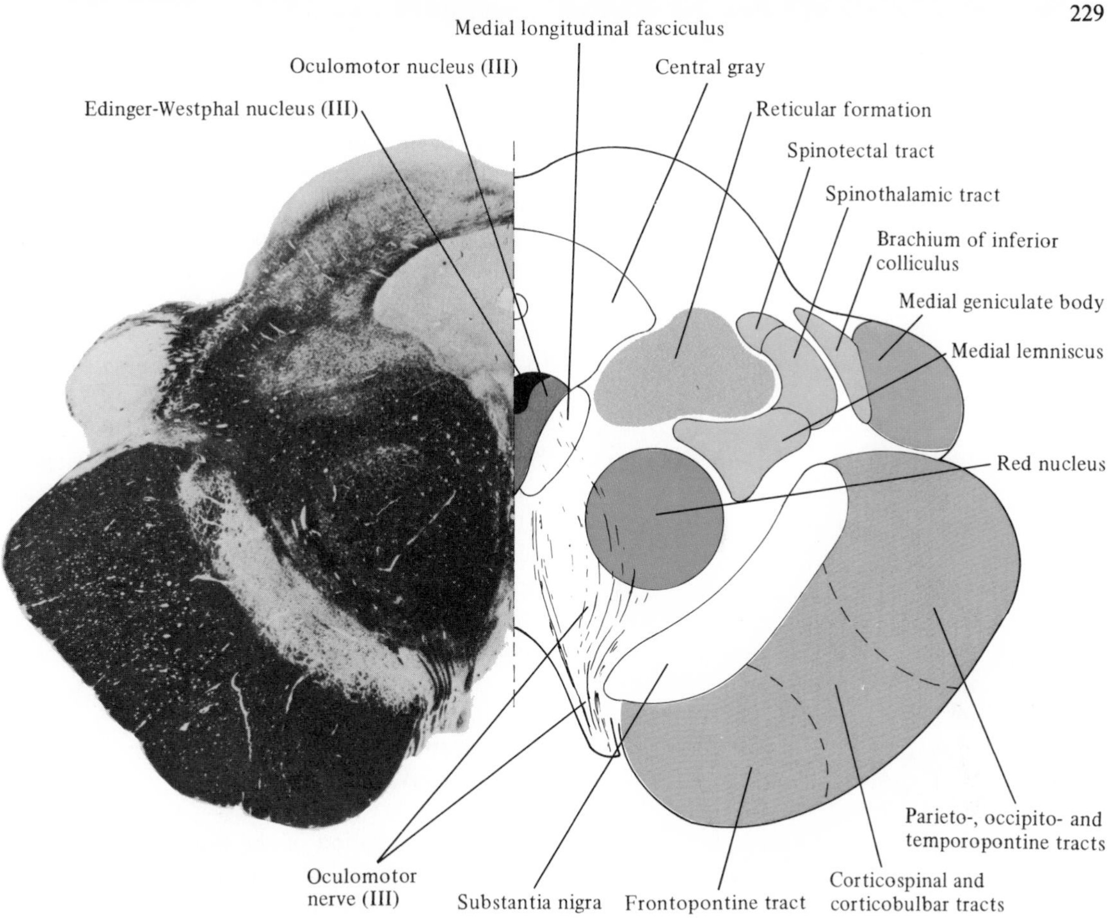

Fig. 129. Cross-Section of Mesencephalon. (The myelin stained left half of the brain stem is reprinted from DeArmond, S. J., M. M. Fusco, and M. M. Dewey, 1976. Structure of the Human Brain, 2nd ed. With permission of Oxford University Press).

pick up information from different sources. This is consistent with physiologic studies, which have shown a widespread convergence of afferent impulses on units in the reticular formation.

Connections

Afferent Connections. The reticular formation receives sensory information via spinoreticular fibers and sensory cranial nerves. It also receives information from the cerebellum, hypothalamus, basal ganglia, and cerebral cortex, especially the premotor cortex.

Efferent Connections. The long ascending and descending pathways originate in the medial magnocellular zone and terminate in various forebrain regions including hypothalamus, midline and intralaminar thalamic nuclei, as well as in all segments of the spinal cord.

Integration between Ascending and Descending Activity

The long efferent pathways originate in the medial zone according to a specific pattern (Fig. 130). Long ascending fibers originate primarily in lower pons and medulla. The areas of maximal origin of descending fibers, i.e., the pontine and medullary reticulospinal fibers (Chapter 7), are displaced rostrally in relation to the areas of origin for ascending pathways. Many of the cells that project in a rostral direction are therefore situated caudal to those projecting to the spinal cord, and there is ample opportunity for interaction between the two systems, especially since the reticular neurons are characterized by a large number of axon collaterals. Some of large cells, further, have axons that dichotomize in a long ascending and descending branch (Fig. 130).

Arrangements of this type provide the anatomic basis for integration of ascending and descending activities. For instance, a change in the level of

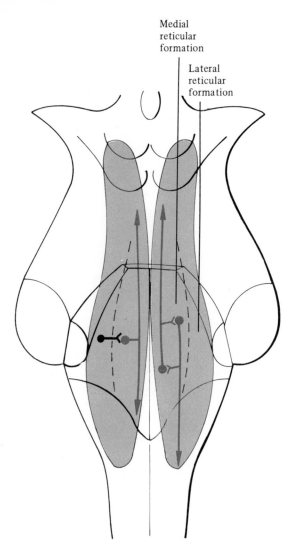

Medial
reticular
formation

Lateral
reticular
formation

Fig. 130. Reticular Formation
The extent of the reticular formation is projected on the dorsal surface of the brain stem. Many of the cells in the medial part of the reticular formation have an axon that gives off a long ascending and a long descending branch (*left side of figure*). Cells giving off long ascending and descending axons are often in a position to influence each other by way of collaterals (*right side of figure*).

consciousness from a drowsy state to extreme degree of attention (ascending activity) is always accompanied by changes in the somatomotor and autonomic spheres (descending activity).

Influences on the Spinal Cord

The reticular formation exerts control over various spinal cord functions, including *somatic motor ac-*

tivities, sensory transmission, and visceral functions, and the activities are highly integrated, e.g., changes in muscular activity are accompanied by alterations in respiratory and cardiovascular functions. The mechanisms by which the reticular formation controls the various activities of the spinal cord are very complicated. Neurons influencing a specific function are often widely distributed in the reticular formation, and it is therefore difficult to identify precisely the areas concerned in the regulation of various functions.

The reticulospinal pathways and their involvement in motor functions are discussed in Chapter 7, and the regulation of respiratory and cardiovascular functions is treated in the context of the autonomic nervous system (Chapter 16). The centrifugal control of sensory input, especially the modulation of pain impulses, has attracted considerable interest in recent years (Chapter 6).

The Ascending Activating System: Sleep and Wakefulness

Electrical stimulation of the brain stem reticular formation or natural stimulation of spinal or cranial sensory nerves produces widespread cortical activation or desynchronization, i.e., the high voltage–slow wave electroencephalogram (EEG) of quiet relaxation is replaced by the low voltage–high frequency EEG of intense wakefulness. The effect is mediated by ascending projections from the reticular formation to the nonspecific midline and intralaminar thalamic nuclei, which project to wide areas of the cerebral cortex. The nonspecific thalamic nuclei are also closely related to so-called specific thalamic nuclei, especially to the ventral anterior nucleus, which provides another link to the cerebral cortex. The widespread corticopetal projections from the basal nucleus of Meynert (Fig. 117) provide yet another route by which ascending stimuli can reach the cerebral cortex.

The concept of the *ascending activating system* is based on physiologic findings of an arousal zone in the brain stem. It is a physiologic concept whose anatomic substrate is represented by areas in the brain stem reticular formation and their ascending pathways to the diencephalon and cerebral cortex.

Physiologic studies and clinical observation have convincingly shown that the reticular formation is of great importance for maintaining a state of wakefulness. When an individual passes from sleep to wakefulness, the EEG changes from a synchronized slow-frequency pattern to a high-frequency desynchronized pattern similar to that seen after stimulation of the brain stem reticular formation. The regulation of the conscious state, however, is an extremely complicated function, in which many parts of the CNS are involved. Different parts of the reticular formation, further, seem to serve different functions in the regulation of consciousness.

Sleep is not merely a passive process of reduced activity in the ascending activating system. It is an active process, in the sense that it derives from neuronal activity in regions that have been referred to as "sleep centers." Areas of special importance for sleep have been identified in the brain stem reticular formation as well as in the thalamus and basal forebrain. The cholinergic and monoaminergic systems (see below) also seem to be involved in the regulation of the sleep–wake cycle and some scientists even speculate that chemical substances in the blood might affect some of the neuronal systems involved in sleep function. How these various brain regions and neuronal systems interact with each other and how they relate to different levels of sleep is not known.

MONOAMINERGIC PATHWAYS

Dramatic progress in neuroscience can often be correlated with the development of new techniques. An excellent example is the introduction in the early 1960s of the fluorescence histochemical methods for the demonstration of monamine-containing cells in the brain. Aided by these methods, scientists have discovered a number of neuron groups, which are located primarily in the brain stem, and which can be characterized on the basis of their neurotransmitter. There are three monoaminergic systems: the 5-hydroxytryptamine (serotonin, 5-HT), noradrenaline, and dopamine neuron systems.

There are some notable anatomic differences between the serotonin and noradrenaline systems on one hand, and the dopamine system on the other. The serotonin and noradrenaline systems are in many ways similar to the neuron systems of the reticular formation. Indeed, their cells of origin are located within or close to the reticular formation and the projections are widely distributed within the CNS. The dopamine cells, on the other hand, are located in the substantia nigra and nearby ventral tegmental area, as well as in some

hypothalamic nuclei, and they project to specific areas of the CNS in an orderly topographic fashion. The nigrostriatal dopaminergic pathway may serve as an example (Fig. 118A).

Serotonergic Pathways

The cells or origin of the serotonin system are mainly located in the *raphe nuclei,* which form an extensive, more or less continuous collection of cell groups close to the midline throughout the brain stem (Fig. 131). The axons of the cells in the rostral group of raphe nuclei are widely distributed in the forebrain. Some of the raphe nuclei project to cerebellum and those located in the medulla oblongata send projections to the spinal cord.

The functions of the serotonergic pathways are not well known. One part of the descending serotonergic fibers, which originates in the raphe magnus nucleus, terminates in the substantia gelatinosa. It has been implicated in pain mechanisms (Fig. 111, Chapter 6). Electrical stimulation of the raphe magnus nucleus has been found to produce powerful analgesia in animals. The ascending serotonin projections seem to favor so-called limbic structures, and it has been speculated that changes in mood and behavior might be closely related to the activity in the ascending serotonin system. The serotonin pathways may also be part of a sleep-inducing system. Experimental studies have shown that inhibition of the serotonin synthesis, or destruction of the raphe nuclei, leads to insomnia, which can be cured by the adminstration of serotonin. Some 5-HT terminals are located on ventricular surfaces and blood vessels, but the physiologic significance is unknown.

Noradrenergic Pathways

Noradrenergic (NA) or norepinephrine (NE) fibers arise from special cell groups in the pontine and medullary reticular formation. One noradrenergic system arises in the lateral reticular formation to innervate hypothalamus, amygdaloid body, and some other areas related to the limbic system via the medial forebrain bundle.

The most well-known of the noradrenergic cell groups is the *nucleus locus ceruleus,* which is located underneath the floor of the fourth ventricle in front of the facial colliculus (Fig. 68). The cells in the nucleus locus ceruleus are heavily pig-

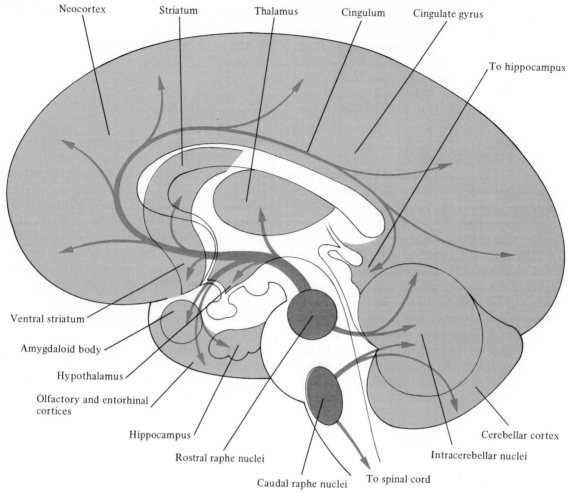

Fig. 131. Serotonergic Pathways

The raphé nuclei form a more or less continuous collection of cell groups close to the midline throughout the brain stem, but for the sake of simplicity they have been subdivided into a rostral and a caudal group in this drawing. The rostral raphé nuclei project to a large number of forebrain structures. The fibers that project laterally through the internal and external capsules to widespread areas of the neocortex are not indicated in this highly schematic drawing.

mented, which gives the area a bluish-gray tint, hence the name (blue place). The projections from locus ceruleus are characterized by a widespread distribution (Fig. 132). Indeed, the nucleus affects practically every major region in the brain and spinal cord in spite of the fact that the number of neurons in the nucleus is rather limited. To accomplish this the individual fibers branch profusely.

The functions of the noradrenergic system have been the subject of much speculation and decades of experimentation. Many of the adrenergic fibers terminate on small blood vessels and capillaries in the brain, which suggests a possible role in the regulation of the cerebral blood flow. It has also

been suggested that the noradrenergic system is an integral part of the ascending activating system, and that the descending pathway from the locus ceruleus to the spinal cord may participate in driving the spinal mechanisms for locomotion. Physiologic and behavioral studies, further, have implicated the noradrenergic system in mood, memory, and hormone regulation, the latter by way of its dense innervation of hypothalamic nuclei.

Dopaminergic Pathways

The dopaminergic pathways have been studied intensively since they were discovered by the aid

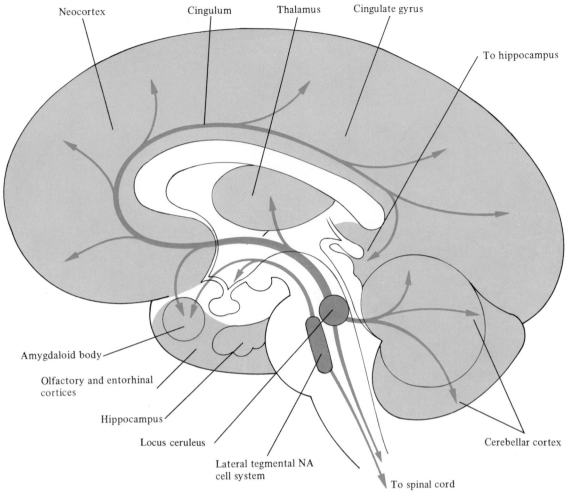

Neocortex   Cingulum   Thalamus   Cingulate gyrus

To hippocampus

Amygdaloid body

Olfactory and entorhinal
cortices

Hippocampus

Locus ceruleus

Lateral tegmental NA
cell system

To spinal cord

Cerebellar cortex

Fig. 132. Noradrenergic Pathways
Locus ceruleus, which is located immediately underneath the floor of the fourth ventricle in the rostrolateral part of pons, is the most important noradrenergic nucleus in the brain. Its projections reach many areas in the forebrain, cerebellum and spinal cord. Noradrenergic neurons in the lateral brain stem tegmentum innervate several structures in the basal forebrain including the hypothalamus and the amygdaloid body.

of the fluorescent histochemical method in the early 1960s. Much of the attention has centered on the nigrostriatal dopamine pathway and its relationship to Parkinson's disease (see Clinical Notes, Chapter 8).

The majority of the dopaminergic cells in the brain are located in the substantia nigra–ventral tegmental area. The axonal projections from these cells form a massive projection, which ascends in the lateral hypothalamus and which distributes to the whole extent of the striatum, including the accumbens and olfactory tubercle (Fig. 133). Other fibers reach the amygdaloid body, the septum, and the frontal cortex.

It is customary to distinguish between a nigro-

striatal and a mesolimbic dopaminergic system. The *nigrostriatal dopaminergic system* originates primarily in the substantia nigra (pars compacta) and terminates in the main, dorsal part of the striatum. Loss of neurons in this system causes Parkinson's disease. The *mesolimbic dopaminergic system* originates to a large extent in the ventral tegmental area in the mesencephalon and it projects to the ventral striatum, septum, amygdala, and the frontal lobe. It has been suggested that excessive activity in the mesolimbic system may occur in some schizophrenic patients.

Another dopamine pathway seems to be of special importance for neuroendocrine functions. This is the *tuberoinfundibular system,* which arises

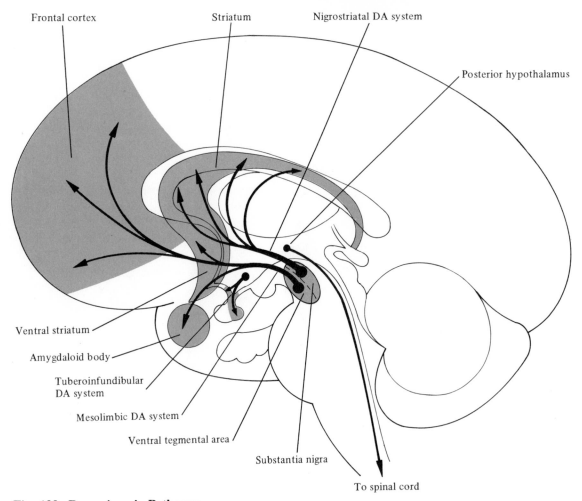

Fig. 133. Dopaminergic Pathways
The nigrostriatal DA system originates in the substantia nigra and terminates in the main dorsal part of the striatum. The ventral tegmental area gives rise to the mesolimbic DA system, which terminates in the ventral striatum, amygdaloid body, frontal lobe, and some other basal forebrain areas. The tuberoinfundibular system innervates the median eminence as well as the posterior and intermediate lobes of the pituitary, and dopamine neurons in the posterior hypothalamus project to the spinal cord.

from cells in the arcuate and periventricular hypothalamic nuclei and innervates the median eminence, and the posterior and intermediate lobes of the pituitary. Dopamine liberated from this system has been shown to have an inhibitory action on the release of prolactin and melanocyte-stimulating hormone from the pituitary. A dopaminergic pathway from the posterior hypothalamus to dorsal and intermediate cell columns of the spinal cord has also been discovered.

CLINICAL NOTES

When a physician sees a patient with a neurologic disorder, one of his first objectives will be to try to determine where the lesion is located. On the basis of a skillful examination of the patient and knowledge of the anatomy of the nervous system, it is usually possible to make a correct anatomic diagnosis, i.e., to determine the location of the pathologic process in the nervous system. Nowhere is this more clearly demonstrated than in the brain stem, where lesions involve cranial nerve nuclei plus long ascending and descending pathways in different combinations. Many brain stem lesions are caused by cerebrovascular disorders. These brain stem syndromes are discussed in Chapter 21.

Disorders of Consciousness

Mental function is often disturbed in patients with neurologic disorder, and it is important to evaluate a patient's mental state as it is expressed in such categories as level of consciousness, emotional reactivity, intellectual ability, and language.

Although it is difficult to define the term consciousness, a person is considered to be in a state of *normal consciousness* if he or she is fully awake and aware of self and environment. Further, the state of consciousness can be said to exist on a continuum with maximal alertness at one extreme and coma at the other. From a medical point of view it is convenient to distinguish between the following stages:

Confusion. A confused person cannot think clearly and is disoriented in time and place.

Somnolence. This is a condition of semiconsciousness; the patient can be aroused by various stimuli, but drifts back to sleep when the stimulus ceases.

Stupor. The patient can be aroused only by repeated and persistent stimulation and may be able to respond briefly to questions or commands.

Coma. The patient appears to be asleep and is in general unable to respond to external or internal stimuli. Reflex responses may or may not be absent depending on the degree of coma.

Consciousness can be disturbed for a variety of reasons, ranging from metabolic disturbances and drug intoxication to head injuries and large space-occupying brain lesions. Many brain regions and biochemical processes are important for consciousness, and it is usually impossible to identify all the pathophysiologic mechanisms by which consciousness is disturbed in a given case. It is appropriate, however, to make a few generalizations.

Metabolic diseases are often accompanied by a reduction in cerebral metabolism or blood flow that affects all neurons, and disturbances in consciousness at the cellular level generally are the result of altered function of both cortical and subcortical neurons. Hypoxia or hypoglycemia are examples of diffuse disease conditions that affect nerve cells both in the cerebral hemispheres and the reticular formation. Intracranial bleeding, tumor, or abscess are examples of conditions that cross-compress the other hemisphere. Alternatively, the space-occupying lesion may produce a transtentorial herniation (see p. 45 and Clinical Examples, Chapter 11) with subsequent compression of the upper brain stem reticular formation. Such herniation often compresses the oculomotor nerve en route.

A major step in the clinical evaluation of an unconscious person is to determine whether the disease is in the two cerebral hemispheres or is primarily in the brain stem itself.

SUGGESTED READING

1. Adams, R. D. and M. Victor, 1981. Principles of Neurology, 2nd ed. McGraw-Hill: New York, pp. 231–247.
2. Brodal, A., 1981. Neurological Anatomy in Relation to Clinical Medicine, 3rd ed. Oxford University Press: New York, pp. 394–447.
3. Hobson, J. A. and M. A. B. Brazier (eds.), 1980. The Reticular Formation Revisited. Raven Press: New York.
4. Lindvall, O. and A. Björklund, 1983. Dopamine- and noradrenaline-containing neuron systems: A review of their anatomy in the rat brain. In P. C. Emson (ed.): Chemical Neuroanatomy. Raven Press: New York, pp. 229–255.
5. Moore, R. Y., 1982. Catecholamine Neuron Systems in Brain. Ann. Neurol. 12:321–327.

11
Cranial Nerves

OLFACTORY (I) AND OPTIC (II) NERVES

OCULOMOTOR (III), TROCHLEAR (IV) AND
ABDUCENS (VI) NERVES
    Functional Anatomy
    Eye Movements and "Gaze Centers"
    Reflexes
    Clinical Notes

TRIGEMINAL NERVE (V)
    Somatosensory Part
    Somatic Motor Part
    Clinical Notes

FACIAL NERVE (VII)
    Somatic Motor Part
    Parasympathetic Part
    Visceral Sensory Part: Taste Pathways
    Clinical Notes

VESTIBULOCOCHLEAR NERVE (VIII)
    Vestibular Receptors
    Vestibular Nerve and Nuclei
    Central Connections
    Eye Muscle Nuclei
    Body Orientation and Posture Reflexes
    Nystagmus
    Clinical Notes

GLOSSOPHARYNGEAL (IX) AND
VAGUS (X) NERVES
    Functional Anatomy
    Reflexes
    Clinical Notes

ACCESSORY NERVE (XI)

HYPOGLOSSAL NERVE (XII)
    Functional Anatomy
    Clinical Notes

CLINICAL EXAMPLES
    Bell's Palsy
    Mediobasal Mesencephalic Syndrome of Weber
    Brain Stem Hemorrhage
    Lateral Medullary Syndrome of Wallenberg
    Cerebellopontine Angle Tumor
    Transtentorial Herniation

SUGGESTED READING

Except for the olfactory (I) and optic (II) nerves, the nuclei of the cranial nerves are located in the brain stem. Three of the cranial nerves are purely sensory (I, II, and VIII), five are motor (III, IV, VI, XI, and XII) and four are mixed (V, VII, IX, and X).

The cranial nerve nuclei, many of which have a columnar appearance, are arranged in an orderly fashion in the brain stem, in the sense that motor nuclei are located medial, and sensory nuclei lateral to the sulcus limitans.

The cranial nerves serve many functions related to the special sense organs, oculomotor activities, mastication, vocalization, facial expression, respiration, and the testing of the cranial nerves is an important part of the neurologic examination. One or several of the cranial nerves are often involved in lesions of the brain stem, and the location of such lesions can usually be determined if the topographic anatomy of the cranial nerves and their nuclei is known.

OLFACTORY (I) AND OPTIC (II) NERVES

The Ist and IInd cranial nerves are not nerves in the usual sense. The olfactory nerve is represented by the central processes of neuroepithelial cells in the olfactory mucosa, and the optic nerve is in reality a central pathway. The visual and olfactory systems are discussed in Chapters 13 and 14.

OCULOMOTOR (III), TROCHLEAR (IV), AND ABDUCENS (VI) NERVES

Functional Anatomy

Somatic Motor Parts

The nuclei of the oculomotor, trochlear, and abducens nerves are located close to the midline. (Fig. 134). The nuclear complex of the third cranial nerve is located in the central gray matter, where it extends from the diencephalic-mesencephalic junction area to the level of the superior colliculus (Fig. 129). It innervates the levator palpebrae superioris and all extrinsic eye muscles except the superior oblique and lateral rectus muscles. The contralateral superior oblique muscle receives innervation from the trochlear nucleus, which is located at the level of the inferior colliculus, and the lateral rectus muscle is innervated by the abducens nucleus in the lower pons.

The trochlear nerve is exceptional in two respects. It is the only cranial nerve that emerges on the dorsal aspect of the brain stem, and it crosses the midline in the anterior medullary velum before its exit.

Parasympathetic Part (III)

A group of preganglionic parasympathetic neurons, the *Edinger-Westphal nucleus,* is part of the oculomotor complex. The cells are situated close to the midline at the level of the superior colliculus (Fig. 129) and their axons proceed in the oculomotor nerve to the *ciliary ganglion,* where they establish synaptic contacts with postganglionic neurons innervating the sphincter pupillae and ciliary muscles. The Edinger-Westphal nucleus is an important component of the light reflex (see below).

Eye Movements and "Gaze Centers"

The eye movements that subserve various visual functions are highly coordinated and finely tuned. They are mostly reflex in nature and occur in response to a variety of stimuli including visual impulses from retina and proprioceptive impulses from the extrinsic eye muscles, as well as messages from the vestibular nuclei, cerebellum, and cerebral cortex. Although the mechanisms responsible for harmonious conjugated eye movements are not fully understood, the following brain stem structures are known to be closely related to eye movements (Fig. 135): The *superior colliculus,* the *paramedian reticular formation,* the *perihypoglossal nuclei,* and the *medial longitudinal fasciculus* (MLF) with its interstitial cell groups, including the *interstitial nucleus of Cajal.*

Superior Colliculus and Pretectal Region

These two structures receive input from the retina, the visual cortex, and the frontal eye field, and are involved in many aspects of visual functions including reflectoric eye and head movements in response to visual stimuli (the so-called visual grasp reflex). The pretectal region, further, is noted especially for its involvement in the pupillary light reflex (see below).

"Gaze Centers"

Neurons in the abducens nucleus and in nearby pontine reticular formation are of special significance for conjugated horizontal eye movements. These neurons, which are sometimes referred to collectively as the *"gaze center" for horizontal eye movements,* secure the coordination between the lateral rectus muscle on one side and the medial rectus muscle on the opposite side. To accomplish this, the neurons must be able to influence part of the oculomotor nuclear complex on the opposite side. They do so via the MLF, which is the most important coordinating pathway for conjugated eye movements and for vestibulo-ocular reflexes.

A *"gaze center" for vertical eye movements* is apparently located in the interstitial nuclei of the rostral MLF and surrounding areas of the mesencephalic reticular formation. These cell groups are closely related to various components of the oculomotor nuclei.

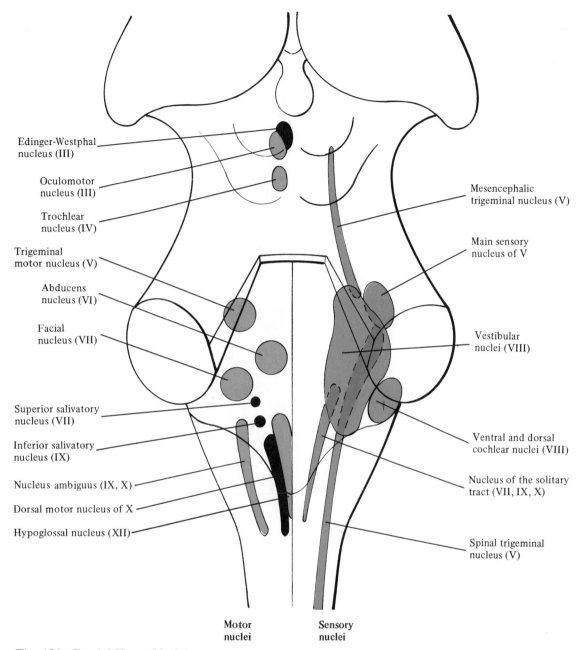

Edinger-Westphal
nucleus (III)

Oculomotor
nucleus (III)

Trochlear
nucleus (IV)

Trigeminal
motor nucleus (V)

Abducens
nucleus (VI)

Facial
nucleus (VII)

Superior salivatory
nucleus (VII)

Inferior salivatory
nucleus (IX)

Nucleus ambiguus (IX, X)

Dorsal motor nucleus of X

Hypoglossal nucleus (XII)

Mesencephalic
trigeminal nucleus (V)

Main sensory
nucleus of V

Vestibular
nuclei (VIII)

Ventral and dorsal
cochlear nuclei (VIII)

Nucleus of the solitary
tract (VII, IX, X)

Spinal trigeminal
nucleus (V)

Motor
nuclei

Sensory
nuclei

Fig. 134. Cranial Nerve Nuclei
The location of the cranial nerve nuclei in the brain stem as viewed from the dorsal side. Motor nuclei (somatomotor, *red;* visceromotor, *black*) are shown to the *left* and sensory nuclei (*blue*) to the *right* (Modified after Herrick.)

Perihypoglossal Nuclei

These highly differentiated cell groups, which lie mainly near the midline just rostral to the hypoglossal nucleus, are closely related to the oculomotor nuclei on one hand, and to the vestibular system and the cerebellum on the other.

Voluntary Eye Movements

Although eye movements are often reflex in nature, they can also be initiated voluntarily through impulses from the *frontal eye field* (area 8) to the superior colliculus or the pontine reticular formation, which in turn are closely related to the various oculomotor centers. The frontal eyefield re-

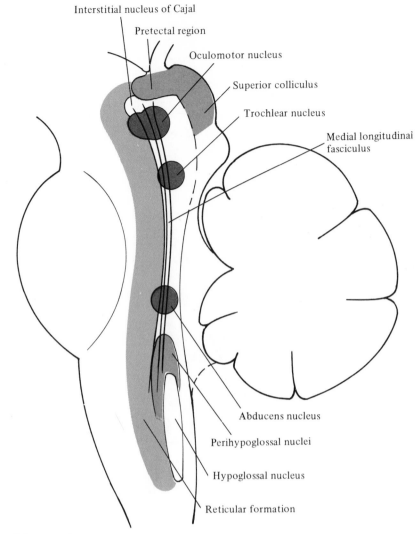

Fig. 135. Centers for Eye Movements
Highly schematic drawing of some of the most important structures concerned with the regulation of eye movements.

ceives impulses from many parts of the CNS including visual association cortex in the occipital lobe.

Reflexes

The *pupillary light reflex* and the *fixation* and *accommodation reflexes* are described in Chapter 13. The *vestibulo-ocular reflex,* i.e., adjustment of eye position in relationship to head movement, is described in relation to the VIIIth nerve.

Clinical Notes

Strabismus and Diplopia

Misalignment of the eyes may be noted by an examiner (as strabismus or squint) or may be apparent to the patient himself (as diplopia or double vision). It may be due to paralysis of one or several of the extraocular muscles. A *IIIrd cranial nerve* lesion results in a deviation of the ipsilateral eye to the lateral side, i.e., lateral or divergent strabismus, because of the unopposed action of the lateral rectus. Ptosis (drooping of the upper lid) and mydriasis (dilation of the pupil) are other characteristic signs. The ptosis is due to paralysis of the levator palpabrae muscle, whereas the dilation of the pupil and paralysis of accommodation is due to the interruption of the parasympathetic fibers in the IIIrd cranial nerve. *Trochlear nerve* lesions are uncommon. They cause vertical diplopia with a compensatory tilt of the head toward the opposite shoulder. Lesions of the *abducens nerve* result in paralysis of lateral movements of the eye, which deviates in a medial direction, i.e., medial or convergent strabismus, because of the unopposed action of the medial rectus muscle.

Ocular palsies may result from lesions of the eye muscle nuclei or from interruption of their respective nerves, two of which (III and VI) extend a considerable distance within the brain stem. Ocular palsies secondary to disorders in the brain stem, e.g., vascular lesions or tumors, are often accompanied by signs of other involvement of parts of cranial nerves or long ascending or descending pathways. The peripheral parts of the nerves are also vulnerable during their extended course through the cavernous sinus to the superior orbital fissure. Peripheral lesions are often attributable to aneurysms in the circle of Willis or tumors on the base of the brain. The oculomotor nerve, closely related to the posterior cerebral artery, is typically involved in a transtentorial herniation (Fig. 30, Chapter 3).

Paralysis of Conjugated Eye Movements

Considering the extensive and complicated mechanisms involved in eye movements, it is not surprising that disturbances in ocular functions may occur as a result of lesions in many parts of the brain. Paralysis of conjugate eye movements, for instance, is a frequent symptom. An acute lesion in the frontal lobe or internal capsule usually causes paralysis of contralateral gaze, and the eyes may deviate toward the side of the lesion. Paralysis of conjugate lateral gaze is also seen following lesions of the "gaze center" for horizontal eye movements in the abducens nucleus or its immediate vicinity. A mesencephalic lesion, e.g., a pineal tumor, may exert pressure on the pretectum and thereby affect the "gaze center" for vertical eye movements, which results in paralysis of upward, or sometimes downward, gaze, especially if the interstitial nuclei of the MLF are involved.

Pupillary Light Reflex

Testing the direct and the consensual reflexes of both eyes is a routine part of the neurologic examination. In a IIIrd cranial nerve lesion, both the direct and the consensual light reflexes are absent on the side of the lesion as the result of paralysis of the pupillary sphincter, but both reflexes are intact in the opposite eye. A blind eye (e.g., optic nerve lesion), on the other hand, does not respond directly to light, but it responds consensually if light is focused on the opposite intact eye.

TRIGEMINAL NERVE (V)

The Vth cranial nerve is a mixed nerve that supplies the skin and mucous membranes of the face with sensory fibers and the masticatory muscles with motor fibers. The sensory part of the nerve, the *portio major,* is much larger than the motor part, the *portio minor.*

Somatosensory Part

Sensory fibers from pseudounipolar cells in the large *semilunar* or *trigeminal (Gasserian) ganglion* on the anterior surface of the petrous bone distribute peripherally in the three main divisions: the *ophthalamic, maxillary,* and *mandibular nerves* (Fig. 136). The central processes of the ganglion cells terminate in the three sensory trigeminal nuclei: the spinal, the main sensory, and the mesencephalic trigeminal nuclei (Fig. 134). Although it is generally held that the *spinal trigeminal nucleus* is concerned with pain and temperature impulses and the *main sensory nucleus* with tactile impulses, the situation is considerably more complicated and not fully understood. It is known, however, that many of the fibers that enter the brain through the main sensory portion give off one branch to the spinal trigeminal nucleus and another to the main sensory nucleus. The spinal nucleus, further, contains several different cell groups characterized by individual specific connections and functional attributes. The caudal part of the spinal trigeminal nucleus, which is continuous with the substantia gelatinosa of the spinal cord, seems to be of special significance for the mediation of pain impulses.

The *mesencephalic trigeminal nucleus* is unique

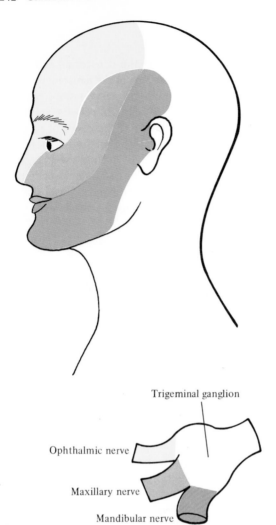

Trigeminal ganglion

Ophthalmic nerve

Maxillary nerve

Mandibular nerve

Fig. 136. Cutaneous Distribution of the Trigeminal Nerve
(Modified after B. Löfström, 1969. Block of the Gasserian ganglion. In "Illustrated Handbook in Local Anaesthesia," (Ed. Ejnar Eriksson) Year Book Medical Publishers, Inc. Chicago.)

in many respects. It is a long slender nucleus that reaches far rostrally to the level of the superior colliculus, and it receives proprioceptive impulses from both the extraocular and the masticatory muscles. Contrary to the general rule, the cell bodies for these sensory fibers are located within the mesencephalic nucleus rather than in the semilunar ganglion. The mesencephalic nucleus, therefore, is in part comparable to a sensory ganglion. Some of the sensory fibers in the mesencephalic root give off collaterals to the trigeminal motor nucleus, thereby providing the anatomic basis for the monosynaptic jaw (*masseter*) *reflex*, i.e., con-

traction of the masseters when the examiner's finger, placed on the patient's chin, is tapped with a percussion hammer.

The central connections of the trigeminal nuclei are discussed in Chapter 6.

Somatic Motor Part

The motor part of the Vth cranial nerve, *portio minor*, which originates in the *trigeminal motor nucleus* in pons, is incorporated in the *mandibular nerve*. The fibers innervate the masticatory muscles (masseter, temporal, pterygoids), anterior belly of the digastric, tensor tympani, and tensor veli palatini. The trigeminal motor nucleus receives both crossed and uncrossed fibers from the cerebral cortex.

The masticatory muscles develop from the mesoderm of the first branchial arch and are related to the digestive tract. The trigeminal motor nucleus, therefore, is sometimes referred to as a special visceral motor nucleus. The facial nucleus and nucleus ambiguus (IX and X) can likewise be referred to as special visceral motor nuclei. However, since the neurons in these three nuclei (trigeminal motor, facial, and ambiguus) resemble other somatic motor neurons, and since they innervate striated rather than smooth muscles, it seems reasonable to refer to them as somatic motor.

Clinical Notes

The nuclei and nerves of the trigeminus have a wide distribution; partial affections of the trigeminal system are therefore quite common. Many disorders, including skull fractures, tumors, and aneurysms, e.g., of the internal carotid artery, may affect the trigeminus. The spinal trigeminal system is typically involved in the lateral medullary (Wallenberg) syndrome (see Clinical Examples).

Corneal Reflex

This reflex, i.e., bilateral blinking elicited by touching the edge of the cornea with a wisp of cotton, is a multisynaptic reflex with the afferent limb in the trigeminal nerve and efferent in the facial nerve. Interruption of the ophthalmic division of the Vth cranial nerve leads to loss of the blink reflex on the affected side. If the cornea is touched on the unaffected side, however, both eyes will close.

Trigeminal Neuralgia (Tic Douloureux)

This is a common disorder of unknown etiology. It occurs in middle or late life and is characterized by paroxysms of sharp, excruciating pain in the distribution of one or more branches of the trigeminal nerve. The slightest tactile stimulus may trigger an attack. Many patients obtain relief from drug therapy, whereas others can be helped by some form of surgical interruption of the trigeminal pathways.

Ophthalmic Zoster

The virus *Herpes zoster* (see Clinical Notes, Chapter 5) may involve any part of the semilunar ganglion. The ophthalmic division is most often affected and can result in corneal scars that may interfere with vision.

FACIAL NERVE (VII)

The VIIth cranial nerve is a mixed nerve with several important functions. It is above all the motor nerve of facial expression, but it also innervates the submaxillary and sublingual glands as well as the lacrimal gland and glands of the nasal cavity, and it conveys taste impulses from the anterior two-thirds of the tongue.

Somatic Motor Part

The highly differentiated facial motor nucleus is located in the caudal part of pons, ventromedial to the spinal trigeminal complex (Fig. 128). The axons detour in a dorsomedial direction around the abducens nucleus before turning ventrally and emerging on the ventrolateral aspect of the brain stem between pons and the olive. The nerve enters the *internal auditory meatus* together with the vestibulocochlear nerve, continuous in the *facial canal,* and leaves the skull through the *stylomastoid foramen.* It branches in a fan-like manner in the region of the parotid gland and innervates the mi-

metic musculature, the stylomastoid, the posterior belly of the digastric muscle and platysma. During its course through the facial canal it gives off a branch to the stapedius muscle.

Parasympathetic Part

Preganglionic parasympathetic fibers from the *superior salivatory nucleus* join the *intermediate nerve.* Since this nerve also contains taste fibers and some cutaneous fibers from the external ear, it is often referred to as the sensory root of the facial nerve.

The parasympathetic fibers, which leave the main nerve during its course in the facial canal, form two major branches: (1) *the greater petrosal nerve,* which innervates the lacrimal and nasopalatine glands (postganglionic neurons in the sphenopalatine ganglion), and (2) *chorda tympani* (postganglionic neurons in the submandibular ganglion), which innervates all salivary glands except the parotid, which receives secretory fibers through the glossopharyngeal nerve.

Visceral Sensory Part: Taste Pathways

Receptors

The sensory cells that receive the stimuli for the four basic taste sensations (sweet, sour, salty, and bitter) are located in *taste buds* on the surface of the *fungiform* and *vallate papillae.* The sensory cells, like the cells of the surrounding epithelium, have a life span of only a few days; they are continuously replaced by new sensory cells, which are derived from the basal cells through mitosis.

Peripheral Pathways

The cell bodies of the fibers that transmit taste impulses from the taste buds of the anterior two-thirds of the tongue are located in the *geniculate ganglion* in the facial canal. The peripheral processes proceed for a short distance in the facial nerve before they enter the *chorda tympani,* which joins the lingual branch of the mandibular nerve (Fig. 137).

Another important taste nerve, the *glossopharyngeal (IX) nerve,* carries impulses from the pos-

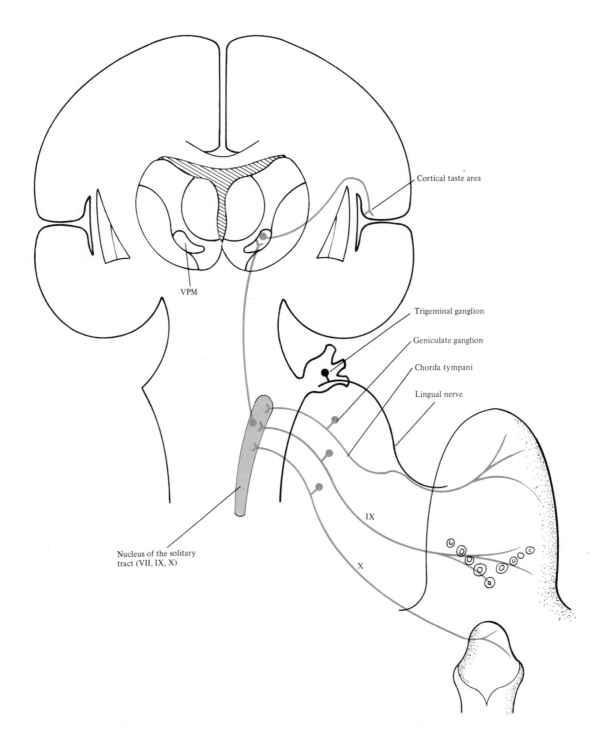

Cortical taste area

VPM

Trigeminal ganglion

Geniculate ganglion

Chorda tympani

Lingual nerve

IX

X

Nucleus of the solitary
tract (VII, IX, X)

Fig. 137. Pathways for Taste

The rostral part of the nucleus of the solitary tract is concerned with the transmission of taste impulses travelling in the facial (VII), glossopharyngeal (IX) and vagal (X) cranial nerves. Impulses from the nucleus of the solitary tract reach the ventral posteromedial nucleus (VPM) before being transmitted to the gustatory cortex in the opercular part of the inferior frontal gyrus on the ipsilateral side. The caudal part of the nucleus of the solitary tract receives viscerosensory impulses through the glossopharyngeal and vagal nerves. These impulses are important for cardiovascular, respiratory and other visceral reflexes.

terior third of the tongue, where a large number of taste buds are located on the sides of the vallate papillae. The *vagus* (*X*), finally, carries some taste impulses from the extreme posterior part of the tongue and the epiglottis.

Central Pathways

The taste impulses transmitted in the above-mentioned three nerves reach the rostral part of the *nucleus of the solitary tract.* The further central connections for taste are complicated. Eventually, the impulses reach both the *hypothalamus* and the *cortical taste area* in the opercular part of inferior frontal gyrus on the ipsilateral side. The impulses that reach the hypothalamus are presumably important in feeding behavior, whereas the gustatory cortex, which is closely related to the somatosensory area for the tongue, subserves conscious sensation of taste.

Disturbances of taste functions are of minor significance compared with many other symptoms that may result from a lesion of the facial nerve. Such lesions give rise to various syndromes depending upon where the lesion is located (see below.)

Clinical Notes

Disorders of the facial nerve are common, and the topographic relationships of the facial canal take on a special significance in the diagnosis of facial nerve lesions. It is often possible to determine the location of the lesion on the basis of existing signs and symptoms.

Lesions of the Facial Nerve (Fig. 138)

A peripheral lesion distal to the chorda tympani (lesion A in Fig. 138) affects only the somatic motor component, i.e., it paralyzes all muscles of facial expression. The sense of taste, however, is intact. A lesion situated in the facial canal peripheral to the geniculate ganglion (lesion B) is likely to include the chorda tympani, in which case taste sensitivity is lost on the anterior two-thirds of the tongue on the ipsilateral side. Since the branch to the stapedius muscle leaves the facial nerve between the geniculate ganglion and the chorda tympani, hyperacusis (painful sensitivity to loud

sound) may also be part of the syndrome. A lesion of the nerve in the proximal part of the facial canal (lesion C) is likely to involve the parasympathetic fibers to the lacrimal gland and usually results in loss of tear secretion in addition to all other symptoms. If the facial nerve is damaged in the internal auditory meatus, the VIIIth cranial nerve is likely to be involved, in which case tinnitus or deafness may be prominent.

The facial nerve can be damaged by many types of lesions including fractures of the petrous bone, middle ear infections, tumors of various kinds (e.g., cerebellopontine angle tumor, see Clinical Examples), and pathologic processes in the pons. The most common facial nerve disorder is *Bell's palsy,* which apparently is due to an inflammatory reaction in the facial canal, often in the course of an upper respiratory infection. If the patient loses the blinking reflex on the affected side, the eye can easily dry out and must be properly protected, especially during sleep. Recovery from Bell's palsy is usually spontaneous (see Clinical Examples).

Supranuclear Facial Paralysis

A supranuclear facial paralysis, e.g., as part of a capsular hemiplegia, is limited to the *lower part of the face.* This fact, which is of great diagnostic value, is explained by referring to the anatomic organization of the corticobulbar fibers to the facial nucleus (Fig. 139). The part of the facial nucleus that innervates the upper half of the face receives corticofugal fibers from the motor cortex of both sides, whereas the component for the lower part of the face receives only a contralateral innervation. A patient with a central facial palsy can close both eyes voluntarily, but in efforts to retract the angles of the mouth (e.g., "social smile") the weakness is revealed on the side contralateral to the lesion. Curiously enough, a hemiplegia patient is able to smile normally when he enjoys a joke. This dissociation between voluntary and emotional innervation indicates that the central fibers controlling the emotional facial expression do not descend in the internal capsule.

VESTIBULOCOCHLEAR NERVE (VIII)

The VIIIth cranial nerve consists of two divisions, the *cochlear* and *vestibular nerve,* both of which

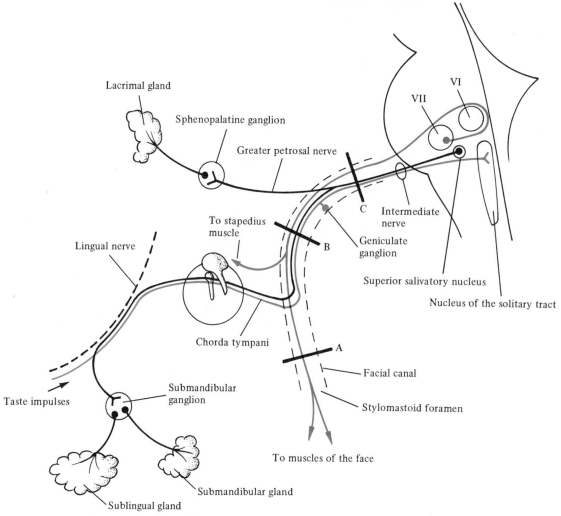

Fig. 138. Lesions of the Facial Nerve
Facial nerve lesions are common, and the symptoms will vary according to the site of the lesion. If the lesion is situated at **A,** i.e., distal to the departure of chorda tympani, there is no loss of taste sensation on the anterior two-thirds of the tongue. A lesion at **B** involves the taste pathway from the anterior two-thirds of the tongue but leaves the tear secretion intact. A lesion at **C** involves all components of the intermediate nerve in addition to the somatomotor component.

carry somatic sensory impulses from specialized receptors in the inner ear (Fig. 140). The two divisions, however, have different functions. The cochlear division carries auditory information from the organ of Corti in the cochlea, whereas the vestibular division transmits propioceptive impulses from the vestibular organ, i.e., the three semicircular canals, the utricle, and the saccule. The cochlear nerve is discussed in Chapter 12.

Vestibular Receptors

The vestibular receptors are represented by hair cells in the three *semicircular ducts* and in the vestibular portion of the labyrinth, which consists of two divisions, the *utricle* and the *saccule.* The utricle and the saccule provide information about changes in the position of the head ("position recorders"), whereas the semicircular canals react to changes in angular movements of the head. The hair cells are located in special areas (Fig. 141A) of the membranous labyrinth, which is filled with endolymph.

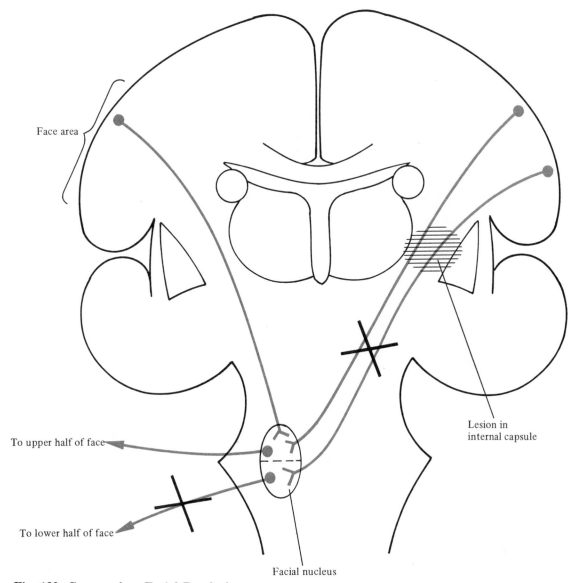

Fig. 139. Supranuclear Facial Paralysis

A supranuclear facial paralysis typically occurs in a capsular lesion. Since the peripheral motor neurons to the upper half of the face receive corticobulbar fibers from both hemispheres a central facial paralysis is evident only in the lower half of the face on the opposite side of the lesion.

The vestibular organs, the maculae, in the saccule and utricle consist of hair cells (Fig. 141B) whose cilia project into a gelatinous mass, the *otolith membrane*. This membrane contains fine crystals of calcium carbonate, the *otoliths*. If the head is tilted, the gravitational force displaces the otolith membrane, and the otoliths stimulate the hair cells. The adequate stimulus is *linear acceleration* (or deceleration).

The hair cells in the semicircular canals are located in dilatations of the canals called ampullae. Each ampulla contains a transversely oriented crista with hair cells (Fig. 141C). The crest is cov-

ered by a gelatinous mass, *the cupula*. Rotational movements of the head tend to deflect the cupula because of the inertia of the endolymph. This, in turn, stimulates the hair cells. The adequate stimulus is a change in speed rather than movement itself, i.e., *rotational acceleration* (or deceleration).

Vestibular Nerve and Nuclei

The bipolar ganglion cells of the vestibular nerve form the *vestibular ganglion* in the bottom of the internal auditory meatus. Their peripheral pro-

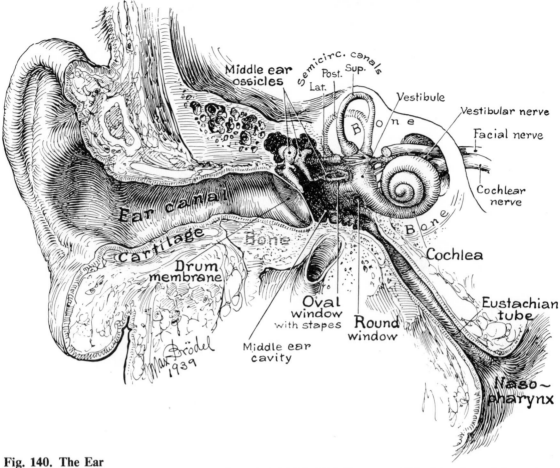

Fig. 140. The Ear
Drawing of the outer, middle, and inner ear. (From Brödel, M. 1946. Three unpublished drawings of the anatomy of the human ear. With permission of W. B. Saunders Co., Philadelphia.)

cesses innervate the sensory cells in the vestibular apparatus, whereas the central processes form the vestibular nerve. The nerve enters the brain stem at the lower border of pons and terminates in the four main vestibular nuclei, the *lateral* (*Deiters*), *medial, superior,* and *inferior nuclei.* The vestibular nuclear complex occupies a rather large area in the lateral part of the brain stem just below the floor of the fourth ventricle (Fig. 134). Although the vestibular apparatus as a whole is of importance for *maintenance of equilibrium* and for *orientation in space,* the different vestibular nuclei have specific connections and functional characteristics.

Central Connections

The information from the vestibular apparatus ultimately influences the motor system by means

of connections between the vestibular nuclei and the following main areas: spinal cord, reticular formation, cerebellum, and eye muscle nuclei (Fig. 142).

Spinal Cord

Although the relationships between the vestibular nuclei and the spinal cord are reciprocal, the vestibulospinal tracts are more prominent than the spinovestibular tracts. The most important descending pathway, the *lateral vestibulospinal tract,* comes from Deiters' nucleus, and it exerts a facilitatory action on the extensor motor neurons. The vestibulospinal tracts belong to the ventromedial descending system in the spinal cord (Chapter 7).

Reticular Formation

Reciprocal connections between the vestibular nuclei and the reticular formation provide the anatomic basis for a close functional cooperation between the two structures. Through its relationship with the reticular formation and its descending reticulospinal pathways, the vestibular system apparently has an alternate route whereby it can influence the motor neurons in the spinal cord (Fig. 142).

Cerebellum

The vestibulocerebellar connections are discussed in Chapter 9. One of the most prominent connections is the one that originates in the "spinocerebellum" and terminates in the lateral vestibular nucleus, which in turn projects to the spinal cord through the lateral vestibulospinal tract. This provides an important route for cerebellar regulation of muscular tone.

Eye Muscle Nuclei

The connections between the vestibular nuclei and the various oculomotor centers by way of the *medial longitudinal fasciculus* (MLF) provide the anatomic substrate for the important *vestibulo-ocular reflex,* i.e., conjugate eye movement in response to vestibular stimulation. The MLF is a complicated bundle, which is located close to the midline underneath the cerebral aqueduct and the floor of the fourth ventricle. It extends from the upper part of the brain stem to the cervical cord, and it is related to the various oculomotor centers, the vestibular nuclei, the motor nuclei of the accessory nerve (XI), and motor neurons of the cervical cord.

The majority of the fibers in the MLF arise from the vestibular nuclear complex, especially from the superior and medial vestibular nuclei (Fig. 142). The fibers from the superior nucleus ascend ipsilaterally and terminate in oculomotor centers of both sides. The fibers from the medial nucleus generally cross over to the opposite side, where some ascend to the oculomotor centers on both sides and others descend to the cervical spinal cord as the *medial vestibulospinal tract.* The descending part of the MLF, therefore, represents yet another pathway whereby the vestibular system can influence the motor apparatus of the spinal cord, especially those parts responsible for the postural adjustment of head and neck in response to vestibular stimulation.

Body Orientation and Postural Reflexes

Maintenance of balance and orientation in space is critically dependent on the vestibular apparatus, which triggers a series of important reflexes including vestibulospinal and vestibulo-ocular reflexes. Many other reflex mechanisms, however, serve to maintain the equilibrium of the body in space. Visual impulses and proprioceptive impulses from muscles, tendons, and joints are of special importance for initiating a number of *body-orienting and postural reflexes.* We are usually unaware of these functions, which are being coordinated primarily by centers in the brain stem.

Nystagmus

Nystagmus, i.e., oscillating movements of the eye, is a frequent manifestation of neurologic disease (see below), and spontaneous nystagmus is always pathologic. However, it can also be induced as part of a neurologic examination, e.g., by irrigating the external auditory meatus with warm or cold water, i.e., *caloric nystagmus.*

Clinical Notes

Vertigo, i.e., a sense of rotation, either of the individual or the environment, is a common symptom in disorders of the vestibular system, especially the labyrinth. The most typical example of labyrinthine vertigo is caused by *Meniere's disease,* which is characterized by abrupt and severe attacks of vertigo, often combined with tinnitus and increasing deafness. *Rhythmic nystagmus,* with alternating slow and quick movements of the eyeballs, is present during the attack, which can last for minutes or hours. The disease is caused by an overproduction of endolymph.

Vertigo can also indicate a lesion of the VIIIth cranial nerve, such as *acoustic neuroma* (see Clinical Examples: Cerebellopontine angle tumor), in which it is often preceded by tinnitus and deafness. A lesion of the vestibular nuclei, on the other hand, usually produces vertigo without loss of hearing.

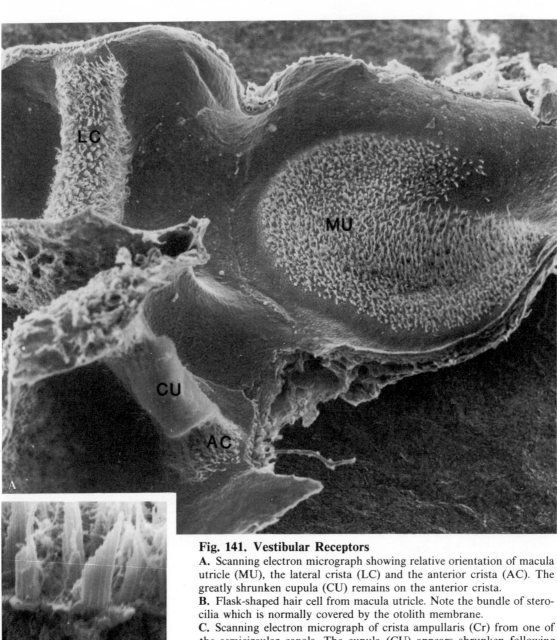

Fig. 141. Vestibular Receptors
A. Scanning electron micrograph showing relative orientation of macula utricle (MU), the lateral crista (LC) and the anterior crista (AC). The greatly shrunken cupula (CU) remains on the anterior crista.
B. Flask-shaped hair cell from macula utricle. Note the bundle of stereocilia which is normally covered by the otolith membrane.
C. Scanning electron micrograph of crista ampullaris (Cr) from one of the semicircular canals. The cupula (CU) appears shrunken following fixation and preparation for scanning electron microscopy.
(The three micrographs were kindly provided by Dr. Ivan Hunter-Duvar, Hospital for Sick Children, University of Toronto, Canada.)

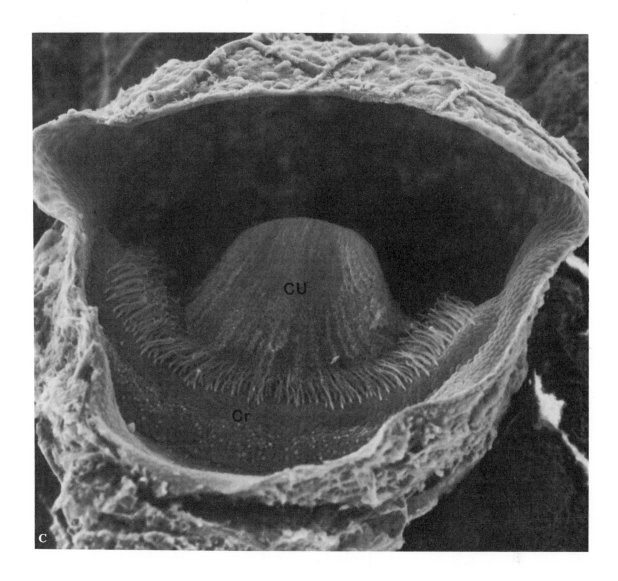

C

GLOSSOPHARYNGEAL (IX) AND VAGUS (X) NERVES

The IXth and Xth cranial nerves are closely related both anatomically and physiologically, and they innervate in part the same structures. The vagus, further, innervates the thoracic and abdominal viscera, and is the most important parasympathetic nerve of the body. The nerves emerge on the lateral side of the medulla dorsal to the olive and leave the skull through the jugular foramen together with the accessory nerve (XI).

Functional Anatomy

Somatic Motor Part

Both the glossopharyngeal and vagus nerves contain fibers that originate in the *nucleus ambiguus* and that innervate the striated muscles of the pharynx. Vagus, in addition, innervates the larynx. The stylopharyngeal muscle is innervated by the glossopharyngeal nerve.

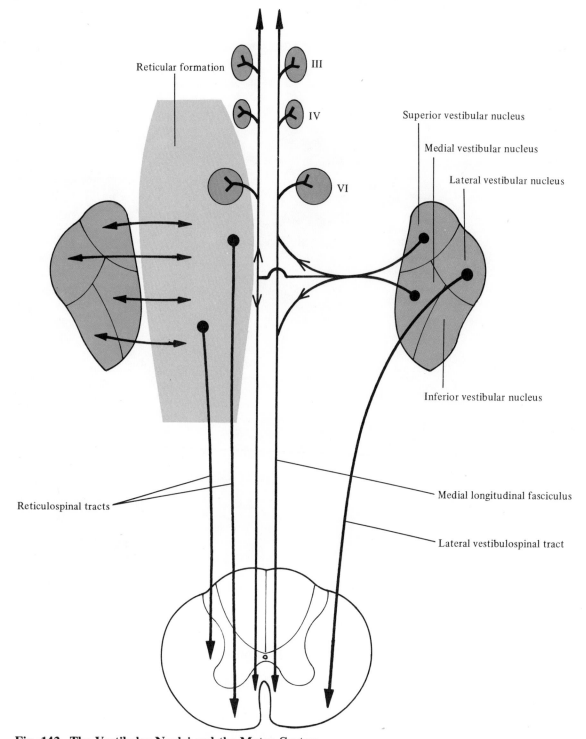

Fig. 142. The Vestibular Nuclei and the Motor System
Highly schematic drawing of the major efferent connections of the vestibular nuclei. The vestibulocerebellar connections have been deleted for didactic purposes.

Parasympathetic Part

Fibers from the *inferior salivatory nucleus* join the glossopharyngeal nerve and supply the parotid gland and pharyngeal glands with secretory fibers. The *dorsal motor nucleus of vagus,* which is located underneath the vagal trigone in the floor of the rhomboid fossa, supplies the thoracic and abdominal viscera with visceromotor and secretory fibers (Fig. 167. Chapter 16).

Sensory Part

Most of the afferent fibers in the glossopharyngeal and vagus nerves convey visceral impulses from the pharynx, soft palate, posterior third of the tongue, tonsils, and tympanic cavity (glossopharyngeal nerve with cell bodies in the petrous ganglion) and from the thorax, abdomen, pharynx, and larynx (vagus nerve with cell bodies in the nodose ganglion). The fibers terminate in the *nucleus of the solitary tract,* which also receives taste impulses from the posterior third of the tongue. Both the IXth and Xth cranial nerves contain somatic sensory fibers from the *external auditory meatus.*

Reflexes

The glossopharyngeal and vagus nerves participate in many important reflexes, e.g., *respiratory and cardiovascular reflexes* (Chapter 16). Swallowing, vomiting, and coughing are other important reflex mechanisms, which in part involve the IXth and Xth cranial nerves.

Swallowing

Stimulation of the pharynx or the back of the tongue initiates swallowing movements, i.e., a series of complicated reflexes that serve to introduce food and drink into the digestive tract. The most important afferent impulses are carried in the glossopharyngeal and vagus nerves to the nucleus of the solitary tract and nearby regions in the reticular formation, which coordinate the mechanisms involved in swallowing. The food is moved into the esophagus by the action of the tongue (hypoglossal nerve) and the palatal and pharyngeal muscles (glossopharyngeal and vagus nerves).

Vomiting

This is a protective mechanism whereby the gastric content is rapidly ejected through contraction of the abdominal muscle coupled with relaxation of the cardiac sphincter and esophagus. The concomitant closure of the glottis prevents aspiration of vomitus into the trachea. Irritation of the mucosa of the upper gastrointestinal tract gives rise to impulses that reach the nucleus of the solitary tract through the glossopharyngeal and vagus nerves. The vomiting response, which consists of a series of complicated somatic and visceral mechanisms, is coordinated by a "vomiting center" in the medulla oblongata. Efferent impulses to motor neurons of the spinal cord are responsible for contraction of the diaphragm and the abdominal muscles, whereas the autonomic innervation through one of the splanchnic nerves contracts the pylorus.

Vomiting can also be triggered by chemical substances in the bloodstream, e.g., apomorphine. The chemosensitive zone is apparently located in or near *area postrema,* which is "outside the blood–brain barrier" and therefore more permeable to many substances in the blood than the rest of the CNS. Area postrema is closely related to the "vomiting center."

Coughing

Irritation of the mucosa in the respiratory pathways elicits a cough response. The afferent impulses travel in the glossopharyngeal and vagus nerves to the nucleus of the solitary tract. The response is mediated through many channels. Motor impulses are mediated through the glossopharyngeal, vagus, and hypoglossal nerves to the pharynx, larynx, and tongue, and other impulses reach the spinal motor neurons that innervate the diaphragm, intercostal, and abdominal muscles.

Clinical Notes

Since both the glossopharyngeal and vagus nerves receive innervation from the cerebral cortex on both sides, supranuclear lesions, e.g., tumors and bleeding in the cerebral hemispheres, do not affect the functions of these nerves if they occur on one side only. Nuclear and intranuclear lesions, however, do give rise to specific symptoms, and since the glossopharyngeal and vagus nerves are closely related both in their intramedullary as well as in the first part of their extramedullary course, they are often affected together by the same lesion.

The main symptoms of a glossopharyngeal nerve lesion is loss of sensibility and taste sensation in the posterior third of the tongue, whereas interruption of the vagus nerve has more widespread, but not necessarily alarming, consequences consisting primarily of transitory difficulties in articulation and swallowing. A bilateral vagus paralysis, on the other hand, is devastating.

Recurrent Laryngeal Nerve Lesion

The recurrent laryngeal nerve (X), which supplies all intrinsic muscles of the larynx except the cricothyroid, is easily damaged by tumors in the neck (e.g., thyroid tumor, metastatic lesions) or by aneurysms of the aortic arch. The voice is initially like a whisper or hoarse. The intact vocal cord, however, usually adapts to the condition with return of fairly normal voice, and the vocal cord paralysis can then be revealed only by a *laryngoscopic examination.*

ACCESSORY NERVE (XI)

The XIth cranial nerve, which is purely motor, innervates the sternocleidomastoid and trapezius muscles. It is customary to divide the XIth cranial nerve into a spinal and a cranial part. The spinal part, which originates in anterior horn cells of the first five cervical segments of the spinal cord, enters the skull through the foramen magnum and joins the cranial part, which comes from the nucleus ambiguus and emerges from the brain together with the vagus nerve. The two parts leave the skull through the jugular foramen. However, since the cranial part soon rejoins the vagus nerve, it is more appropriate to refer to the cranial part as an aberrant vagus fascicle.

HYPOGLOSSAL NERVE (XII)

Functional Anatomy

The hypoglossal nucleus, which is located underneath the hypoglossal trigone in the floor of the fourth ventricle, innervates the muscles of the tongue. The fibers emerge from the medulla between the pyramid and olive as a series of 10–12

rootlets, which quickly come together as the hypoglossal nerve. The nerve leaves the skull through the hypoglossal canal.

Fibers from the first and second cervical nerves join the hypoglossal nerve and form the *ansa hypoglossi* together with the third cervical nerve. Branches from the ansa innervates the infrahyoid muscles.

Clinical Notes

Damage to the hypoglossal nerve results in paresis or paralysis of the ipsilateral half of the tongue. The paralysis can be easily demonstrated by asking the patient to protrude the tongue, which deviates toward the side of the lesion.

Although a hemiparalysis of the tongue can also result from a lesion of the hypoglossal nucleus, *nuclear lesions* are usually bilateral because of the close proximity of the right and left nucleus. *Chronic bulbar palsy* is a serious motor disorder that results from progressive degeneration of the motor nuclei in the medulla oblongata. A gradually worsening dysarthria and difficulties in swallowing are typical symptoms.

Since the hypoglossal nucleus receives corticobulbar fibers only from the contralateral hemisphere, a patient with *capsular hemiplegia* also suffers from a hypoglossal paralysis on the hemiplegic side.

CLINICAL EXAMPLES

Bell's Palsy

A 25-year-old healthy female was recovering from a mild upper respiratory infection when she awoke one morning and noticed that the right side of her face felt "pulled." While washing her hair that morning, she was bothered by the soap that kept coming into her right eye. Many sounds in her environment seemed excessively loud in her right ear.

Examination the next day showed moderate weakness of all facial muscles on the right side of her face. She could not taste well on the anterior surface of the right half of the tongue.

On the assumption that this patient suffered from Bell's palsy, i.e., acute peripheral facial paralysis, she was treated with steroids and her condition improved slowly.

Six weeks later a routine examination revealed that when she depressed her right eyelid the corner of her right mouth elevated slightly. In addition, she reported that tasting certain spices caused tearing from her right eye. The sense of taste on the right anterior surface of her tongue remained impaired.

1. This patient did indeed suffer from an acute neuropathy of the facial nerve. What part of the nerve was damaged?

2. When a damaged peripheral nerve regenerates, frequently the reinnervation does not totally follow the original pathways (aberrant reinnervation). What is the evidence for aberrant reinnervation in this case, and which branches of the facial nerve were involved in the process?

Discussion

Bell's palsy, or peripheral facial paralysis of unknown etiology, accounts for about 80% of all cases of facial palsy. It frequently follows exposure to cold on one side of the face or a mild viral respiratory infection.

Facial paralysis and taste deficit indicate that both the motor and sensory roots of VII are involved, and the hyperacusis reveals that the nerve was damaged proximal to the branch innervating the stapedius muscle (see Fig. 138).

As the damaged nerve recovered and reinnervation took place, the patient developed synkinesis or abnormal associated movements. In addition, there must have been damage at the level of the geniculate ganglion where parasympathetic fibers from the nervous intermedius leave the ganglion and travel in the greater superficial petrosal nerve. This is witnessed by the fact that the patient developed the "crocodile tear phenomenon" in which strong taste sensations produce involuntary lacrimation on the same side as the Bell's palsy. The phenomenon is believed to arise from regenerating autonomic fibers that should have reinnervated the salivary glands, but instead reinnervated the lacrimal glands.

Mediobasal Mesencephalic Syndrome of Weber

A 40-year-old man was suffering from headache and visual disturbance. One month earlier he had developed both horizontal and vertical diplopia and a drooping right eyelid (ptosis). He experienced progressive difficulty focusing his right eye at the same time as the left side of his body became weaker.

Examination confirmed that his right pupil was widely dilated. The direct light reflex was abolished in the right eye but a normal consensual response was present in the left eye. His right eye, further, was externally rotated and could not be brought across the midline or moved vertically. Ptosis was also evident on the right side. His left eye had full excursions in all directions, and the remainder of his cranial nerve functions were normal.

Motor examination showed a moderate left hemiparesis with increased stretch reflexes and Babinski's sign on the left.

A CT brain scan demonstrated an enhancing spherical lesion along the right ventral surface of the mesencephalon, and a subsequent angiography showed a large aneurysm arising from the right posterior communicating artery near its origin from the right posterior cerebral artery.

1. What cranial nerve is damaged in this patient and does the location of the aneurysm explain the involvement of that nerve?

2. Why does he have a left hemiparesis?

3. You receive a phone call from the patient's family physician, who tells you that 6 months ago the patient's right pupil was 3 mm larger than his left pupil, but his right extraocular functions were all normal and he did not have any hemiparesis. Does this make sense?

Discussion

The combination of ipsilateral third nerve paresis and contralateral hemiparesis is known as Weber's syndrome and is indicative of unilateral dysfunction of mediobasal mesencephalon (Fig. 185). Although this syndrome was originally described in cases of midbrain infarction, the most common cause of Weber's syndrome is a mass lesion at the base of the midbrain, usually an enlarging posterior communicating artery aneurysm.

As the mass lesion expands the third nerve is compressed, resulting initially in pupillary dilation and then ocular motor paresis. If the mass continues to expand the adjacent cerebral peduncle is compressed, leading to a contralateral hemiparesis.

The pupillomotor fibers from the Edinger-Westphal nucleus are often the first fibers to be affected in a compression of the third nerve. The observation of pupillary dysfunction in the absence of extraocular dysfunction, therefore, makes good sense.

Brain Stem Hemorrhage

A 68-year-old woman with poorly controlled hypertension suddenly slumped to the ground and lost consciousness while shopping. She required assistance with respiration in the ambulance.

On examination in the Emergency Room, her blood pressure was 200/120. She appeared comatose with her eyes closed, and had no spontaneous movements. Her respiratory rate was depressed, and she was intubated and artificially ventilated. The neurologic examination showed pinpoint size pupils, and her corneal reflexes were absent bilaterally. Irrigation of either external ear canal with ice water caused no deviation of her eyes, i.e., her vestibulo-ocular reflex was absent. Her gag (pharyngeal) reflex was very weak. She responded with bilateral and symmetric extensor (decerebrate) posturing to painful stimuli, and Babinski's sign was present bilaterally.

An emergency enhanced CT scan was performed (see Fig.)

1. Where is the lesion?

2. Why were her pupils pinpoint in size?

3. Irrigation of ice water into the external ear canals (ice water calorics) is a commonly utilized tool to assess the connections between the vestibular and oculomotor nuclei. Why did her eyes not respond to this maneuver?

4. Occasionally, patients will survive this type of vascular catastrophe for varying periods of time, and they may even be able to respond to some written or spoken commands. Typically, the only response they are capable of making is elevating the eyelids or look upwards or downwards, but not laterally. This condition is sometimes known as the "locked in syndrome." Why should such patients be able to raise their eyelids voluntarily or look in a vertical direction?

Discussion

The lesion is a large, fairly symmetric hemorrhage in the pons. Intracranial hemorrhages typically occur in persons with chronic, poorly controlled hypertension in four characteristic locations: the lenticular nucleus, thalamus, pons, or cerebellum. In large pontine hemorrhages, the deficit is devastating because all long ascending and descending

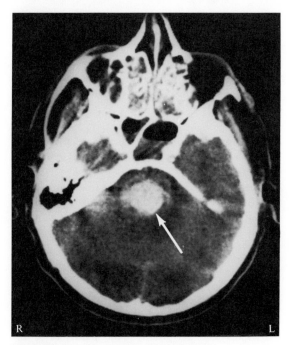

Fig. CE11A. Brainstem Hemorrhage
The CT scan was kindly provided by Dr. V. Haughton.

pathways including corticobulbar and corticospinal tracts are interrupted.

Patients with pontine hemorrhage have pinpoint pupils because the descending sympathetic fibers to the ciliospinal center are damaged with concomitant paralysis of the dilator pupillae muscles. However, the parasympathetic innervation (Edinger-Westphal nuclei and the third cranial nerves in the mesencephalon) to the pupillary constrictor muscles are not involved.

Damage to the vestibular nuclei or their connections with the oculomotor nuclei, i.e., the medial longitudinal fasciculus (Fig. 142), eliminates ice water caloric responses.

In the "locked in" syndrome, the mesencephalic centers for levator palpebrae superioris (third cranial nerve nuclei) and for vertical gaze are preserved. The supranuclear pathways innervating these structures are also intact. Thus, such patients are able to raise their eyelids and look up and down voluntarily, if consciousness is preserved. The pontine centers for lateral gaze, however, are damaged (see Fig. 135).

Lateral Medullary Syndrome of Wallenberg

A 65-year-old female with mild hypertension was suddenly struck with severe vertigo and inability to walk.

On examination her vision was normal. Extraocular movements were intact, but she had continuous lateral nystagmus, which increased when looking to her left. Her right corneal reflex could not be elicited by stroking the right cornea, but blinking occurred bilaterally when the left cornea was stimulated. Facial sensation to pain and temperature on the right was absent, but there was no facial weakness. Hearing was intact. There was weakness of her soft palate and the gag reflex was diminished. Horner's syndrome was present on the right side of her face. She had lost pain and temperature sensitivity over the left side of her body, but the muscle strength in her limbs seemed normal. Her balance was very poor and she drifted to the right upon sitting or standing. However, her limbs were not ataxic.

1. Where is this patient's lesion?

2. Why did the patient not blink in response to stimulation of the right cornea, and why could a response be elicited in both eyes by stimulating the left cornea?

3. What artery supplies the area of the brain involved in this patient's lesion?

Discussion

The patient has suffered an infarction involving the dorsolateral quadrant of her right rostral medulla (see Fig. 184). The areas involved and their corresponding clinical deficits include the vestibular nuclei and vestibulocerebellar connections (vertigo, nystagmus, and titubation), descending sympathic fibers (Horner's syndrome), descending tract and nucleus of V (ipsilateral facial sensory loss), spinothalamic tract (contralateral body pain and temperature loss), and frequently the nucleus ambiguus and the root fibers of IX and X (paralysis of soft palate and diminished gag reflex).

The corneal reflex was abolished on the right side because of damage to the spinal trigeminal nucleus on the right side. Stimulation of the left cornea, however, produces bilateral blinking and eye closure because the efferent limb of the reflex arc (facial nerve) is still intact on both sides.

Although Wallenberg's syndrome has often been said to be caused by occlusion of the posterior inferior cerebellar artery (PICA), recent investigations have shown that the syndrome is almost always caused by occlusion of the vertebral artery. Depending on the site of occlusion, the deficits may vary considerably from case to case. Most patients with this syndrome have a good prognosis and recover with little deficit.

Cerebellopontine Angle Tumor

A 65-year-old woman was first seen by her local physician 3 months prior to admission for evaluation of hearing loss on the right side. Her physician found fluid behind the right tympanic membrane and prescribed a decongestant, but the hearing did not improve significantly. About two months later, she noticed that the coordination in her right hand was reduced and was referred for neurologic evaluation.

On examination her vision, pupils, optic fundi, and extraocular movements were normal. Stimulation of her right cornea with a wisp of cotton did not elicit blinking or closure of the eyes, whereas stimulation of the left cornea produced blinking not only of the left eye but also of the right (consensual response). She did not taste salt or sugar well on the anterior surface of her tongue on the right side, but there was no significant weakness of her right facial muscles. She had a sensorineural type of hearing loss on the right side. The remainder of her cranial nerve examination was normal.

She had mild generalized weakness with some difficulty in maintaining muscle contractions in the right arm, and the muscle tone was reduced in the right arm and leg. The finger-to-nose test revealed a moderate ataxia in her right arm. She had difficulty with tandem gait and tended to veer off to the right side.

An axial CT scan (see figure next page) was obtained in order to provide an image through the posterior fossa.

1. Which cranial nerves are involved?

2. Why was the sense of taste on the right side of the tongue affected?

3. What type of lesion is most likely responsible for the symptoms?

4. What is the dark circular structure medial to the lesion? What parts of the brain lie directly above and below this structure?

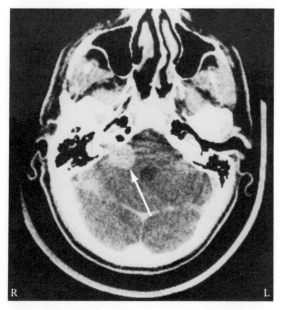

Fig. CE11B. Cerebellopontine Angle Tumor
The CT scan was kindly provided by Dr. V. Haughton.

5. What is the Y-shaped structure at the end of the arrow (away from the arrow head)?

Discussion

This patient's neurologic deficits involve the right Vth and VIIIth cranial nerves, as well as the intermediate nerve (VII) including especially the taste fibers to the anterior part of the tongue. Apparently, some of the cerebellar connections are also affected by the lesion.

The examination suggests an intracranial extra-axial lesion where the above-mentioned cranial nerves are very close to one another and to one of the cerebellar peduncles[1] (see Fig. 37). This places the lesion at the base of the skull along the clivus at the mid- to lower pons level, where the lesion would press on the middle cerebellar peduncle. There are two types of tumors that commonly arise in this location, acoustic neurinomas (or Schwannomas) and meningiomas. This patient had an *acoustic neurinoma,* which typically begins in the internal auditory canal and then grows me-

dially, involving the VIIIth, Vth, and VIIth cranial nerves, usually in that order.

An enhancing mass lesion at the porus acusticus is deforming the right side of the fourth ventricle, represented by the nearly circular dark area in the midline. The arms of the Y-shaped structure are the membranes of the tentorium cerebelli and the vertical portion of the Y is the falx cerebri. At the junction of the falx and tentorium (center of the Y) there is a widened area of enhancement, which represents the straight sinus. Note also that the right external auditory canal (the left-hand side of the picture) is widened and outlined in toto. In addition, one can see nasal turbinates and adjacent maxillary sinuses.

Transtentorial Herniation

An 8-year-old boy was admitted to the hospital because of coma. He was one of many children in a family of itinerant farm workers. He had a history of frequent middle ear infections (otitis media), for which he received irregular medical care. One month before admission he developed a repeat attack of acute otitis media in his right ear, which resulted in localized right ear pain and fever. A physician prescribed an antibiotic which the patient took for only 2 days, after which his fever and pain lessened. He was well for the next week, but then began to complain of right-sided headaches that became progressively worse. On the morning of admission he was found by his parents to be very sleepy, could not be easily aroused, and was brought to the hospital.

On examination in the Emergency Room he was found to be comatose. He did not respond to visual stimuli (threats). His right pupil was dilated to 5 mm. and did not react to light, and papilledema was present in both eyes. His gag (pharyngeal) reflex was present, but reduced in intensity. With painful stimulation, he showed bilateral extensor posturing (decerebrate posturing), and it was noted that the right extremities were as weak as the left. He showed no spontaneous movements. Babinski's sign was present bilaterally. Near the end of the examination it was noted that the left pupil had become dilated and fixed, and both eyes showed lateral deviation.

An emergency CT brain scan demonstrated a large hypodense hemisphere lesion which caused a 10 mm. shift of the midline structures from right to left (see Fig. C). The picture is consistent with

---

1. Although the disappearance of the corneal reflex on the side of the lesion is often said to be due to compression of the fifth cranial nerve, a tumor in this location may also interfere with the corneal reflex by compressing the spinal tract of trigeminus.

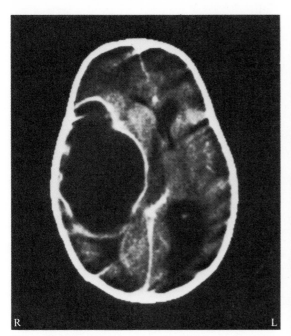

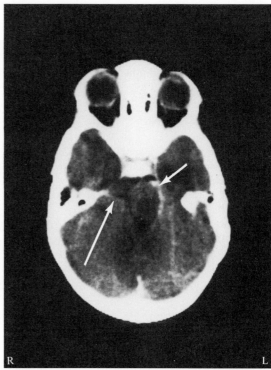

C

Fig. CE11C and D. Transtentorial Herniation
The CT scans were kindly provided by Dr. V. Haughton.

D

a very large brain abscess. On a lower CT scan
(Fig. D) part of the right temporal lobe (long arrow) was seen to press against the mesencephalon.
A linear enhancement, probably representing the
tentorial margin, is seen along the left lateral border of the mesencephalon (short arrow). An area
with decreased density, which could be consistent
with an infarct, was also seen within the central
substance of the mesencephalon just below the
inferior colliculi.

1. What part of the right temporal lobe is pressing
against the mesencephalon, and what membrane structure did it have to pass over to do so?
2. Which cranial nerve is related to the ocular abnormalities first seen in his right eye, and how did this
cranial nerve become damaged?
3. Why did the patient have papilledema?
4. Why was the patient paretic on the right side of
his body?

Discussion

This unfortunate boy demonstrates a common
clinical syndrome that results from a rapidly expanding mass lesion in the supratentorial compartment. In this case, a brain abscess, which ap-

parently arose from the middle ear infection,
developed in the right hemisphere. The abscess
grew so rapidly that the surrounding brain tissue
was unable to accommodate the increased volume,
resulting in a rapid rise in intracranial pressure.
Once a critical pressure had been reached, the medial part of the temporal lobe, including the uncus
and parahippocampal gyrus, herniated through the
tentorial notch and pressed against the lateral aspect of the mesencephalon on the right side (see
Fig. 30).

Damage to the IIIrd cranial nerve on the side
of the herniation caused ipsilateral pupillary dilation and later complete oculomotor paralysis. The
nerve, apparently, is either compressed by the herniating tissue or trapped between the posterior cerebral artery and the superior cerebellar artery as
the brain stem is displaced downward (see Fig.
32).

Bilateral papilledema is caused by increase in
intracranial pressure.

If the herniation is particularly severe, the mesencephalon is pressed laterally against the contralateral edge of the tentorium, which may result
in a hemorrhagic infarct. The bleeding and the
pressure on the base of the left cerebral peduncle

may cause damage to the corticospinal tract, which could explain the paresis ipsilateral to the side of the herniation (false localizing sign). Ultimately, both oculomotor nerves become paralyzed.

Transtentorial herniation is always a very seri-ous matter regardless of the cause. Hemorrhagic infarction of the brain stem due to increased intra-cranial pressure is rarely, if ever, compatible with survival.

SUGGESTED READING

1. Baloh, R. W. and V. Honrubia, 1979. Clinical Neurophysiology of the Vestibular System. F. A. Davis: Philadelphia.

2. Brodal, A., 1965. The Cranial Nerves. Anatomy and Anatomico-Clinical Correlations, 2nd ed. Blackwell: Oxford.

3. Brodal, A., 1981. Neurological Anatomy in Relation to Clinical Medicine, 3rd ed. Oxford University Press: New York, pp. 448–575.

4. Sears, E. S. and G. M. Franklin, 1979. Diseases of the Cranial Nerves. In: The Science and Practice of Clinical Medicine, Vol. 5: Neurology (R. N. Rosenberg, ed.). Grune & Stratton: New York, pp. 471–494.

12
Auditory System

EXTERNAL AND MIDDLE EAR
   Middle Ear Ossicles: A Mechanical
     Transformer
   Middle Ear Muscles and Middle Ear Reflex

INNER EAR
   The Cochlea
   Organ of Corti and Mechanism of Transduction
   Tonotopic Organization: Pitch Discrimination
   Innervation of the Auditory Receptors

CENTRAL AUDITORY PATHWAYS
   The Cochlear Nuclei
   Trapezoid Body, Lateral Lemniscus, and
     Auditory Radiation
   Superior Olivary Complex: Localization of
     Sound in Space
   Auditory Cortex

FUNCTIONAL ASPECTS
   Pitch Discrimination
   Intensity Discrimination
   Sound Localization
   Centrifugal Modulation of Auditory Input

CLINICAL NOTES
   Test of Hearing
   Otosclerosis
   Acoustic Neurinoma
   Hereditary Deafness

SUGGESTED READING

The auditory system has a great analytical capacity. The pitch and intensity of sound can be determined with great accuracy, and the ear can differentiate between sounds of different quality, i.e., different voices and musical instruments. The anatomic substrate for these amazing functions consists of an intricate receptor apparatus, the cochlea, in the inner ear, and a series of complicated pathways and CNS structures that have been extensively studied in recent years.

Hearing and speech constitute some of the most important means of communication, and deafness is a great handicap in social behavior. It is a gigantic medical problem because 10% of the population suffer from significant hearing loss.

The internal ear is related to hearing and equilibrium, and its sensory organs, the cochlea and the vestibular apparatus, are innervated by the vestibulocochlear nerve (VIII). The vestibular apparatus and the vestibular division of the VIIIth cranial nerve is described in relation to the other cranial nerves in Chapter 11.

The cochlear division is part of the auditory system, which informs us about sounds in the environment. Sound is propagated as pressure waves, and the *pitch* of the sound is determined by the frequency of the sound waves, expressed in cycles per second (cps).[1] The *intensity* of the sound is related to the amplitude of the waves, and it is measured in decibels (db).[2]

EXTERNAL AND MIDDLE EAR

The external ear, the *auricle* (pinna) and the *external auditory canal* (meatus), direct the sound waves to the *tympanic membrane,* or eardrum, which serves as a boundary between the external and the middle ear (Figs. 140 and 143). The air-filled cavity of the middle ear, the *tympanic cavity,* which contains the three ossicles, is connected to the pharynx through the *eustachian tube.* The tube is normally closed, but it opens during swallowing, thereby permitting equilibration of air pressure on the two sides of the eardrum.

Middle Ear Ossicles: A Mechanical Transformer

The three ossicles, the *malleus* (hammer), *incus* (anvil), and *stapes* (stirrup), form a bridge between the eardrum and the oval window of the inner ear (Fig. 143), and they are joined in such a way that they transmit the oscillations of the eardrum to the footplate of the stapes, which is attached to the oval window by an annular ligament. By channeling the energy of vibration of the large

eardrum to the much smaller area of the oval window, the ossicular chain produces the additional force required to set the fluid of the cochlea in motion.

Middle Ear Muscles and Middle Ear Reflex

The position and tension of the auditory ossicles can be regulated by two muscles, the *tensor tympani* and *stapedius,* which attach to the malleus and the stapes, respectively. The tensor tympani is innervated by the motor trigeminal nucleus and the stapedius by the facial nucleus. The muscles respond in a reflectoric manner to various stimuli, especially to loud noise.

The reflectoric contraction of the middle ear muscles, known as the *acoustic middle ear reflex,* decreases the sound transmission through the middle ear by making the ossicular chain more rigid. The middle ear reflex is a protective mechanism against excessive stimulation, which can easily cause damage to the sensitive receptors or hair cells in the inner ear. The reflex may, in addition, have more subtle functions designed to improve speech discrimination in noisy environments. For instance, the reflex is more efficient in the low-frequency range, and it may therefore reduce the masking of high frequencies by low-frequency sounds.

INNER EAR

The Cochlea

The auditory part of the inner ear, the *cochlea,* is shaped like a snail shell (Fig. 144), and it contains perilymph like the other spaces of the *bony labyrinth,* the vestibule, and the semicircular canals. The *osseus cochlea* is coiled around a bony core, the *modiolus,* which contains the ganglion cells of the cochlear portion of the VIIIth cranial nerve. Inside the osseus cochlea is the *membranous cochlea* or *cochlear duct,* which contains endolymph, and which is attached to a thin bony shelf, the *spiral lamina,* which winds around the modiolus like the threads of a screw. Since the cochlear duct is broadly attached to the lateral wall of the osseus cochlea as well, it divides the bony canal into an upper compartment, *scala vestibuli,* and a lower compartment, *scala tympani* (Fig. 145A).

---

1. The human ear can detect sound waves with frequencies between 20–16,000 cps or Hz (Hertz). The human ear has the greatest sensitivity for sounds around 1000 Hz. The greater the frequency, the higher the pitch.
2. Normal conversation at 3 feet is usually carried on with an intensity of 60–70 db. The noise from a jet engine at close range has an intensity of 120–140 db, which is close to the limit of the human ear. Since the intensity scale is logarithmic, the jet engine noise has an intensity that is many thousand times higher than the normal conversation voice.

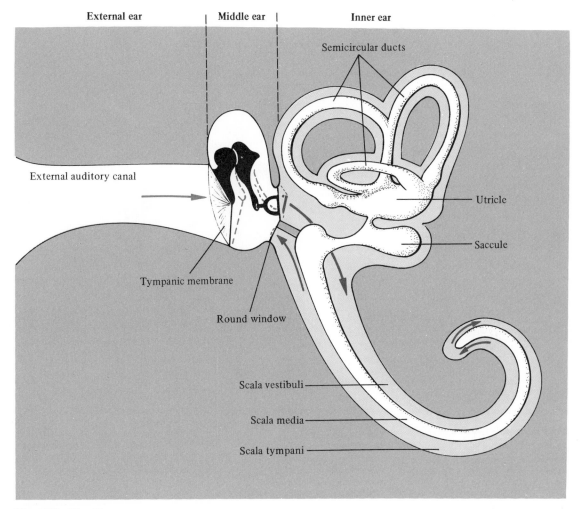

Fig. 143. The Ear

Diagram of the external, middle, and inner ear. The middle ear ossicles, the malleus, incus, and stapes, are *black*. The extreme positions to which the ossicles can be moved by oscillations of the eardrum as a result of incoming sound waves are indicated by *red*. The cochlea has been partly uncoiled to show the fluid movement in the perilymph (*red arrows*). The fluid motions that originate at the oval window by movement of the stapes are dissipated at the round window (Modified from Klinke, R. Physiology of Hearing. In: Fundamentals of Sensory Physiology (Ed. R. F. Schmidt), 1978. Springer-Verlag, New York, Heidelberg, Berlin).

The cochlear duct, which lies between the two bony compartments, is referred to as *scala media.* Since the cochlear duct ends as a closed sac, there is an opening, *helicotrema,* at the apex of the cochlea, where the scala tympani and scala vestibuli communicate with each other.

Organ of Corti and Mechanism of Transduction

The organ of Corti (Fig. 145), which contains the auditory receptors, is located on the upper surface of the *basilar membrane*. This membrane, which forms the floor of the cochlear duct, is a crucial component in the mechanism that finally transduces the mechanical energy of the sound waves to chemoelectrical potentials. The sound vibrations that enter the scala vestibuli and the perilymph at the oval window produce displacement of the basilar membrane before they finally dissipate back to the middle ear by movements of the membrane covering the round window. Oscillations of the basilar membrane produce a shearing force on the cilia of the receptor cells, which are in firm contact with the nonoscillating gelatinous

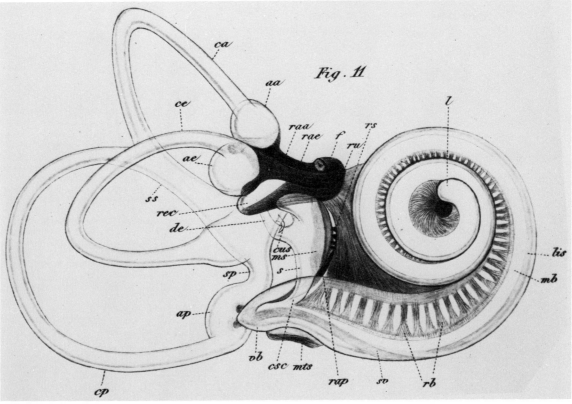

Abbreviations

rec = Utricular recess	cp = Posterior semicircular duct	mb = Basal membrane
aa = Anterior ampulla	cus = Utriculosaccular canal	l = Cupula
ae = External ampulla	s = Sacculus	raa = Ramulus of the anterior ampulla
ap = Posterior ampulla	de = Eudolymphatic duct	rac = Ramulus of the lateral ampulla
ca = Anterior semicircular duct	csc = Ductus reuniens	rap = Ramulus of the posterior ampulla
ce = Lateral semicircular duct	vb = Vestibular caecum	rs = Ramulus of the saccules
	sv = Stria vascularis	f = Facial nerve
	lis = Spinal ligament	ms = Macula of the sacculus

Fig. 144. The Inner Ear

Drawing of the inner ear in a 5-month human embryo (From Gustav Retzius, 1884, Das Gehörorgan der Wirbelthiere, Vol. II, Samson & Wallin, Stockholm).

Fig. 145. The Organ of Corti   ▷

A. Drawing of a cross section through one turn of the cochlea (Courtesy of J. Kálmánfi)

B. Diagrammatic cross section through the cochlear duct with the organ of Corti and closeup views of an inner and an outer hair cell. Afferent nerve fibers are indicated by fully drawn lines and by dots where transected; terminal swellings are undotted. The efferent nerve fibers are stippled and shown as open circles when transected. Their terminal swellings are finely dotted. The intraganglionic and inner spiral bundles are composed of efferent fibers; the outer spiral bundle of afferent fibers. Note the inverse relationship of afferent and efferent nerve terminals on inner and outer hair cells. (From Brodal, A., 1981. Neurological Anatomy, Third edition. With permission of the author and Oxford University Press.)

C. Scanning electron micrograph of the organ of Corti of a guinea pig. The tectorial membrane has been removed in order to illustrate the stereocilia, which are normally imbedded in the tectorial membrane. (Micrograph courtesy of G. Bredberg. From Nolte, J., 1981. The Human Brain. With permission of C. V. Mosby Company, St. Louis, Toronto-London.)

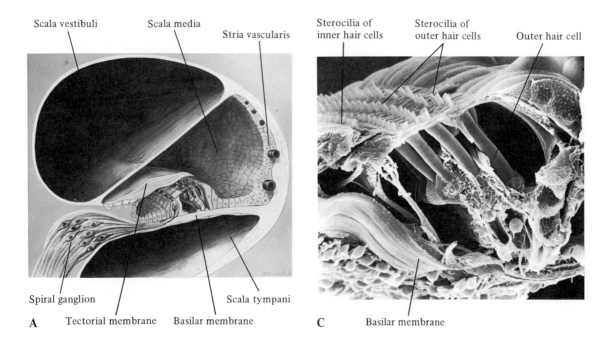

A

Scala vestibuli
Scala media
Stria vascularis
Spiral ganglion
Tectorial membrane
Basilar membrane
Scala tympani

C

Sterocilia of inner hair cells
Sterocilia of outer hair cells
Outer hair cell
Basilar membrane

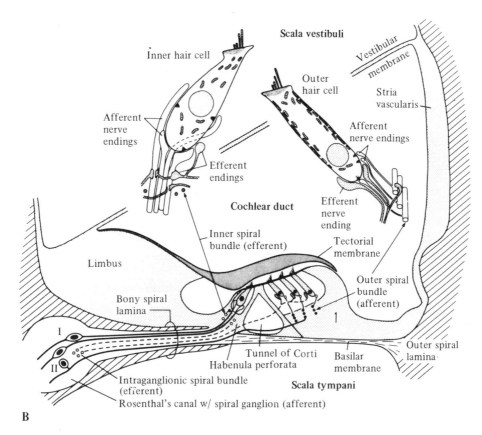

Scala vestibuli
Inner hair cell
Outer hair cell
Vestibular membrane
Stria vascularis
Afferent nerve endings
Efferent endings
Afferent nerve endings
Cochlear duct
Efferent nerve ending
Inner spiral bundle (efferent)
Tectorial membrane
Limbus
Bony spiral lamina
Outer spiral bundle (afferent)
I
II
Tunnel of Corti
Habenula perforata
Basilar membrane
Outer spiral lamina
Scala tympani
Intraganglionic spiral bundle (efferent)
Rosenthal's canal w/ spiral ganglion (afferent)

B

tectorial membrane. The tilting of the stiff cilia, apparently, is the adequate stimulus for the auditory receptor cells.

Tonotopic Organization: Pitch Discrimination

A very important feature of the displacement mechanism of the basilar membrane is the fact that different parts of the membrane respond with maximal efficiency to different frequencies. High-frequency sounds produce maximal displacement of the basal part of the membrane, whereas progressively lower frequencies involve more and more apical parts of the membrane. The reason for this is primarily related to the fact that the elastic fibers that form the membrane are relatively short at the base of the cochlea, but become progressively longer toward the apex. In other words, the basilar membrane is wider at the apex of the cochlea than at the base.

The basilar membrane is lined with two groups of hair cells along the length of the cochlear duct: a single row of *inner hair cells* and several rows of *outer hair cells.* The two types of hair cells can be distinguished morphologically, and show striking differences in patterns of innervation (see below). Therefore, they are likely to serve different functions, but little is known in this regard. Since different parts of the basilar membrane stimulate a specific set of inner and outer hair cells, the spatial representation of frequency, i.e., tonotopicity, is preserved in the transduction mechanism. Indeed, the principle of tonotopic organization characterizes the entire central auditory pathway (see below).

Innervation of the Auditory Receptors

The hair cells are innervated by afferent fibers of the cochlear nerve and by efferent fibers of the olivocochlear bundle.

The *cochlear nerve* is formed by the central processes of the bipolar ganglion cells, which are located in the spiral ganglion of the modiolus. The nerve passes through the internal auditory canal together with the vestibular and facial nerves and enters the brain stem at the pontomedullary junction (Fig. 37 in dissection guide). The peripheral processes of the spiral ganglion cells proceed to the organ of Corti, where the large majority of fibers (about 90%) innervate the relatively small population of inner hair cells.

The neural events that are transmitted to the CNS through the cochlear nerve can be modulated by a centrifugal fiber system, the *olivocochlear bundle.* The axons of this pathway originate in the *superior olivary complex* in the pons (Fig. 128, Chapter 10) and terminate on the base of the hair cells. The function of the olivocochlear bundle is most likely to increase the "signal-to-noise" ratio by suppressing unwanted auditory signals.

CENTRAL AUDITORY PATHWAYS

The Cochlear Nuclei

The cochlear nerve enters the *ventral cochlear nucleus* on the ventrolateral side of the inferior cerebellar peduncle. The nerve fibers bifurcate within the nucleus, and one branch terminates within the ventral nucleus, whereas the other branch proceeds to the *dorsal cochlear nucleus* on the dorsolateral aspect of the inferior cerebellar peduncle.

The cochlear nuclei contain many different cell types, which can be distinguished on the basis of their electrophysiologic properties and specific connections. The most important principle of organization, however, is the fact that the cochlear nerve fibers terminate in a strict *cochleotopic* or *tonotopic* pattern within the various subdivisions of the cochlear nucleus. This tonotopicity, which is based on a spatial organization of the neurons involved, is maintained throughout the central auditory pathways.

Trapezoid Body, Lateral Lemniscus, and Auditory Radiation

The central auditory connections from the cochlear nuclei to the auditory cortex in the temporal lobe are rather complicated, and they are illustrated schematically in Fig. 146. The axonal projections from the ventral cochlear nucleus form the *trapezoid body,* which crosses over to the other side of the brain stem in the ventral part of tegmentum and then ascends as the *lateral lemniscus* on the opposite side. Fibers from the dorsal cochlear nucleus reach the opposite side via the *dorsal acoustic stria.* Although some of the fibers in the

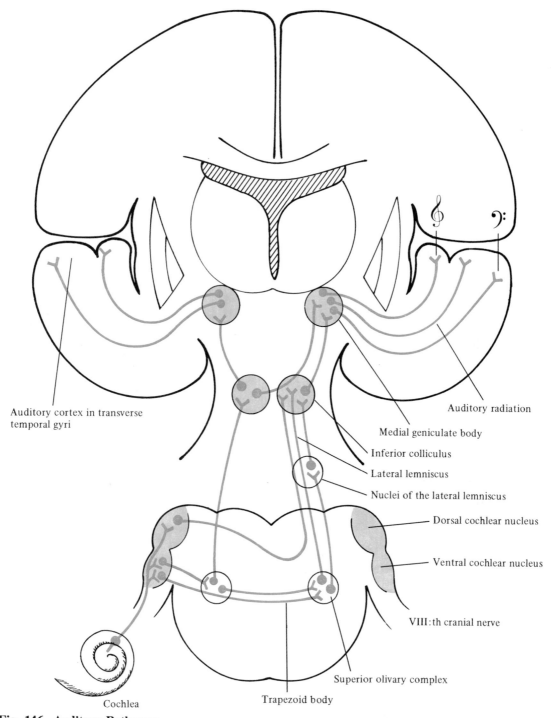

Auditory cortex in transverse
temporal gyri

Auditory radiation

Medial geniculate body

Inferior colliculus

Lateral lemniscus

Nuclei of the lateral lemniscus

Dorsal cochlear nucleus

Ventral cochlear nucleus

VIII:th cranial nerve

Superior olivary complex

Trapezoid body

Cochlea

Fig. 146. Auditory Pathways
Highly schematic diagram of the central auditory pathways. The centrifugal fibers, including the olivocochlear
bundle from the superior olivary complex to the organ of Corti, are not shown.

lateral lemniscus pass through the *inferior colliculus* to the *medial geniculate body* (Fig. 151), most of them establish synaptic contacts with inferior collicular cells, which in turn project through the brachium of the inferior colliculus to the medial geniculate body, the last relay in the auditory path to the cerebral cortex. The *auditory radiation,* i.e., the fibers from the medial geniculate body to the auditory cortex on the upper bank of the superior temporal gyrus, pass through the sublenticular part of the internal capsule.

The cochlear nuclei, inferior colliculus, and medial geniculate body are not merely relays in the auditory pathway; they represent complicated *integration centers* where information from many sources interact. The situation is further complicated by the fact that many other brain stem nuclei, e.g., the *superior olivary complex* and the *nuclei of the lateral lemniscus,* are intercalated in the auditory pathways. Undoubtedly, a considerable amount of information processing occurs before the auditory signals finally reach the auditory cortex.

Some of the secondary auditory fibers ascend in the lateral lemniscus without crossing the midline in pons, which means that the auditory cortex on one side receives impulses both from the contralateral and the ipsilateral ear. It should also be noted that a significant number of the fibers from the inferior colliculus project to the contralateral rather than the ipsilateral medial geniculate nucleus. Taken together, these anatomic features explain why restricted unilateral lesions of the ascending auditory pathways are of little consequence to hearing.

Superior Olivary Complex: Localization of Sound in Space

One of the cell groups in the superior olivary complex is of special importance for *sound localization.* The nucleus is populated by transversely oriented bipolar neurons with a lateral and a medial dendrite. The lateral dendrite receives auditory input from one ear and the medial dendrite from the other ear. These neurons, apparently, are sensitive to the time difference of auditory stimuli, which is one of the cues used to localize sound in space.

Auditory Cortex

The auditory cortex is located in the *transverse temporal gyri* (Heschl's gyri) and surrounding areas of the *planum temporale*[3] on the upper bank of the superior temporal gyrus. The auditory region, which is represented by Brodmann's cortical areas 41 and 42, is almost completely hidden in the depth of the lateral fissure. The tonal frequencies, represented by functional *frequency columns,* are organized in a *tonotopic pattern* with the highest frequencies represented in the medial part of planum temporale. Other sound variables, e.g., intensity and location, are apparently also represented by functional columns in the auditory cortex.

A wealth of association fibers connects the auditory cortex with a number of surrounding cortical regions, i.e., *auditory association areas,* located primarily on the dorsal and lateral aspects of the superior temporal gyrus, e.g., area 22 and Wernicke's area (Fig. 179).

FUNCTIONAL ASPECTS

The detection and analysis of sound involve very complicated mechanisms, which to some extent are reflected in the complicated anatomy of the auditory system. Many of the functional aspects of hearing are directly related to our ability to recognize and appreciate speech, and they are therefore of vital importance in our everyday life. The ability to discriminate between different frequencies and intensities of sound, or to localize the source of a sound, are important aspects of hearing.

Pitch Discrimination

A tonotopic organization, i.e., a spatial representation of tonal frequencies, is one of the most striking characteristics of the auditory pathway. The spatial separation of tones with different frequencies occurs in the cochlea, where the basal part of the organ of Corti is stimulated by high-frequency

---

3. Planum temporale, which contains part of Wernicke's speech area (Chapter 19), is usually much larger on the left side of the brain. This is most likely related to the linguistic dominance of the left hemisphere.

tones, whereas progressively lower frequencies involve more and more apical parts of the organ. A strict cochleotopic pattern is then preserved throughout the different relays in the auditory path to the cerebral cortex, where high-pitch tones are represented in the medial part of the auditory cortex close to the insula, whereas low-frequency sounds are represented in the lateral part, close to the lateral surface of the brain.

Although the auditory cortex is tonotopically organized, it does not seem to be absolutely essential for frequency discrimination. The analytic capacity of the auditory system, however, extends beyond the pure discrimination of tonal frequencies; we can effectively distinguish between different voices and different musical instruments and it is likely that the auditory cortex and its related association areas become increasingly involved in more subtle aspects of sound discrimination.

Intensity Discrimination

This type of discrimination, apparently, is dependent both on the number of auditory receptors stimulated and on the discharge rate in the individual nerve fibers. The cerebral cortex is not essential for intensity discrimination.

Sound Localization

This important function is dependent foremost on binaural representation in some of the auditory structures of the brain. A sound that comes from a specific direction will usually reach the two ears with slight time difference and with somewhat different intensity, and these two factors are important cues in sound localization. Consequently, deafness in one ear sharply reduces the ability to localize sound.

The central neural mechanisms responsible for localization of sound in space are not completely known; nor is it known to what extent the cerebral cortex is involved. It has been shown, however, that one of the cell groups in the *superior olivary complex* is populated by bipolar cells, with a medial and lateral dendrite. The two dendrites, further, receive input from opposite ears, which makes it possible for the neurons to register interaural time or intensity differences. The superior olivary complex and other structures with similar

features would seem to be likely candidates for functions related to sound localization.

Centrifugal Modulation of Auditory Input

A descending pathway from the auditory cortex to the medial geniculate body, the inferior colliculus, and the other auditory brainstem nuclei parallels the ascending auditory pathway. The final link in this centrifugal pathway is the *olivocochlear bundle* from the superior olivary complex to the auditory receptors in the organ of Corti. The functions of the centrifugal pathway are most likely to increase the "signal-to-noise" ratio and to sharpen the auditory information in different ways.

CLINICAL NOTES

Deafness is a problem of gigantic proportions. Ten percent of the population have hearing defects serious enough to interfere with the understanding of speech. Two types of deafness can be distinguished: (1) *conductive deafness* and (2) *sensorineural deafness.* The first type is related to defects in conductive mechanisms in the middle ear resulting from conditions such as otitis media and otosclerosis. Sensorineural deafness is caused by disease in the cochlea or its central connection, the auditory nerve (VIIIth cranial nerve). CNS lesions seldom cause abnormalities in hearing, since supranuclear auditory pathways are bilateral.

Tinnitus, i.e., noise (ringing, humming, whistling, etc.) in the ears, is a common symptom in disorders of the middle and inner ear, but it can also occur in disease of the VIIIth cranial nerve, e.g., acoustic neurinoma (see below). Even wax in the ears can cause tinnitus.

Tests of Hearing

Many simple procedures can be used to test hearing. A rough estimate can be obtained by recording the distance at which the patient is able to hear a whisper or a watch tick with one ear while the other ear is covered.

The *Rinne* test can be used to differentiate between conductive and sensorineural deafness. The stem of a vibrating tuning fork of 256 or 512 Hz frequency is placed on the mastoid process (bone conduction) until it is no longer heard by the patient, at which time the fork is held at the external auditory canal (air conduction). Since air conduction should be greater than bone conduction, the sound can be heard for about twice as long if the air conduction is intact (normal Rinne test). However, the sound cannot be heard if the air conduction is severely impaired by a middle ear disease (abnormal Rinne test). In partial nerve deafness the Rinne test is normal but both the bone and air conduction is quantitatively decreased.

More elaborate tests can be performed with sophisticated *audiometers*, which can present frequencies and intensities through the whole range of hearing.

Otosclerosis

This is the most common cause of conductive deafness in the adult. The disease usually starts in the second or third decade and is characterized by progressive ossification of the annular ligament around the base of the stapes, which eventually becomes fixed in its position in the oval window. Surgical procedures to replace the stapes usually result in a significant improvement in hearing.

Acoustic Neurinoma

The most common form of cerebellopontine angle tumor (see Clinical Examples, Chapter 11) is the acoustic neurinoma, which originates from Schwann's cells of the sheath surrounding the VIIIth cranial nerve in the internal auditory canal. The first symptom is usually tinnitus followed by hearing defects, loss of corneal reflex (Vth cranial nerve), and cerebellar signs.

Hereditary Deafness

Genetic abnormalities can cause a number of syndromes in which deafness is a prominent feature. Other defects associated with hereditary deafness include malformations of the external ear; albinism; ocular abnormalities; mental deficiencies; or neurologic abnormalities including progressive ophthalmoplegia, polyneuropathy, and cerebellar ataxia.

SUGGESTED READING

1. Brodal, A., 1981. Neurological Anatomy in Relation to Clinical Medicine, 3rd ed. Oxford University Press: New York, pp. 602–639.
2. Miller, J. M. and A. L. Towe, 1979. Audition: Structural and acoustical properties. In T. Ruch and H. D. Patton (eds.): Physiology and Biophysics, 20th ed. W. B. Saunders: Philadelphia, pp. 339–434.
3. Morest, D. K., 1975. Structural organization of the auditory pathways. In D. B. Tower (ed.): The Nervous System, Vol. 3: Human Communication and Its Disorders (E. L. Eagles, vol. ed.). Raven Press, New York, pp. 19–30.
4. Mountcastle, V. B., 1980. Central nervous mechanisms in hearing. V. B. Mountcastle, (ed.) Medical Physiology, 14th ed., Vol. 1. C. V. Mosby: St. Louis, Missouri, pp. 457–480.
5. Schubert, E. D., 1980. Hearing: Its Function and Dysfunction. Springer-Verlag: Wien, New York.

13
Visual System

THE RETINA
  Photoreceptors and Retinal Neurons
  Retinal Topography

VISUAL PATHWAYS
  Optic Nerve, Chiasm, and Tract
  Optic Radiation and Visual Cortex

FUNCTIONAL CONSIDERATIONS
  The Different Functions of Rods and Cones
  Topographic Organization of the Visual
    Pathway
  Brain Mechanisms of Vision
  Reflexes

CLINICAL NOTES
  Ophthalmoscopy: The Fundus Oculi
  Papilledema ("Choked Disc")
  Lesions of the Visual Pathways

CLINICAL EXAMPLE
  Internal Carotid Artery Aneurysm

SUGGESTED READING

The phenomenal development that has taken place in our understanding of the nervous system during the last few decades is due in large part to the discovery of sensitive methods for experimental investigations. This is especially well demonstrated in regard to the visual system, which has revealed many of its secrets to those who have used the methods wisely. The form and function of the retina, its fine structure and the biochemical processes involved in photoreception, have been elucidated. The central visual connections have been traced in great detail, and we are beginning to understand how the visual cortex processes the incoming signals. It is not unreasonable to believe that the day will come when the neural mechanisms underlying the perception of three dimensional forms and movements can be explained.

But the visual system takes on an added importance in clinical neurology. The visual pathways extend from the frontal end of the brain to the occipital pole, and they are therefore often involved in brain lesions. The pathways, furthermore, are highly organized and lesions in different parts produce characteristic symptoms, which often makes it possible to locate the pathologic process.

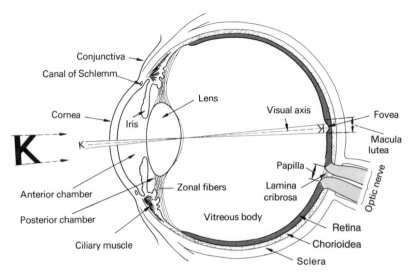

Fig. 147. The Eye
Horizontal section through the right eye. Retina is indicated with *red*. (From O. J. Grüsser and U. Grüsser-Cornehls. Physiology of Vision. In: Fundamentals of Sensory Physiology (Ed. R. F. Schmidt) Springer-Verlag. New York—Heidelberg, Berlin.)

The eye has many features in common with a camera. It is a hollow, transparent structure covered by a thick, fibrous coat, the *sclera* (Fig. 147). The rostral part of the coat, the *cornea,* is transparent and serves as the "window" of the eye. Together with the *lens,* the cornea forms part of the refractive system, which focuses light rays on the sensitive part of the eye, the *retina.* The *iris* controls the amount of incoming light by regulating the size of the *pupil;* it is analogous to the "f-stop" setting of a camera. Although the optic system of the eye is similar to that of a camera, the functions of the eye are considerably more intricate, and the comparison is especially weak in regard to the retina, which is infinitely more complicated than a film plate.

THE RETINA

Photoreceptors and Retinal Neurons

The sensory part of the eye, the retina, is an evaginated part of the forebrain and it is attached to the brain through a fiber tract referred to as the optic nerve. The visual receptors, the *rods* and *cones* (Fig. 148) are located in the deep portion of the retina in close contact with the *pigmented epithelium.* The pigment cells regulate the content of visual pigment in the outer segments of the receptor cells, where the receptor response is triggered. The two types of photoreceptors serve some-

what different functions. The rods are more sensitive to light than the cones and they enable us to see in dim light whereas the cones mediate color vision in brighter light. The cones, further, enable us to see sharp images, and the *fovea centralis,* i.e., the area of highest visual acuity, is populated by cones only. The line of vision, i.e., the *optic* (visual) *axis,* extends from the object, seen through the center of the pupil, to the fovea centralis. The relative distribution of rods and cones is characteristic in the sense that the concentration of cones decreases, while the concentration of rods increases, toward the periphery of the retina.

As a specialized part of the CNS, the retina contains several major classes of neurons besides the receptor cells (Fig. 149). *Bipolar neurons* transmit the impulses from the receptor cells to the *ganglion cells,* whose axons converge toward the *optic disc,* where the approximately 1 million optic nerve fibers leave the eye. The visual information transmitted from receptors via bipolar cells to ganglion cells is being modulated by interneurons, i.e., *horizontal* and *amacrine* (axonless) *cells,* which primarily provide for lateral transmission of information within the individual layers of the retina.

The capacity for special resolution is in part related to the extent of convergence in the pathway from receptor to ganglion cell. For instance, many of the cones in the region of the fovea centralis make synaptic contact with one bipolar cell, which

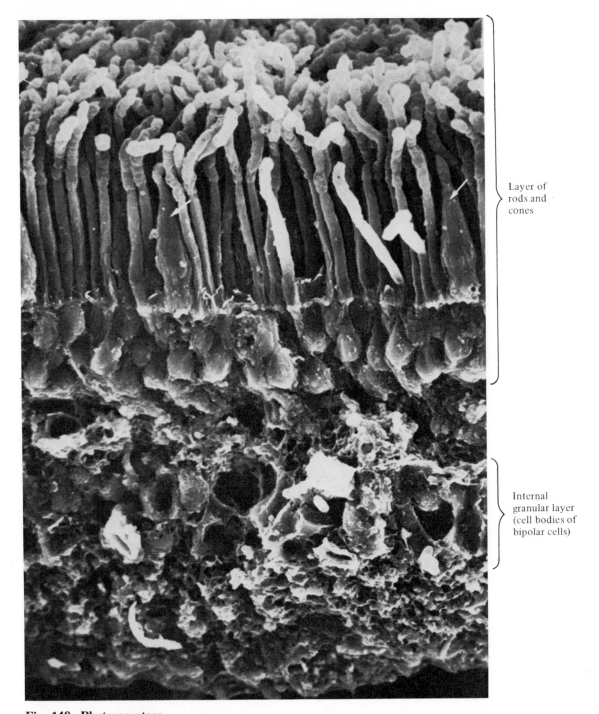

Layer of
rods and
cones

Internal
granular layer
(cell bodies of
bipolar cells)

Fig. 148. Photoreceptors
Scanning electron micrograph of a fractured retina from a Rhesus monkey. Note that most of the photoreceptors shown here are rods. Only a few cones (arrows) are seen. (From Fujita, T, K. Tanaka and J. Tokunaga, 1981. SEM Atlas of Cells and Tissues. With permission of the authors and Igaku-Shoin, Tokyo–New York. Micrograph courtesy of Dr. T. Masutani, Department of Anatomy, Fukuoka University School of Medicine, Japan.)

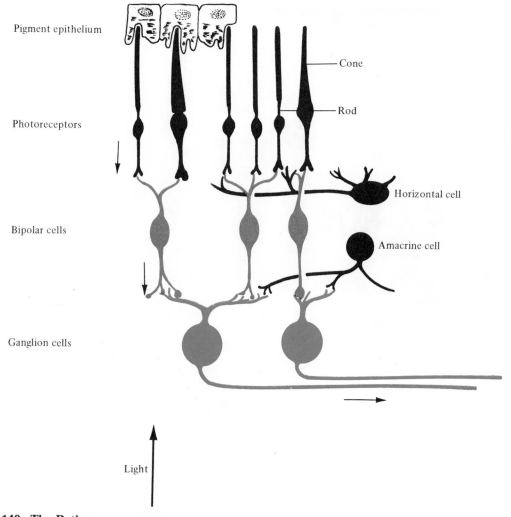

Pigment epithelium

Cone

Rod

Photoreceptors

Horizontal cell

Bipolar cells

Amacrine cell

Ganglion cells

Light

Fig. 149. The Retina
Highly schematic figure of the organization of retina. The photoreceptors as well as the interneurons, i.e., the horizontal and amacrine cells, are shown in *black*. Bipolar cells, *red;* ganglion cells, *blue.*

in turn is related to one ganglion cell. In regard to the rods, on the other hand, there is often convergence of impulses from several photoreceptors to one ganglion cell, and the convergence is especially pronounced in the peripheral part of the retina. The elaborate connections between the different retinal neurons indicate that a considerable amount of analysis of visual information takes place already in the retina.

Retinal Topography

The retina around the posterior pole of the eyeball, i.e., the *fundus oculi* (see Clinical Notes and Fig. 155), can be observed with the aid of an ophthalmoscope. The *optic disc* or *papilla* is a round or

slightly oval pale area of the retina where the optic nerve fibers leave the eye. The retinal vessels, which reach the eye through the optic nerve, radiate from the center of the disc. Since the region of the optic disc does not contain any receptor cells, it is referred to as the *blind spot* of the retina.

The blind spot in the right eye can be demonstrated by closing the left eye and fixating the right eye at a distant object. Hold a pencil at arm's length in front of the right eye and move it laterally from the line of fixation. The pencil disappears when its image passes across the blind spot.

The *fovea centralis,* i.e., the area of highest visual acuity, is a small pit in the center of the *macula lutea* (the yellow spot), which is slightly deeper in tint than the surrounding fundus. The

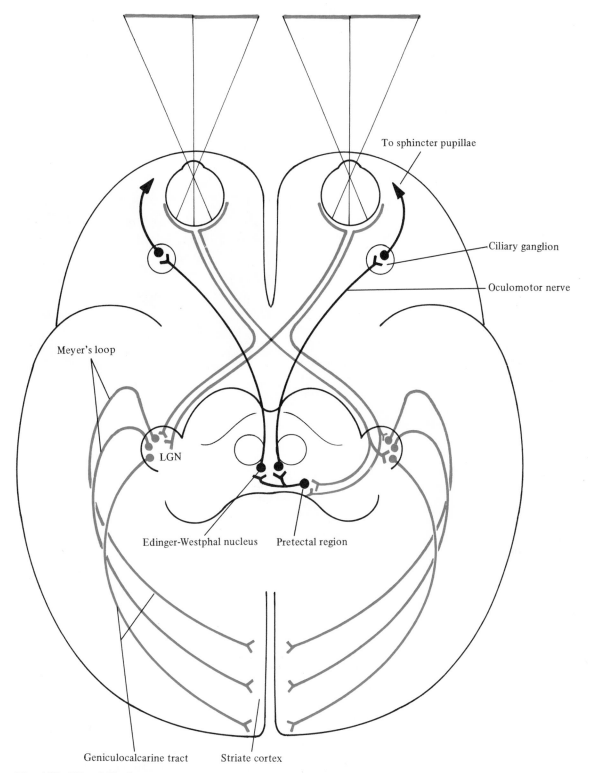

To sphincter pupillae

Ciliary ganglion

Oculomotor nerve

Meyer's loop

LGN

Edinger-Westphal nucleus   Pretectal region

Geniculocalcarine tract   Striate cortex

Fig. 150. Visual Pathways
The pathway for the pupillary light reflex is also illustrated.

fovea usually appears as a bright reflex about three disc diameters on the temporal side of the optic disc.

VISUAL PATHWAYS

Optic Nerve, Chiasm, and Tract

The *optic nerve* perforates the sclera and proceeds in a caudal direction to the *optic chiasm,* where the fibers from the nasal halves of each retina cross over to the *optic tract* on the opposite side (Fig. 150). Since the fibers from the nasal half of each retina decussate in the optic chiasm, each optic tract contains the fibers from the temporal retina of the ipsilateral eye and the nasal retina of the contralateral eye. In other words, each optic tract contains information from the contralateral visual field.

The optic tract sweeps around the cerebral peduncle to the *lateral geniculate nucleus,* LGN (Fig. 151) where most of the fibers terminate in a precise retinotopic pattern. Other fibers terminate in the superior colliculus and the pretectal region, which are important areas for control of eye movements (Fig. 135, Chapter 11) and the pupillary light reflex (Fig. 150).

The optic nerve is an integral part of the CNS, rather than a peripheral nerve, and it is surrounded by dura, arachnoid, and pia mater as is the rest of the CNS. The subdural and subarachnoid spaces of the brain, therefore, are continuous along the optic nerve, and an increase in intracranial pressure is readily transmitted along the optic nerve to the optic disc, where it manifests itself as papilledema (see Clinical Notes).

Optic Radiation and Visual Cortex

Neurons in the LGN give rise to the optic radiation or *geniculocalcarine tract,* which projects to the *primary visual cortex* (area 17) in the region of the calcarine sulcus in the occipital lobe. The optic radiation proceeds through the retro- and sublenticular parts of the internal capsule. The fan-like arrangement of its fibers can usually be appreciated during the blunt dissection of the brain (Fig. 46 in dissection guide). The fibers that carry impulses from the inferior retinal quadrants sweep around the temporal horn of the lateral ventricle (Fig. 152) before they proceed in a caudal direction to

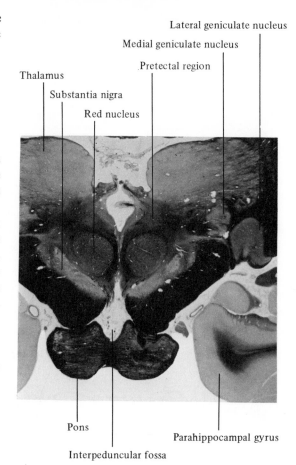

Lateral geniculate nucleus
Medial geniculate nucleus
Pretectal region
Thalamus
Substantia nigra
Red nucleus
Pons
Parahippocampal gyrus
Interpeduncular fossa

Fig. 151. Lateral Geniculate Nuclei
Myelin-stained section through the upper brain stem of the human brain. The section, which is close to level H in Fig. 73, cuts through the posterior part of diencephalon, the mesencephalon as well as the basal part of pons.

the inferior lip of the calcarine sulcus (Fig. 153). The part of the optic radiation that makes a detour into the temporal lobe is referred to as Meyer's loop. The fibers carrying information from the upper retinal quadrants proceed more directly through the deep parts of the parietotemporal lobes to the upper lip of the calcarine sulcus. Although the optic radiation is spread out in a fan-like manner, its fibers are orderly arranged, and localized lesions tend to give rise to well-demarcated homonymous defects, scotomas, in the opposite visual field (see Clinical Notes).

Primary visual cortex, which is located primarily on the medial aspect of the occipital lobe (Fig. 153), contains a horizontal stripe, *the line of Gennari,* which can be seen by the naked eye. The

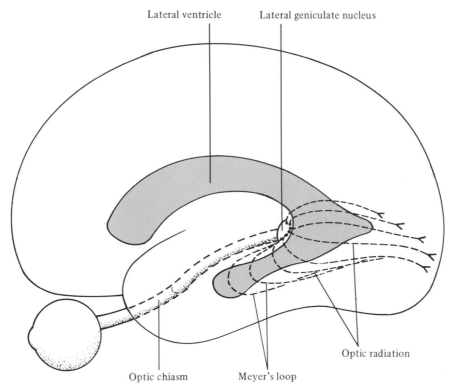

Fig. 152. Optic Radiation
Diagram illustrating the sweep of the optic radiation on the outside of the lateral ventricle. The ventral part of the radiation, Meyer's loop, makes a detour into the temporal lobe before it proceeds in a caudal direction to the calcarine sulcus. Note how the visual pathways extend from the eyeballs to the occipital lobes in the back of the head. (Modified from Sanford, H. S., H. L. Bair, 1939. Visual disturbances associated with tumors of the temporal lobe. Arch. Neurol. Psychiatry (Chicago), 42: 21–43)

line, which is located in layer IV, is composed of heavily myelinated fibers, and its presence has given the primary visual cortex the name *striate cortex*. Since the fibers from the nasal halves of each retina cross in optic chiasm, each cortex receives information only from the opposite visual field (Fig. 150).

Although the striate area represents the end station for the optic radiation, it is by no means the end of the visual pathway. The primary visual cortex is closely associated with surrounding cortical areas, the *para-* and *peristriate areas* (Brodmann's areas 18 and 19), which are of special importance for higher visual functions. In fact, also these areas do receive direct input from the lateral geniculate nucleus.

FUNCTIONAL CONSIDERATIONS

The Different Functions of Rods and Cones

The rods are characterized by great sensitivity and they are used in dim light and in peripheral vision. Further, they do not differentiate colors, and the visual world becomes gray in twilight. Cones, on the other hand, perceive the differentiation of colors; they operate only in bright light and they provide for great acuity.

It is somewhat surprising to realize that the light must pass through the various layers of the retina before it reaches the photoreceptors, which are situated adjacent to the pigment epithelium. In the region of the fovea centralis, however, all blood vessels and most neuronal elements are pushed aside to reduce the dispersion and absorption of the light reaching the cones in the fovea.

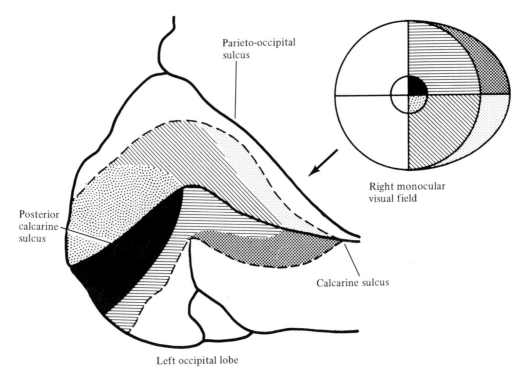

Fig. 153. Striate Cortex
The projection of the right visual field on the visual cortex in the left occipital lobe. Note that the central part of retina, i.e., the area of highest visual acuity, is represented by a much larger cortical area than the peripheral parts of the retina. There is also an inversion of the quadrants. (From Popper, K. R. and J. C. Eccles, 1951, The Self and Its Brain. With permission from Springer, Berlin-Heidelberg)

It is beyond the scope of this text to discuss the complicated biochemical aspects of photoreception. Suffice it to say that the photoreceptors contain light-sensitive pigments, which are being decomposed as a result of absorption of light energy by the receptors. This releases energy, which is transformed into nerve impulses.

Topographic Organization of the Visual Pathway

The visual pathway from the retina to the primary visual cortex is highly organized in the sense that there is a point-to-point localization of each part of the retina throughout the system. Thus, the primary visual cortex is characterized by a precise retinotopic organization, and it is sometimes referred to as the "cortical retina." However, the topographic projection of the retina is nonlinear in the sense that the central part of the retina, which is the region of highest discrimination is represented by a relatively much larger cortical area than the peripheral parts of the retina (Fig. 153). This reflects a very important principle of cortical organization. The amount of cortical tissue devoted to a specific region of the body, including the retina, is related to the functional importance of the region rather than to its size.

Figure 153 illustrates a few more points worth remembering. First, the macula projects to the posterior part of the calcarine cortex, whereas the peripheral parts of the retina project to its anterior part. Second, the upper part of the visual field is represented below the calcarine fissure, and the lower part above the fissure.

Brain Mechanisms of Vision

By closing the eyes for a moment and reflecting on the fate of a blind person, one is suddenly reminded of what life would be like without vision. The eye is our most important special sense organ, and this fact alone has made the visual system one of the most popular research objects in the brain. Thanks to generous research support and a phenomenal surge in the development of neuroanatomic and neurophysiologic research techniques, scientists have been able to learn more about the brain mechanism of vision during the last 30–40 years than during all of the previous years of recorded scientific activities.

The Retina and LGN

Considering the histology and synaptic organization of the retina and LGN, it seems safe to conclude that a considerable amount of information processing must take place in these structures, and physiologists have made many significant discoveries by recording the activities of individual cells in response to various types of visual stimuli.

Receptive fields. The receptive field of a cell in the visual system is the area of the retina in which a particular stimulus can influence the electrical activity of the cell. The retinal ganglion cells have fairly simple receptive fields, many of which are organized in a concentric manner with a circular central area surrounded by a ring-shaped outer zone. Illumination of the central area results in either excitation ("on"-center cell) or inhibition ("off"-center cell), whereas illumination of the surrounding zone (the "surround") has the opposite effect. The most effective stimulus for many of the retinal ganglion cells, therefore, is a circular spot of light of a particular size in a specific part of the visual field. An evenly illuminated area has no effect on the ganglion cells since simultaneous illumination of both center and surround tends to cancel out. The retinal ganglion cells are concerned with the contrast between different areas in the visual field[1] rather than with the specific level of illumination. The cells of the LGN have receptive fields similar to those of the retinal ganglion cells, i.e., with the center-surround configuration. Since the receptive fields of the LGN cells, like those of the ganglion cells, are circular-symmetric, orientation becomes an important feature

1. The term "visual field" should not be confused with receptive field. The "visual field" refers to the area within which an object is more or less distinctly seen by the eye in a fixed position.

only when the information reaches the cerebral cortex (see below).

That the cells in the retina can be stimulated by only one eye is easily appreciated. This, however, is the case also for the cells in the LGN. LGN is a laminated structure with six different layers, and anatomic studies have shown that the input from the two eyes are segregated. Three of the six layers receive input from one eye and the three remaining layers receive input from the other eye. Further, since most of the LGN cells receive input from the retina and send their axons to the visual cortex, there is no significant mixing of inputs from the two eyes in LGN. In other words, possibility for binocular convergence does not exist in LGN. Only when the visual information reaches the visual cortex do fibers carrying information from the two eyes converge on single cells.

Visual Cortex

When the signals reach the primary visual cortex (area 17), some major transformations take place. First, most of the cortical cells are *orientation specific,* i.e., they respond to lines of a specific orientation, rather than to spots of light; some cells even respond to lines that are moving in a specific direction. Second, many of the cells are characterized by *binocular convergence,* i.e., they respond to stimulation of both eyes. The above-mentioned functions of the primary visual cortex, i.e., orientation specificity and binocular convergence, most likely represent early stages in the brain's analyses of visual forms and perception of depths. The physiologic properties of the visual cortex are reflected in its architecture, in the sense that cells with common functional properties are grouped together in vertically organized columns (see below).

Although information that reaches the primary visual cortex at any one site does spread throughout the thickness of the cortex, the lateral spread of information is limited to a few millimeters. In other words, the primary visual cortex is analyzing the visual world in a piecemeal fashion. This, no doubt, represents an early stage in the path toward visual perception, and the primary visual cortex is by no means the end station for visual impulses. Area 17 is closely associated with higher visual areas in surrounding parts of the occipital and parietotemporal lobes, which apparently are involved in increasingly more complicated functions

Fig. 154. "Ocular Dominance" Columns

A. Dark-field autoradiograph of a section from the primary visual cortex (area 17) of macaque monkey following an injection of tritiated proline into one eye. The label was taken up by cell bodies in the retina and transported to the LGN. Following transneuronal transport into LGN cells, the label reached the visual cortex via the optic radiation. The "ocular dominance" columns are confirmed by the presence of periodic bright patches. Note that the banded projections are limited to layer IV, where most of the geniculocalcarine fibers terminate. (Micrograph courtesy of Dr. Torsten Wiesel. From Hubel, D. H. and T. N. Wiesel. Brain Mechanisms of Vision. Scientific American, September 1979, Vol. 241, No. 3.)

B. "Ocular dominance" columns demonstrated with the 2-deoxyglycose method in a rhesus monkey with the right eye occluded. The "ocular dominance" columns, i.e., the alternate dark and light striations, extend throughout the entire thickness of the cortex rather than being limited to layer IV, as in **A.** This is related to the fact that the 2-deoxyglycose method reveals the entire column of cells activated by one eye regardless of number of synapses involved. (Micrograph courtesy of Dr. Louis Sokoloff. From Sokoloff. Localization of functional activity in the central nervous system by measurement of glycose utilization with radioactive deoxyglycose. J. of Cerebral Blood Flow and Metabolism. 1981, Vol. 1, 7–36. With permission from Raven Press, New York.)

related to the perception of colors, three-dimensional forms, and movements.

"Ocular Dominance" and "Orientation" Columns. Columnar organization seems to be an important feature of many cortical areas, and two types of functional columns have been identified in the striate cortex. One type, the "ocular dominance" column (Fig 154), is related to eye preference of the cortical neuron. Although most cortical neurons respond to an appropriate stimulus regardless of which eye it is presented to, they usually prefer one eye over the other. Neurons that respond more effectively to stimuli in the right eye form functional columns that alternate with functional columns related primarily to the left eye. The anatomic basis for this spatial variation in eye preference can be demonstrated with a variety of techniques including the autoradiographic tract-tracing method (Fig. 154A) and the 2-deoxyglycose method (Fig. 154B). Another type of column is characterized by orientation sensitivity, i.e., "orientation" column.

Reflexes

Pupillary Light Reflex

The size of the pupil is determined by the activity in the parasympathetic innervation of the pupillary sphincter, and to a lesser degree by the sympathetic innervation of the vessels of the iris and the dilator pupillae. The size variations are induced by different factors, e.g., by change in illumination, by stress and during accommodation (see below).

The well-known phenomenon of pupillary constriction in response to bright light is called the *direct light reflex.* The afferent link in the reflex arc is represented by fibers that reach the pretectal region through the optic nerve and the optic tract

(Fig. 150). Neurons in the pretectal region (Fig. 151) connect with the parasympathetic Edinger-Westphal nucleus, which innervates the pupillary sphincter via the ciliary ganglion. Since fibers cross over from one side to the other both in the optic nerves (at the optic chiasm) and in the pretectal area, the unexposed pupil constricts as well, i.e., the reflex is a *crossed* or *consensual light reflex.* The evaluation of the pupillary light reflexes is an important part of the neurologic examination.

Fixation and Accommodation Reflexes

The fixation of the eyes on an object, the *fixation reflex,* and the adaptation of the eyes for near vision, the *accommodation reflex,* are dependent on complicated reflex arcs that apparently involve the visual projections to the occipital cortex and subsequent corticofugal projections to the superior colliculus and the pretectal region.

CLINICAL NOTES

Since vision is the most important of the special senses in the human, blindness is a very serious handicap. Most visual disturbances are caused by refractive errors or diseases of the eye, and an ophthalmologic disorder, therefore, should be excluded before a neurologic deficit is considered.

Cataract and glaucoma are two of the most common non-neurologic causes of blindness. *Cataract* is a loss of the transparency of the lens or its capsule. Since the cornea is the main refracting medium in the eye, the lens can be surgically removed and the loss of refractive power can usually be compensated for by eyeglasses or by an artificial lens. *Glaucoma* is characterized by increased intraocular pressure caused by restricted re-entry of

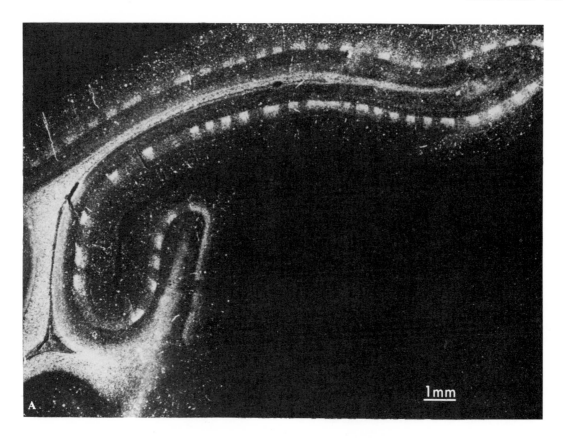

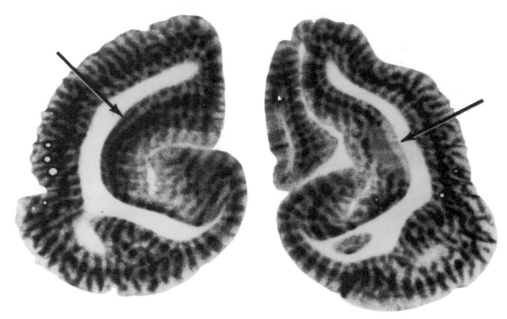

the aqueous humor into the bloodstream. Continuous high pressure in the eye fluid causes destruction of the optic nerve fibers with visual field defects, and it is therefore important to make a correct diagnosis at an early stage.

Ophthalmoscopy: The Fundus Oculi

The ophthalamoscopic examination of the fundus is an extremely important part of the neurologic examination; indeed, every physician should be able to examine the fundus since many systemic diseases, e.g., diabetes mellitus, hypertension, and arteriosclerosis, produce characteristic changes in the retina.

The *normal fundus* is shown in Fig. 155A. The optic disc stands out sharply because of its pale appearance and well-defined margin. The retinal vessels radiate from the center of the disc and divide repeatedly as they spread over the fundus.

A disease in the optic nerve may cause *optic atrophy,* which is characterized by a very pale or even chalk-white disc. Changes in the retinal vessels are seen primarily in arteriosclerosis and hypertension. The picture of *hypertensive retinopathy,* which is especially dramatic, contains arterial constriction, obliteration of the veins at the arteriovenous crossings, and retinal exudates. In more advanced stages it may even be pronounced swelling of the disc, i.e., *papilledema,* which is indistinguishable from that seen in a patient with increased intracranial pressure.

Papilledema ("Choked Disc")

Swelling of the optic papilla (Fig. 155B) is one of the most important signs of increased intracranial pressure, which is a common sequel of expanding intracranial processes, including brain tumor, bleeding, and infection. Although increased intracranial pressure is not the only cause of papilledema, it is by far the most important. Pronounced venous congestion, bleeding, and exudates appear in later stages of papilledema.

The optic nerve, like the brain, is surrounded both by dura mater and pia–arachnoid, which are continuous with the meningeal spaces surrounding the brain. Increased CSF pressure in the skull, therefore, is immediately transmitted to CSF along the optic nerve, which interferes with venous outflow and probably also lymphatic drainage of the retina.

Lesions of the Visual Pathways

Since the visual pathways extend all the way from the eyeball in front to the occipital lobe in the posterior part of the hemisphere, they can be interrupted by lesions in many parts of the brain. Further, the visual pathways are highly organized, and lesions in different parts of the visual pathways produce characteristic visual field defects, which make it possible in many cases to determine the location of the lesion. Countless disorders can affect the visual pathways, but some should be noted in particular. Pituitary tumors, meningiomas, and aneurysms of the carotid artery or the circle of Willis often affect the optic chiasm or nearby regions of the optic nerve or tract. Intracerebral tumors and bleeding can easily encroach on the optic radiation.

Since lesions interrupting various parts of the visual pathways cause specific visual field defects, *examination of the visual fields* constitutes a very important part of the neurologic examination. The fields of vision can be accurately delineated by *perimetry,* but they can be estimated in a matter of seconds by the *confrontation method.* With one eye covered, the patient is instructed to fix his gaze on one of the examiner's eyes and report when he first sees a small object, e.g., a pencil, which the examiner moves into the patient's field of vision. By bringing the pencil into the visual field from many directions it is often possible to detect a significant visual field defect. Partial defects within the field of vision are called *scotomas.* Visual defects, further, are always named according to the visual field loss and not to the corresponding part of the nonfunctional retina.

Lesions of the Optic Nerve

Prechiasmal lesions cause monocular abnormalities, which can vary from *complete blindness* (lesion A in Fig. 156) to various types of *scotomas.* If the lesion of the optic nerve is complete, the afferent fibers for the pupillary light reflex will be interrupted, and the pupil will not react to light stimulation. However, the pupillary response can be elicited by stimulating the opposite eye (consensual reflex).

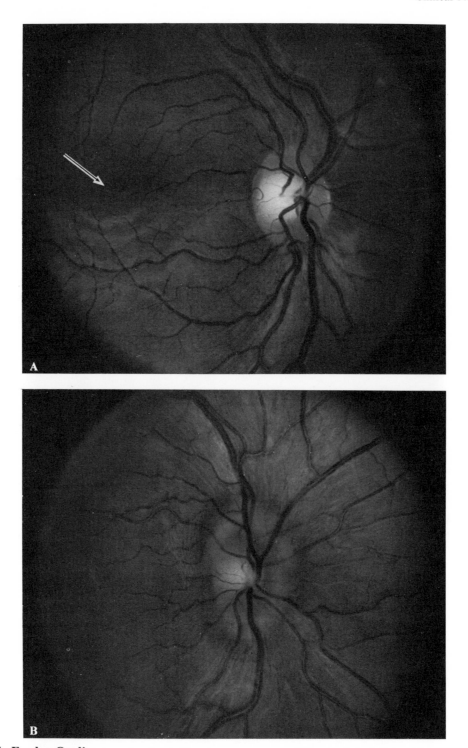

Fig. 155. Fundus Oculi
A. Normal fundus. Note the sharp border of the optic disc. The arrow points to fovea centralis.
B. Papilledema with congestion of the disc and blurring of its margins. Note also that the optic cup (the central whitish area) is reduced in size compared with the normal optic cup. (The photographs were kindly provided by Dr. S. Newman.)

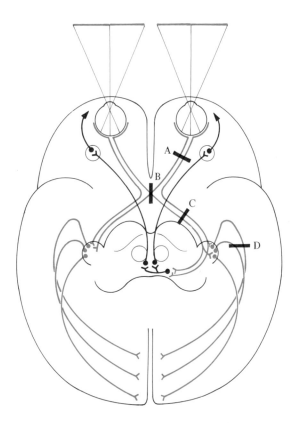

Visual field defects

L   R

A. Monocular blindness

B. Bitemporal hemianopsia

C. Homonymous hemianopsia

D. Upper quadrantanopsia

Fig. 156. Lesions of the Visual Pathways
Diagram illustrating some of the most typical lesions of the visual pathways. Whereas complete lesions at **A, B** and **C** give rise to field defects as indicated by the figure, lesions of the optic radiation produce homonymous field defects that are often incomplete and asymmetric. A homonymous superior quadrantanopsia may occur in temporal lobe lesions involving Meyer's loop **(D).**

Lesions of the Optic Chiasm

A chiasmal lesion, which interrupts the midline decussating fibers, produces a typical *bitemporal hemianopsia*[2] (lesion B in Fig. 156). If such a lesion is caused by a pituitary tumor, the defect usually starts as an *upper bitemporal quadrantanopsia,* since the tumor first exerts pressure on the inferior part of the chiasm, where the fibers from the lower regions of the nasal halves of the two retinae cross. An aneurysm in the anterior cerebral or the anterior communicating artery is likely to produce a *lower bitemporal quadrantanopsia.*

Lesions in the Optic Tract and Optic Radiation

Like the chiasmal lesion, the postchiasmal lesion produces bilateral field defects, but the typical symptom is a *homonymous* defect, i.e., a defect that affects the corresponding halves of the two visual fields. A lesion of the whole optic tract results in a *complete homonymous hemianopsia* (lesion C in Fig. 156), whereas lesions of the optic radiation are more apt to be partial due to the widespread extent of the geniculocalcarine fiber system and to produce *incomplete homonymous hemianopsia.* For instance, a temporal lobe lesion may interrupt Meyer's loop, the inferior portion of the optic radiation, and thereby produce a *contralateral upper quadrantanopsia* (lesion D in Fig. 156). Such lesions are hardly ever as regular as depicted in D.

Vision is sometimes preserved in the area of the macula lutea, i.e., *macular sparing.* This phenomenon is usually seen in vascular lesions of the occipital lobe. It is often explained on the basis of overlapping blood supply (from middle and posterior cerebral arteries) in the occipital pole, where macula is represented. Occipital lobe lesions and *visual agnosia* are discussed in Chapter 19.

---

2. Hemianopsia (hemianopia) means blindness in one-half of the visual field of one or both eyes.

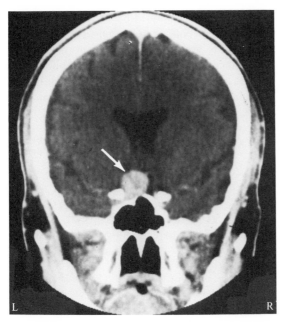

Fig. CE13A. Internal Carotid Artery Aneurysm
The CT scan was kindly provided by Dr. V. Haughton.

CLINICAL EXAMPLE

Internal Carotid Artery Aneurysm

A 49-year-old woman had been bothered by mild headache for half a year and she had lately started to complain about pain in and around her left eye. She sought medical attention when she experienced a gradual deterioration of vision in the left eye.

When seen by the neurologist, she had almost complete blindness in her left eye and a superior temporal quadrantanopsia in the right eye. The pupillary light reflex could not be elicited by light stimulation of her left eye, but a consensual reflex was obtained by stimulating the opposite eye.

A CT scan in a coronal plane (Fig. CE13 above) was obtained after intravenous infusion of contrast. The enhancing mass lesion (arrow) is resting on the base of the skull immediately above the sphenoid sinus. Note the asymmetric lateral ventricles.

1. It is impossible to tell whether this lesion is of vascular (i.e., aneurysm) or neoplastic (i.e., tumor) origin. The spherical shape and generally smooth border suggest that it is an aneurysm. Assuming that this is the case, what artery did it arise from?

2. At what point in the optic pathway can a single lesion cause monocular blindness and contralateral quadrantanopsia? Is this lesion in the appropriate place to cause such a defect?

3. A single CT cut cannot reveal the entire rostrocaudal extent of this lesion. If it were to extend an additional 2–3 cm in posterior direction, what other important structure located at the base of the brain could be damaged?

Discussion

This lesion represents a "giant" aneurysm of the internal carotid artery. Most intracranial aneurysms arise in arteries that are related to the anterior portion of the circle of Willis and they are usually around 1 cm in diameter when they start to produce symptoms. This aneurysm, which has a diameter of about 2 cm, probably arises from the internal carotid artery near the origin of the ophthalmic artery (supraclinoid aneurysm).

A lesion in this region is likely to involve the optic nerve and chiasm. Compression of the rostral part of the chiasm, from the lateral and ventral side, apparently involves the "knee-fibers," which would explain the superior temporal quadrantanopsia in her right eye (see figure below). Compres-

Fig. CE13B. Internal Carotid Artery Aneurysm
Diagram of the arrangement of visual fibers in the chiasm. The ventrally located fibers crossing in the chiasm make a loop into the terminal portion of the opposite optic nerve. This explains why a lesion that primarily involves the optic nerve on one side may cause superior temporal quadrantanopsia in the opposite eye. Further, since the "knee fibers" come close to the lateral surface of the chiasm after the crossing, lateral pressure on the chiasm usually causes visual field defects of both eyes.

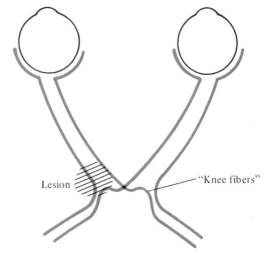

sion of the optic nerve on the left side causes blindness in her left eye. A lesion in this location could conceivably involve the oculomotor nerve, but this was not the case in this patient.

The sella turcica, pituitary gland, infundibular stalk, and hypothalamus all lie in the immediate neighborhood of the lesion. Therefore, if the aneurysm were to expand further, signs of hypothalamic or hypothalamohypophysial dysfunction are likely to appear. This aneurysm is occupying and distending a portion of the subarachnoid space and, if ruptured, would give rise to a subarachnoid bleeding, which is a very serious condition.

Suggested Reading

1. Adams, R. D. and M. Victor, 1981. Principles of Neurology, 2nd ed. McGraw-Hill: New York, pp. 165–175.
2. Brodal, A., 1981. Neurological Anatomy in Relation to Clinical Medicine, 3rd ed. Oxford University Press: New York, pp. 578–601.
3. Dowling, J. E., 1979. Information processing by local circuits: The vertebrate retina as a model system. In F. O. Schmitt and F. G. Worden (eds.): The Neurosciences, Fourth Study Program, MIT Press, Cambridge, Massachusetts, pp. 163–181.
4. Hubel, D. H. and T. N. Wiesel, 1977. Ferrier lecture: Functional architecture of macaque monkey visual cortex. Proc. R. Soc. Lond. [Biol.] 198: 1–59.
5. Hubel, D. H. and T. N. Wiesel, 1979. Brain mechanisms of vision. Scientific American 241(3): 130–144.

14
Olfactory System

OLFACTORY EPITHELIUM
   Olfactory Receptor Cells

OLFACTORY PATHWAYS
   Olfactory Nerve
   Olfactory Bulb
   Olfactory Tract and Its Projection Areas

FUNCTIONAL ASPECTS
   Microsmatic Man
   Functional Significance of Higher Order
     Olfactory Connections
   Centrifugal Pathways: Central Modulation of
     Olfactory Stimuli

CLINICAL NOTES
   Anosmia
   Testing the Sense of Smell
   Uncinate Seizures

CLINICAL EXAMPLE
   Olfactory Groove Meningioma (Subfrontal
     Meningioma)

SUGGESTED READING

The central olfactory pathways constitute a rather small part of the human brain, and olfaction is undoubtedly of less clinical significance than vision and hearing. Nevertheless, the sense of smell is of considerable importance in our everyday life; it plays a significant role in food intake, in reproductive and endocrine functions, and in certain social behaviors of many mammalian species including man. Both repugnant odors and sweet perfumes have a powerful effect on mood and behavior.

OLFACTORY EPITHELIUM

The olfactory epithelium occupies about a 2.5 cm²
area in each nasal cavity, where it covers the upper
concha and adjacent part of the nasal cavity (Fig.
157A). Because the epithelium is located in the
upper part of the nasal cavity, only part of the
air reaches the olfactory receptor cells in normal
inspiration. Sniffing, which produces extra air cur-
rents in the nasal cavity, may therefore be necessary to bring enough odorous molecules in contact
with the olfactory epithelium, especially if the odor
is weak. The epithelium consists of olfactory receptor cells that are surrounded and supported by
epithelial secretory cells called supporting cells
(Fig. 158). The olfactory epithelium is covered by
a secretion produced by the olfactory glands of
Bowman and the supporting cells.

Olfactory Receptor Cells

These are represented by several million bipolar
sensory neurons whose axons project to the olfactory bulb. The peripheral process or dendrite of
the receptor cell contains a knob-like enlargement,
the *olfactory vesicle,* from which several 100–200
μm long hair-like *cilia* project into the mucus covering the epithelium (Fig. 157B). Although the
actual transduction mechanism is unknown, it
seems clear that the highly specialized cilia, whose
distal parts lie in parallel with and close to the
surface of the mucus, are excited by odorous molecules in the air. To reach the cilia, the chemicals
in the air must be dissolved in the fluid that surrounds the cilia.

There are strong indications that the olfactory
receptor cells are renewed continuously throughout life. This constant turnover may reflect an adaptation on part of the olfactory sensory neurons,
which seem especially vulnerable to injuries from
the environment. The reconstitution is accomplished through a process in which immature sensory cells (basal cells) in the deep part of the olfactory epithelium are transformed into mature
receptor cells. This neurogenetic process, which
is unique in the mature nervous system, raises
some important questions related to the coding
of olfactory stimuli. Because the phenomenon implies a continuous development, not only of receptor cell bodies in the olfactory epithelium but also
of their axons projecting to the olfactory bulb,
one wonders if the newly formed axons are related

to a specific site in the glomerular layer or if their
central connections are randomly made? If a certain group of receptor cells are responsive to a
specific odor, which may well be the case, the axons of newly generated receptor cells must find
their way to a specific set of glomeruli.

OLFACTORY PATHWAYS

Olfactory Nerve

The thin unmyelinated axons, *fila olfactoria,* of
the receptor cells form about 20 slender bundles
that pass through tiny openings in the cribriform
plate of the ethmoid bone to reach the olfactory
bulb (Fig. 158). These bundles represent the first
cranial nerve, *the olfactory nerve.* As the bundles
pass through the cribriform plate they are surrounded by tubular sheaths of the meninges. The
subarachnoid space, therefore, is in more or less
direct continuity with the lymphatic system in the
nasal cavity, which makes it relatively easy for a
nasal infection to spread to the meninges and the
brain.

Olfactory Bulb

The olfactory bulb is the rostral expanded part
of the olfactory stalk, which extends forward underneath the frontal lobe from its attachment to
the brain in front of the anterior perforated substance. The large mitral cells (blue in Fig. 158)
are the major relay neurons in the olfactory bulb
and their main function is to transmit olfactory
stimuli from receptor cells to centrally located
brain regions. The synaptic contacts between the
incoming olfactory nerve fibers and the dendrites
of the mitral cells take place in specialized structures called glomeruli. A glomerulus is a more
or less spherical structure, partially or wholly encapsulated by glial processes, and characterized
by a wealth of synaptic contacts. Many thousands
of receptor cells synapse with the dendritic
branches of one or only a few mitral cells within
a glomerulus; this means that there is a high degree
of convergence of olfactory receptors onto mitral
cells.

Interneurons and Reciprocal Synapses

The transmission of olfactory impulses from receptor cells to mitral cells is only one aspect of the
complicated interactions that take place in the olfactory bulb. Physiologic studies indicate that a

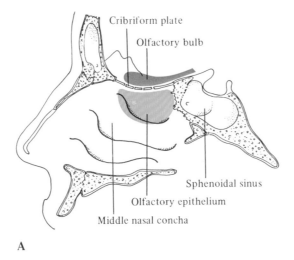

Cribriform plate

Olfactory bulb

Sphenoidal sinus

Olfactory epithelium

Middle nasal concha

A

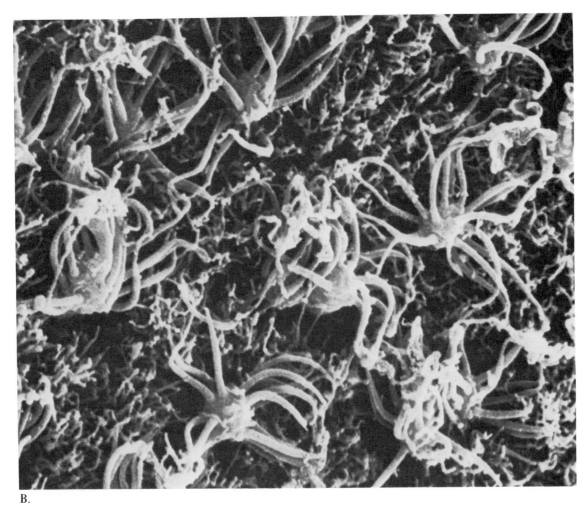

B.

Fig. 157. The Olfactory Epithelium

A. The olfactory epithelium (*light red*) is located in the upper part of the nasal cavity. The olfactory bulb (*dark red*), which is located in the anterior cranial fossa, is separated from the olfactory epithelium by the cribriform plate of the ethmoid bone.

B. Scanning electron micrograph of the olfactory epithelium in the human. 15–18 cilia radiate into the overlying mucus from each olfactory vesicle. (From Fujita, T., K. Tanaka and J. Tokunaga, 1981. SEM Atlas of Cells and Tissue. Igaku-Shoin, Tokyo–New York. With permission of the authors and the publisher.)

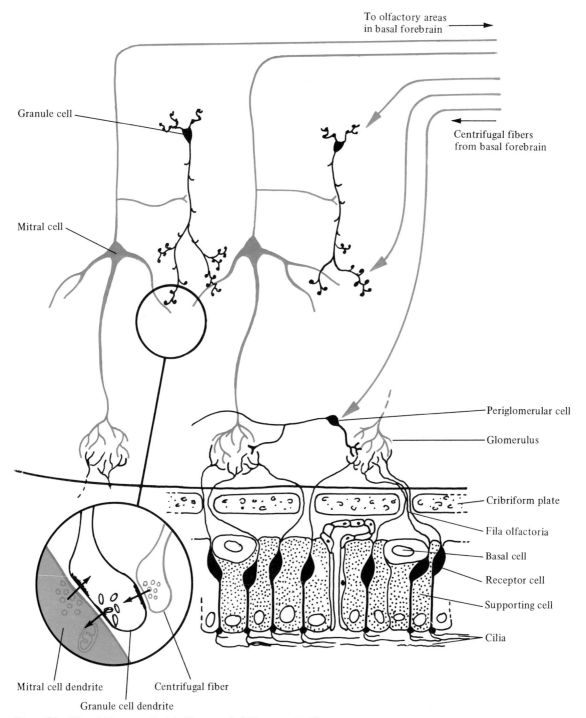

To olfactory areas
in basal forebrain

Granule cell

Mitral cell

Centrifugal fibers
from basal forebrain

Periglomerular cell

Glomerulus

Cribriform plate

Fila olfactoria

Basal cell

Receptor cell

Supporting cell

Cilia

Mitral cell dendrite

Centrifugal fiber

Granule cell dendrite

Fig. 158. The Olfactory Epithelium and Olfactory Bulb
Schematic drawing of the main neuronal elements of the olfactory bulb and their relationship to the olfactory receptor cells and the olfactory tract. The *inset* in the *lower left corner* shows a dendrodendritic synapse connection between a mitral cell dendrite (*blue*) and a granule cell dendrite (*black*). Note that the centrifugal fiber (*red*) from the basal forebrain forms an axodendritic synapse with the spine of the granule cell dendrite.

considerable amount of information processing occurs in the bulb. A large number of inhibitory interneurons are present in the bulb, the most common being the *granule* and *periglomerular cells.* The interneurons (black in Fig. 158), which modulate and control the transmission of olfactory impulses at several points within the bulb, are in turn influenced by collateral branches from mitral cells as well as by centrifugal pathways from a number of regions in the basal forebrain and brain stem.

The reciprocal *dendrodendritic synapse* for recurrent inhibition in the CNS was first discovered in the olfactory bulb, between the dendrites of mitral and granule cells (see inset in Fig. 158). The mitral cell excites the granule cell through one portion of the reciprocal synapse, whereupon the granule cell inhibits the same mitral cell through the other portion. This type of self-inhibition has now been described in many other parts of the nervous system. In view of the fact that one granule cell is related to several mitral cells, the inhibitory action released by a mitral cell can also affect nearby mitral cells; this is an example of lateral inhibition.

The layers of the olfactory bulb. The different cellular elements in the bulb are arranged in the following layers, beginning with the surface (Fig. 158):

1. *The fiber layer* is the most superficial layer; it consists of the incoming olfactory nerve fibers.

2. *The glomerular layer* consists of several rows of glomeruli that are surrounded by periglomerular cells.

3. *The plexiform layer* is characterized primarily by the dendritic branches of mitral cells and granule cells, and the numerous synaptic contacts that occur between them.

4. *The mitral layer,* which contains large mitral cells, is not well-defined in the human.

5. *The granular layer* contains a large number of small interneurons, the granule cells. The granule cell resembles the amacrine cell of the retina in that it lacks a morphologically distinct axon. The proximal dendrites of the granule cell branch locally in the granular layer, and a superficial spiny dendrite usually extends into the plexiform layer.

Olfactory Tract and Its Projection Areas

The axon of the mitral cells form the olfactory tract, which courses through the olfactory stalk to olfactory areas in the basal forebrain (Fig. 159). The olfactory areas include the *anterior olfactory nucleus* at the base of the olfactory stalk, and the *olfactory tubercle,* which is represented by the most anterolateral part of the *anterior perforated space.* The most important olfactory area is the *primary olfactory cortex* (prepiriform cortex), which forms a continuous field in part of the frontal and the temporal lobes. The frontal olfactory cortex is located adjacent to that part of the olfactory tract (often referred to as the lateral olfactory tract) that is near the limen insulae. At the limen insulae, the olfactory tract turns sharply in a medial direction, and its fibers fan out over the dorsomedial surface of the temporal lobe in the region of the *uncus* of the parahippocampal gyrus. This is the temporal olfactory cortex, which also includes the cortical amygdaloid nucleus. Most of the temporal olfactory cortex is located on the dorsal surface of the uncus and cannot be seen from the ventral side (Fig. 159).

Although most textbooks refer to a lateral, an intermediate, and a medial olfactory tract, this nomenclature is somewhat confusing. Practically all olfactory bulb projection fibers to the olfactory cortex are concentrated in the lateral olfactory tract. An intermediate olfactory tract cannot usually be located on the ventral surface, but crosssections through the anterior perforated space invariably demonstrate a fiber bundle that joins the anterior commissure from the ventral side. This bundle originates in the anterior olfactory nucleus on one side and projects to the anterior olfactory nucleus and olfactory bulb on the opposite side. Although some fibers from the olfactory tract deviate medially to reach the medial part of the anterior olfactory nucleus there is no significant accumulation of olfactory bulb projection fibers to justify the term medial olfactory tract. Nor is there any indication from experiments in primates that medially running fibers reach the septal area, the diagonal band, or any other structure medial to the anterior perforated space.

Considering these facts, it is appropriate to discontinue referring to a medial and an intermediate olfactory tract. Instead the lateral olfactory tract can be referred to as the *olfactory tract.*

In comparison with other sensory systems, a review of the olfactory pathways reveals some unique features. First, whereas there are at least three neurons that link the periphery to the cerebral cortex in other sensory systems, the olfactory pathway is characterized by a two-neuron chain.

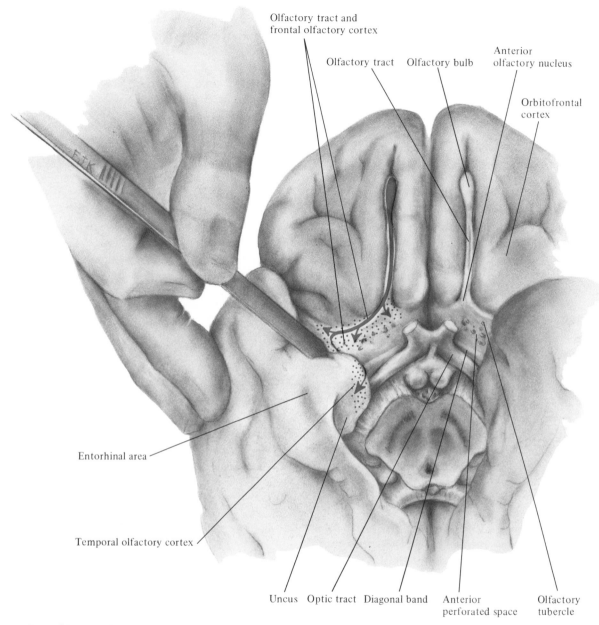

Olfactory tract and
frontal olfactory cortex

Olfactory tract   Olfactory bulb

Anterior
olfactory nucleus

Orbitofrontal
cortex

Entorhinal area

Temporal olfactory cortex

Uncus   Optic tract   Diagonal band   Anterior
perforated space

Olfactory
tubercle

Fig. 159. The Olfactory Tract and Its Projection Areas
The key areas of the olfactory system are easily identified on the basal surface of the brain. The temporal lobe
has been deviated laterally to show the lateral extention of the olfactory tract, which makes a sharp bend in
the region of the limen insulae to reach the uncus of the parahippocampal gyrus.

Second, the first-order neurons in the olfactory
path are represented by the bipolar receptor cells,
whose central processes form the first cranial
nerve. Third, the second-order neurons, the mitral
cells, project directly to the cerebral cortex rather
than to the thalamus.

FUNCTIONAL ASPECTS

Microsmatic Man

On the basis of the development of the olfactory
system, vertebrates can be divided into *macros-
matic* (= those with a keen sense of smell), and
microsmatic (= those with a poorly developed

sense of smell). Although it is common practice to refer to man as a microsmatic mammal, one must nevertheless remember that the olfactory sense organ is capable of discriminating among thousands of different substances on the basis of their smell, and it can detect odors of which there are only traces in the atmosphere. As shown by perfumers and wine tasters, the efficiency of the olfactory sense can be greatly improved by training. Therefore, even if man is not critically dependent on the olfactory system for his survival, it is questionable if his sense of smell should be considered poorly developed.

The olfactory receptors are similar to taste receptors in that they are stimulated by chemicals dissolved in liquids, and both types of receptors are important for food selection. Much of what we perceive as the flavor of food is in fact related to the sense of smell. This becomes evident when a person suffers from a head cold, in which case excessive mucus prevents odors from reaching the olfactory receptors, and the food seems to have lost most of its "taste."

Functional Significance of Higher Order Olfactory Connections

Although both the olfactory bulb and primary olfactory cortex are likely to be of importance for the perception of smell, we know very little about the functional significance of the different primary olfactory areas in the forebrain. Some recent studies, however, indicate that the *orbitofrontal cortex* may be of specific significance for the discrimination of odors. The pathways between the primary olfactory cortex and orbitofrontal cortex are not known in detail, but possibilities for interaction apparently exist both via cortical association fibers and by way of the mediodorsal thalamic nucleus.

Centrifugal Pathways: Central Modulation of Olfactory Stimuli

Some of the most interesting discoveries in recent years are related to the centrifugal fiber systems to the olfactory bulb (red arrows in Fig. 158). Such pathways originate in widespread regions of the basal telencephalon, the hypothalamus, and the brain stem. The activities in these pathways may serve to control and modulate the transmis-

sion of incoming olfactory stimuli, and they may play a role in the reduction of perceptual intensity, which occurs during prolonged exposure to an odorous substance.

CLINICAL NOTES

Anosmia

Lesions of the olfactory pathways may result in the loss of the sense of smell, i.e., *anosmia*. Unilateral anosmia is usually not noticed by the patient, whereas bilateral anosmia is readily apparent because food loses much of its flavor. As a matter of fact, the patient usually complains of loss of taste rather than of smell. The most common cause of anosmia is a nasal infection. However, more serious conditions, such as fractures of the ethmoid bone or orbitofrontal tumors, may also result in anosmia, and it is therefore important to know how to test the sense of smell.

Testing the Sense of Smell

Commonly known nonirritating odoriferous substances, such as chocolate, coffee, or tobacco can be used to test the sense of smell. The odor is applied to one nostril at a time by letting the patient sniff the test substance at the same time as he closes the other nostril. Even if the patient may not be able to identify the test substance, the olfactory nerves are usually intact as long as an odor can be detected. It is thus important that the test substance used be nonirritating since a positive response can occur due to irritation of the nasal mucosa, innervated by an intact trigeminal nerve.

Uncinate Seizures

Lesions that involve the primary olfactory cortex can give rise to olfactory hallucinations, usually in the form of a disagreeable odor. This is occasionally the first sign of a focal epileptic discharge in the temporal lobe. The hallucination, which is often accompanied by chewing or smacking movements and a feeling of unreality, indicates that the irritation is located in the uncus of the parahippocampal gyrus or the adjoining regions. The syndrome is referred to as an uncinate seizure, which

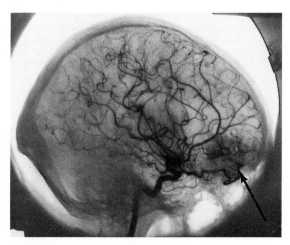

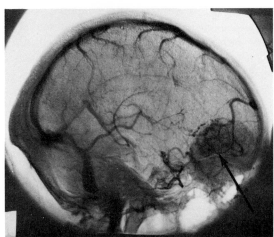

A. Olfactory Groove Meningeoma (Arterial Phase)

B. Olfactory Groove Meningioma (Venous Phase)

Fig. CE14A and B.
The angiograms were kindly provided by Dr. L. Morris.

is one of the group of convulsive disorders known as complex partial epilepsy (Chapter 19).

CLINICAL EXAMPLE

Olfactory Groove Meningioma (Subfrontal Meningioma)

A 70-year-old female suffering from senile dementia was admitted for new onset of seizures. The above arteriograms were obtained.

1. Where is the lesion?
2. Which cranial nerve functions might be affected by this lesion?

Discussion

The arteriograms demonstrate a lesion that extends from the inner table of the skull into the substance of the frontal lobe. The arteriogram (Fig. A: arterial phase) shows that the tumor is supplied primarily by branches of the ophthalmic artery (arrow). In the venous phase (Fig. B), a significant amount of contrast has accumulated in the abnormal blood vessels of the tumor (tumor stain) and the extent of the kidney-shaped tumor, which is lying on the base of the skull in the anterior fossa (arrow) can be easily appreciated. The angiographic appearance is typical of a meningioma. These are usually benign tumors that arise from arachnoid cells and become symptomatic by exerting pressure on surrounding brain substance and/or cranial nerves.

This tumor most likely arose from arachnoid cells along the cribriform plate, hence the name olfactory groove meningioma. One of the earliest and most important symptoms resulting from such a meningioma is unilateral or bilateral anosmia due to compression of the olfactory nerves or tracts (Fig. 157). Visual disturbances occur if the optic nerves become involved.

SUGGESTED READING

1. Doty, R. L., 1976. Mammalian Olfaction, Reproductive Processes, and Behavior. Academic Press: New York.
2. Eslinger, P. J., A. R. Damasio, and G. W. Van Hoesen, 1982. Olfactory dysfunction in man: A review of anatomical and behavioral aspects. Brain and Cognition. 1: 259–285.
3. Heimer, L., G. W. Van Hoesen, and D. L. Rosene, 1977. The olfactory pathways and the anterior perforated substance in the primate brain. Int. Journal Neurol. 12: 42–52.

15

Hypothalamus and the Hypothalamohypophysial System

ANATOMIC ORGANIZATION
  Boundaries and Subdivisions
  Hypothalamic Nuclei
  Major Fiber Systems

FUNCTIONAL ASPECTS
  Hypothalamic Control "Centers"
  Hypothalamohypophysial Relationships
  The Hypothalamus and the Autonomic
    Nervous System

CLINICAL NOTES
  Hypothalamohypophysial Disorders:
    A Diversity of Symptoms
  Hypothalamic Syndromes
  Psychosomatic Disorders

CLINICAL EXAMPLE
  Pituitary Adenoma

SUGGESTED READING

The hypothalamus is a primary regulator of autonomic and endocrine functions. Indeed, Sir Charles Sherrington, the eminent English neurophysiologist, called the hypothalamus "the head ganglion of the autonomic nervous system."

Most of the hypothalamic nuclei have ill-defined boundaries, and specific functions have been assigned to only a few of them. The hypothalamus is characterized by numerous connections with other parts of the CNS, especially with the cerebral cortex, the hippocampus, and the amygdaloid body. There are also direct connections between the hypothalamus and various autonomic centers in the brain stem and the spinal cord. Through its intimate neuronal and vascular relationships with the pituitary, the hypothalamus controls the release of the pituitary hormones.

In the early part of this century, little was known about either the anatomic organization or the functional significance of the hypothalamus. However, much important information about the hypothalamus has been obtained through extensive animal experimentation and clinical studies during the last 50 years. The complicated anatomy of this area of CNS has been clarified and it is now well-established that the hypothalamus is a primary regulator of autonomic and endocrine functions. It controls or modifies a variety of homeostatic processes that include respiration, circulation, food–water intake, digestion, metabolism, and body temperature. A properly functioning hypothalamus is crucial for the harmonious growth of the body, for differentiation of sexual characteristics, and for sexual and reproductive activities. Because the hypothalamus is crucially involved in the integration of the various autonomic and somatomotor reactions that accompany different emotional expressions, it is often included in the "limbic system."

ANATOMIC ORGANIZATION

Boundaries and Subdivisions

Despite its many important functions, the hypothalamus weighs only about 4 g in the adult human. It is located at the base of the diencephalon below the thalamus on each side of the third ventricle. The boundary between the thalamus and the hypothalamus is indicated on a midsagittal section by a distinct groove, the *hypothalamic sulcus* (Fig. 39 in dissection guide). The *lamina terminalis* indicates the rostral boundary of the hypothalamus, and an imaginary line that extends from the posterior commissure to the caudal limit of the mammillary body represents the caudal boundary (Fig. 38). Dorsolaterally, the hypothalamus extends to the medial edge of the internal capsule (Fig. 73D in dissection guide). Although the hypothalamic boundaries are easily described, it is important to realize that the hypothalamus does not form a well-circumscribed region of the CNS. On the contrary, it is continuous with the surrounding parts of the CNS. For instance, the hypothalamus is continuous rostrally with the septal area in the mediobasal parts of the telencephalon and with various components of the anterior perforated substance. Its anterior part is continuous laterally with the substantia innomina (Figs. 117 and 161), whereas the caudal part is continuous with the

central gray matter and the tegmentum of the mesencephalon.

The basal surface of the hypothalamus is characterized by the *mammillary bodies* caudally and the *optic chiasm* rostrally (Fig. 37). Between these two structures is a gray swelling, the *tuber cinereum,* which is hidden behind the hypophysis in Figs. 37. This tapers ventrally into a funnel-shaped structure, the *infundibulum,* which represents the most proximal part of the *neurohypophysis.* The infundibulum and the infundibular part of the adenohypophysis together form the *hypophysial stalk.* The infundibular region constitutes an important link between the hypothalamus and the pituitary; it is often referred to as the *median eminence.* The *lateral eminence* in the lateral part of the tuber cinereum is a rounded prominence produced by a group of superficially located nuclei, the *lateral tuberal nuclei* (Fig. 160C).

The conspicuous landmarks on the ventral surface of the brain can be used to divide the hypothalamus into three parts (Fig. 160): the supraoptic (rostral), the tuberal (middle), and the mammillary (caudal) part. It is also customary to subdivide each half of the hypothalamus into a medial and a lateral longitudinal zone. A large part of the cell-rich medial zone, where the neurons form more or less well-defined nuclei, is directly involved in the control of the pituitary. Although there are some prominent nuclei also in the basolateral part of the hypothalamus, a large part of the lateral zone cannot be easily subdivided into nuclei, and is, therefore, referred to as the lateral hypothalamic area. The loosely scattered cells of the lateral hypothalamic area have long overlapping dendrites, similar to the cells of the reticular formation. Some of these neurons send axons directly to the cerebral cortex and others project down into the brain stem and spinal cord.

Hypothalamic Nuclei

The most well-known hypothalamic nuclei are illustrated as if projected on the wall of the third ventricle in Fig. 160 A, and they are shown in cross-sections through the rostral, middle, and caudal parts of the hypothalamus in Figs. B, C, and D. Although some of the cell groups, e.g., the supraoptic and paraventricular nuclei, are easily identified as separate units (Fig. 161), others cannot be sharply delimited from the surrounding substance.

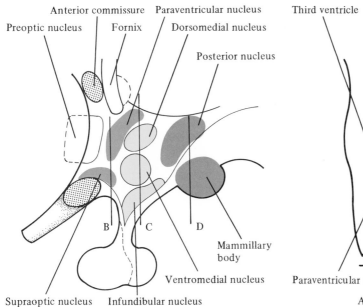

A. Diagram with labels: Anterior commissure, Preoptic nucleus, Fornix, Paraventricular nucleus, Dorsomedial nucleus, Posterior nucleus, B, C, D, Mammillary body, Ventromedial nucleus, Supraoptic nucleus, Infundibular nucleus

A.

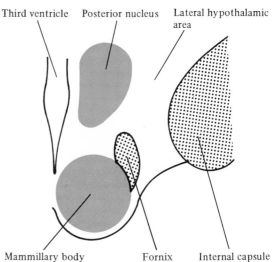

B. Diagram with labels: Third ventricle, Fornix, Stria terminalis, Internal capsule, Supraoptic nucleus, Optic tract, Lateral hypothalamic area, Anterior hypothalamic area, Paraventricular nucleus

B. Anterior hypothalamus

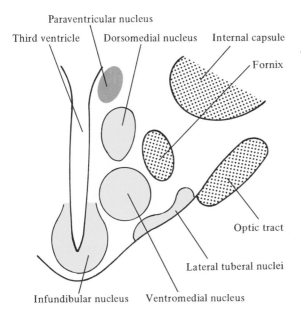

C. Diagram with labels: Paraventricular nucleus, Third ventricle, Dorsomedial nucleus, Internal capsule, Fornix, Optic tract, Lateral tuberal nuclei, Infundibular nucleus, Ventromedial nucleus

C. Middle hypothalamus

D. Diagram with labels: Third ventricle, Posterior nucleus, Lateral hypothalamic area, Mammillary body, Fornix, Internal capsule

D. Posterior hypothalamus

Fig. 160. Hypothalamic Nuclei
A. Diagram of the ventricular surface of the hypothalamus showing the approximate location of the most important hypothalamic nuclei (Modified from W. E. Le Gros Clark, 1936, J. Anat. (Lond.)).
B, C, and D. Cross-sections through the anterior **(B)**, middle **(C)** and posterior **(D)** hypothalamus.

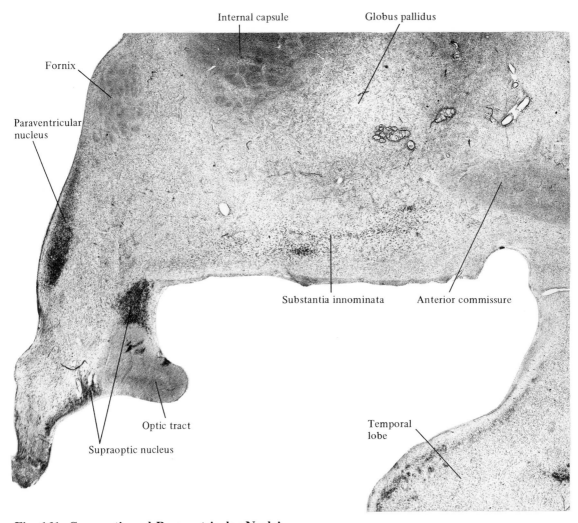

Fig. 161. Supraoptic and Paraventricular Nuclei
Nissl-stained cross-section through the anterior hypothalamus of a human brain showing the circumscribed supraoptic and paraventricular nuclei.

Anterior Group (Fig. 160 B)

Important nuclei in this group are the *preoptic* and the *suprachiasmatic nuclei.* Animal experiments have shown that the preoptic nucleus and the adjoining regions of the anterior hypothalamus are involved in the integration of several homeostatic functions including temperature regulation and maternal behavior. The suprachiasmatic nucleus, which is located just dorsal to the optic chiasm, receives direct input from the retina. The nucleus seems to play an important role in a system whereby visual stimuli can modulate neuroendocrine mechanisms.

Included in the anterior group are also the two prominent and highly vascularized *supraoptic* and *paraventricular nuclei,* whose large cells send their axons to the posterior lobe of the pituitary (*supraopticohypophysial tract*). The paraventricular nucleus, furthermore, projects to brainstem and spinal cord autonomic centers.

Middle Group (Fig. 160 C)

This group contains the *dorsomedial,* the *ventromedial,* and the *infundibular (arcuate) nuclei,* which surround the ventral part of the third ventricle. The ventromedial nucleus occupies a strategic position in the hypothalamus. It has widespread afferent and efferent connections with many other regions of the CNS, including the brain stem. Axons from cells in the infundibular nucleus, and

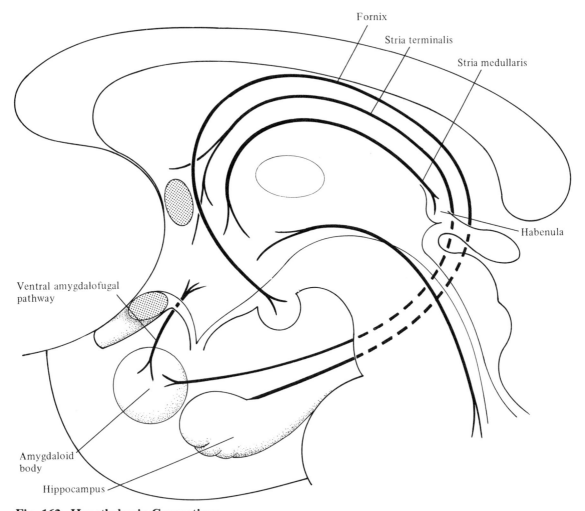

Fornix

Stria terminalis

Stria medullaris

Habenula

Ventral amygdalofugal
pathway

Amygdaloid
body

Hippocampus

Fig. 162. Hypothalamic Connections
Only some of the most prominent pathways have been indicated in this schematic drawing.

surrounding parts of the basomedial hypothalamus, form a diffuse projection system, the *tubero-infundibular tract,* that terminates on the hypophysial portal vessel system. This provides for a neurovascular link between the hypothalamus and the anterior pituitary (see below). The *lateral tuberal nuclei* are situated close to the surface in the lateral tuberal region, where they produce a prominent bulge, the *lateral eminence.*

Posterior Group (Fig. 160 D)

The posterior part of the hypothalamus consists of the *posterior hypothalamic nucleus* and the *mamillary body.* The posterior hypothalamic nucleus is a large but poorly defined cell group that

is continuous with the central gray matter of the mesencephalon. The mamillary body, which is a focal point for several prominent fiber bundles, consists of a large medial and a smaller lateral nucleus. It is surrounded by a capsule of heavily myelinated fibers.

Major Fiber Systems (Fig. 162)

The study of hypothalamic fiber connections has been hampered by many factors, especially by the fact that the hypothalamus is located at the base of the brain and, therefore, difficult to reach for experimental purposes. Nevertheless, with the aid of modern tract-tracing techniques it has become apparent that hypothalamus is intimately related to many regions both in the forebrain (e.g., the amygdaloid body, hippocampus and cerebral cortex), the brain stem, and the spinal cord.

Fornix

The *fornix* is a large fiber bundle that originates in the hippocampal formation and projects to the septal area, the anterior thalamus, and the hypothalamus. It can be exposed by blunt dissection of the lateral wall of the third ventricle (Fig. 163 B) and followed to the mammillary body, where many of its fibers terminate. Other fibers leave the main bundle along its course through the hypothalamus. These are distributed to the infundibular and the ventromedial hypothalamic nuclei. The fornix also contains fibers that carry impulses from the septal area to the hippocampus.

Stria Terminalis

The *stria terminalis* is the main pathway that reciprocally connects the amygdaloid body and the medial hypothalamus. Similar to the fornix, the stria terminalis makes a dorsally convex detour behind and above the thalamus on the path to the hypothalamus. It can be identified in the floor of the lateral ventricle, where it accompanies the thalamostriate vein in the groove that separates the thalamus from the caudate nucleus (Fig. 59). In the region of the anterior commissure the stria terminalis divides into different components, which distribute their fibers to the medial hypothalamus and areas in the basal part of the telencephalon. Because of its widespread distribution to the medial hypothalamus, the stria terminalis is an important pathway for the amygdaloid modulation of hypothalamohypophysial functions.

The amygdaloid body is also related to the lateral hypothalamus through a diffuse system of fibers, the *ventral amygdalofugal pathway.*

Stria Medullaris

The *stria medullaris* is another prominent fiber bundle, which can be easily identified on the mediodorsal side of the thalamus (Fig. 59). Many of the fibers in this bundle connect the lateral preoptic–hypothalamic region with the habenular complex. However, like most other hypothalamic pathways, the stria medullaris is a complicated bundle that contains many different fiber components that have various origins and terminations.

Dorsal Longitudinal Fasciculus

The *dorsal longitudinal fasciculus* is a component of an extensive periventricular system of descending and ascending fibers. It connects the hypothalamus with the mesencephalic central gray region. There are also direct connections from the hypothalamus to preganglionic autonomic nuclei in the brain stem and the spinal cord.

"Medial Forebrain Bundle"

The *"medial forebrain bundle"* is one of the most famous hypothalamic fiber bundles, but at the same time one of the most incomprehensible. The term was introduced by the German neurologist Edinger to denote a widespread and loosely arranged system of longitudinally running fibers in the lateral hypothalamic area of highly olfactory oriented animals. Some of its components are long axons that arise from olfactory areas and from monoaminergic cell groups in the brain stem. Other components are diffusely organized ascending and descending links similar to those found in the brain stem reticular formation. Some of the components are collaterals of other well-known pathways, such as the stria medullaris or the mammillary peduncle. Although it may be convenient to continue using the term "medial forebrain bundle" for this multitude of different and often loosely arranged fiber systems, one should remember that the term is used to designate a heterogenous group of axons that run the length of the lateral hypothalamus. Because of the great number of different origins and terminations of its different components, the term "medial forebrain bundle" has little meaning from a connectional point of view.

Hypothalamohypophysial Pathways

The hypothalamus is closely related to both the neuro- and the adenohypophysis. The *supraopticohypophysial tract* (Fig. 164A), which contains axons from the large neurosecretory cells in the

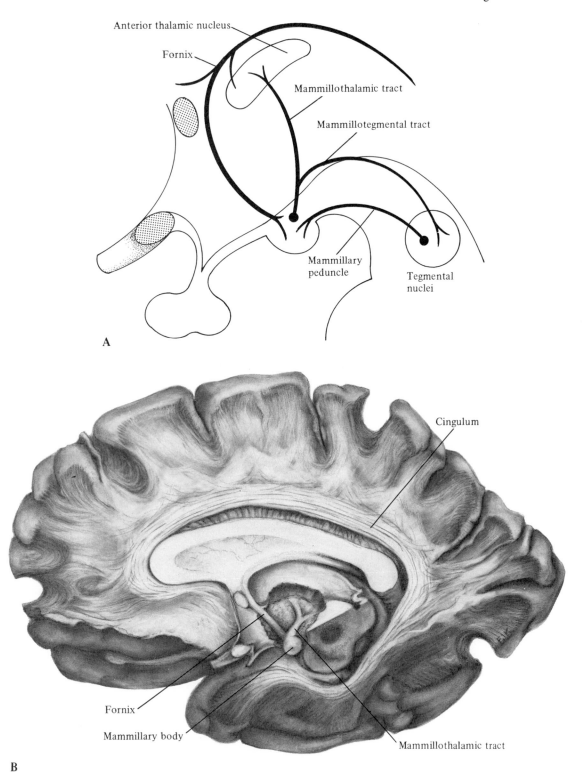

Fig. 163. Connections of the Mammillary Body
A. Highly schematic drawing of the main fiber connections of the mammillary body.
B. Blunt dissection of the human brain from the medial side. The gray substance of the hypothalamus has been removed to expose the fornix and the mamillothalamic tract. The medial parts of the hemisphere has also been removed to show the cingulum.

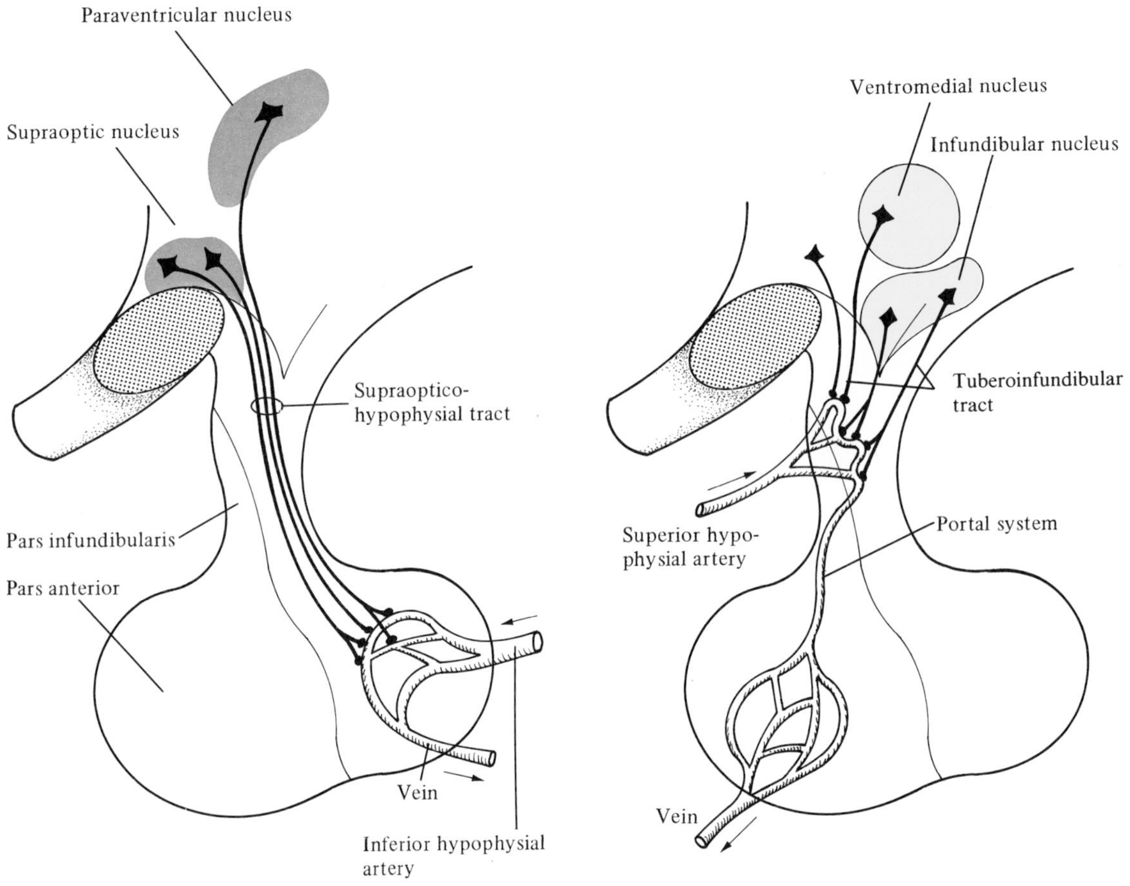

Fig. 164. Hypothalamohypophysial Pathways
A. Supraopticohypophysial tract.
B. Tuberoinfundibular tract and the hypophysial portal system.

supraoptic and paraventricular nuclei, terminates in the posterior lobe of the pituitary. Other neurosecretory fibers originate in different parts of the basomedial hypothalamus and project to the infundibulum. This is the tuberohypophysial or *tuberoinfundibular tract* (Fig. 164B), whose axons terminate upon the capillary loops of the *hypophysial portal system*. The tuberoinfundibular tract and the portal system together form a neurovascular chain between the hypothalamus and the adenohypophysis (see below).

Fiber Connections of the Mammillary Body

The mammillary body is different from the rest of the hypothalamus in several regards. It is surrounded by a capsule of heavily myelinated fibers, and it is not as closely related to autonomic and endocrine functions as the rest of the medial hypo-

thalamus. The exceptional position of the mammillary body is reflected in its prominent fiber connections with the hippocampus formation, the anterior thalamus, and the midbrain (Fig. 163).

The afferent pathways to the mammillary body are represented by the *fornix* (see above) and by the *mammillary peduncle*. The last bundle originates in the tegmental nuclei in the midbrain and terminates primarily in the lateral mammillary nucleus. Most of the efferent fibers leave the mammillary body in a dorsal direction as the *mammillothalamic tract* (Fig. 163 B), which proceeds in the internal medullary lamina to the anterior thalamic nucleus. Collaterals of the mammillothalamic fibers form the less conspicuous *mammillotegmental tract,* which primarily projects to the tegmental cell groups that give rise to the mammillary peduncle.

Cholinergic and Monoaminergic Pathways Related to the Hypothalamus

Several classes of transmitter substances have been identified in the CNS, and some of the neurons that produce acetylcholine and different monoamines project to the hypothalamus. In fact, some cholinergic and monoaminergic cells are even located within the hypothalamus. These neurotransmitter systems undoubtedly play important roles in hypothalamic and neuroendocrine functions.

An *ascending cholinergic pathway,* which originates in the substantia nigra and the ventral tegmental area, has a widespread distribution in the forebrain, including the hypothalamus.

The monoaminergic systems originating in the brain stem have a wide distribution in the forebrain, and some of the projection systems, e.g., the *mesolimbic dopamine pathway* and the *ventral ascending noradrenergic* and *serotonergic pathways,* pass through the lateral hypothalamic area. The ascending noradrenergic and serotonergic systems distribute a significant number of fibers to both the lateral and the medial hypothalamus on their way to more rostral regions. There are also intrinsic hypothalamic monoaminergic systems of special importance for neuroendocrine mechanisms. One example is the *tuberoinfundibular dopaminergic system,* which arises from dopamine-containing cells in the infundibular or arcuate nucleus and projects to the median eminence.

a nodal region for several pathways or systems of special importance for the function in question. Such a region is essential for the proper performance of a specific function, and if the area is damaged, the function will be disturbed. But one should keep in mind that the function can usually be influenced from other parts of the brain as well.

It is beyond the scope of this book to give an account of all the physiologic mechanisms in which hypothalamus is involved, and the following discussion will mainly serve to focus attention on the remarkable diversity of hypothalamic functions. For instance, the hypothalamus is well-known for its regulation of the endocrine system. These regulatory activities are dependent on intimate nervous and vascular relations between the hypothalamus and the pituitary. Through its efferent projections to various autonomic centers in the brain stem and the spinal cord, the hypothalamus is directly involved in the modulation of visceral functions. The integrative functions of the hypothalamus often involve the somatic nervous system as well. Such activities as eating, drinking, and sexual behavior, for instance, are in large part coordinated and controlled by the hypothalamus. The region is also of importance for consciousness and for sleep–wake behavior. The hypothalamus, finally, is critically involved in the integration of affective behavior in general; it represents "the final common path" in emotional expression and is therefore often included in the concept of the "limbic system" (Chapter 17).

FUNCTIONAL ASPECTS

Hypothalamic Control "Centers"

The presence of a certain degree of functional topography in the hypothalamus has promoted the concept of hypothalamic "centers," e.g., "temperature center," "hunger center," and "satiety center," and "centers" for cardiovascular, respiratory, and gastrointestinal functions. With a few exceptions, the "centers" are morphologically poorly defined, and they cannot usually be correlated with specific hypothalamic nuclei, but the efferent responses they induce are usually highly differentiated and complex.

The significance of a hypothalamic "center" for a specific function is reflected not only in its internal structure and histochemical features, but also in its relationships with other brain regions; it is

Hypothalamohypophysial Relationships

Neurosecretion

The hypothalamic control of the pituitary is dependent on a process called neurosecretion, which means that the activity involves the secretion of hormones into the bloodstream. The hypothalamic hormones are produced by neurosecretory cells located in the *"hypophysiotrophic area."* Some hypothalamic hormones are carried by axonal transport to the posterior lobe of the pituitary by way of the *supraopticohypophysial tract.* The *tuberoinfundibular tract* and the *portal vessels* together form a neurovascular transport system that carries hypothalamic hormones, sometimes called releasing factors (RF), to the anterior lobe where they regulate the release of the various anterior lobe hormones. The entire endocrine system, therefore, is under the control of the hypothalamus. Thus, the hypothalamohypophysial relationships are of great scientific and clinical interest.

Hypothalamus and the Neurohypophysis: Release of ADH and Oxytocin

The neurohypophysis, which consists of the infundibulum and the neural lobe,[1] is an outgrowth of the diencephalon, and it receives axonal projections from large neurosecretory neurons in the *supraoptic and paraventricular nuclei* of the hypothalamus. These axons form the *supraopticohypophysial tract* (Fig. 164 A). They carry neurosecretory material containing *antidiuretic hormone* (ADH), or *vasopressin*, and *oxytocin* to the neural lobe, where the axon terminals release the hormones into capillaries.

Most of the axons in the supraopticohypophysial tract originate in the highly vascularized supraoptic nucleus, whose cells produce both ADH and oxytocin. The release of ADH is controlled by various mechanisms. An increased amount of ADH is released in response to a rise in the osmotic pressure of the blood circulating through the nucleus or in the surrounding extracellular fluid. ADH, in turn, increases the resorption of water in the distal tubules of the kidneys. Inhibitory influences are exerted by vagal afferents from receptors in the atrial walls of the heart, stimulated by increased filling of the cardiovascular system.

Oxytocin, which is also produced both in the paraventricular and the supraoptic nucleus, promotes the contraction of the smooth muscles of the uterus and the mammary glands.

Hypothalamus and the Adenohypophysis: Regulation of the Endocrine Glands

The anatomic basis for the hypothalamic control of the anterior lobe[2] of the pituitary is rather complicated. Neurosecretory cells in the *infundibular*

nucleus, the *ventromedial nucleus,* and neighboring regions of the basomedial hypothalamus produce releasing factors (RF) or inhibiting factors (IF), which regulate the secretion of the trophic hormones from the anterior lobe of the pituitary. To reach the anterior lobe, the hormones are carried by axoplasmic transport through the axons of the *tuberoinfundibular tract* (Fig. 164 B) and discharged into capillary loops (portal capillaries) in the median eminence. The hormones are then transported through the *hypophysial portal veins* to a second capillary net in the anterior lobe, where they influence the secretion of the various adenohypophysial hormones, such as thyrotropin (TSH), adrenocorticotropin (ACTH), follicle-stimulating hormone (FSH), luteinizing hormone (LH), growth hormone (GH), melanocyte-stimulating hormone (MSH), and prolactin.

Although the hypothalamic neurons that produce the different hormones have not yet been clearly identified, there seems to be a certain degree of topography in the localization of the neurons responsible for the production of the various hormones. For example, neurons in the medial preoptic region seem to be of critical importance for stimulating the production of LH, whereas a more widespread region in the basomedial hypothalamus is directly involved in the control of ACTH release.

In regard to the neuroendocrine regulation in general, it is important to realize that the hypothalamic cell groups involved in different endocrine functions receive a variety of stimuli through their afferent connections with other brain regions, especially the amygdaloid body, the hippocampus, and various regions in the brain stem. Hypothalamic neurons are also subjected to hormonal feedback control. Such feedback mechanisms are often quite complicated in the sense that they involve not only the neurosecretory hypothalamic neurons but also hormone-sensitive cells in other brain regions, which are in a position to modulate hypothalamic activity.

The Hypothalamus and the Autonomic Nervous System

Basic autonomic reflexes are established on the brain stem and spinal cord level, and many vital activities, including respiration and cardiovascular and gastrointestinal functions, are to a large extent reflectoric in nature and can be carried out without

---

1. The neural lobe or pars nervosa is often equated with the posterior lobe. Strictly speaking, however, the posterior lobe also includes the rudimentary intermediate part of the adenohypophysis.
2. The anterior lobe or pars anterior is the main part of the adenohypophysis. Another part, pars infundibularis (tuberalis), covers the anterior part of the infundibulum. The third part, pars intermedius, which is rudimentary in the human, is included in the posterior lobe.

suprabulbar control. Nevertheless, a balanced activity in the visceral organs requires central modulation, and most of the central control of various sympathetic and parasympathetic centers in the brain stem and spinal cord occurs by way of the hypothalamus and its descending pathways. Generally, the hypothalamic control functions are not related to isolated autonomic responses, but to organized patterns of autonomic events, often closely coupled to endocrine adjustments. Indeed, the integrative functions of hypothalamus often require the coordination of a series of autonomic, endocrine, and somatic responses. The control of body temperature is a good example. Emotional responses, e.g., the *defense reaction* and *emotional fainting,* are also integrated at the hypothalamic level.

Regulation of Body Temperature

Warm-sensitive receptors are located in the preopticoanterior hypothalamic area, sensing the temperature of the arterial blood passing this richly vascularized region. The region is sometimes referred to as the *"heat loss center,"* because it initiates a series of processes that result in heat loss in response to increased body temperature. The "heat loss center" sends impulses to a region in the caudal part of hypothalamus where the different mechanisms for heat loss, including *peripheral vasodilation* and *sweating,* are integrated. There is also a mechanism for the preservation of heat in the caudal hypothalamus. In response to a drop in the surrounding temperature, cells in the caudal hypothalamus integrate a series of events, including *peripheral vasoconstriction, piloerection, increased metabolism,* and *shivering* to preserve the heat. The initial impulses in this case come from cold-sensitive receptors, which are located in the skin rather than within the hypothalamus.

The Defense Reaction and Emotional Fainting

The *defense reaction* (fight–flight response) is typical for all mammals, including man, who are faced with a threatening situation. It is characterized by an intense stimulation of the adrenergic fibers to the cardiovascular system, which results in an increase in cardiac output, heart rate, and blood pressure. Since the sympathetic cholinergic vasodilation fibers to the skeletal muscles are also stimulated, the increased cardiac output is immediately taken up in the skeletal muscle blood flow, thereby preparing the muscles for a fight or flight response if needed. The sympathetic response is reinforced by an increased liberation of adrenaline and noradrenaline from the adrenal medulla.

Emotional fainting is the antithesis of the defense reaction. It is characterized by a feeling of weakness and dizziness in response to an emotional situation characterized by a strong vasovagal reaction. A similar response can be seen in some animals and it is known as the "playing dead" reaction or "playing possum" since it is especially well known in the opossum, who suddenly drops as if dead when confronted with imminent danger.

The defense reaction and emotional fainting are two of the most dramatic examples of a series of emotional responses in the human. Although these responses are integrated at the hypothalamic level, they are triggered and modulated by other forebrain regions, e.g., the cerebral cortex and the amygdaloid body.

CLINICAL NOTES

Hypothalamohypophysial Disorders: A Diversity of Symptoms

The hypothalamus and the pituitary influence a large number of both endocrine and nonendocrine functions and it is difficult to give a systematic account of the number and variety of possible symptoms in hypothalamohypophysial disorders. Damage to different parts of the hypothalamohypophysial system may result in various neuroendocrine disturbances. Autonomic dysfunctions in the respiratory, the cardiovascular, and the gastrointestinal systems are commonly seen, as are disturbances in temperature regulation, water balance, sexual behavior, and food intake. Hypothalamic lesions can also change the level of consciousness, the sleep–wake cycle, and emotional behavior. It is no doubt easy to appreciate that the functional disturbances that accompany hypothalamohypophysial disorders may have serious consequences for the patient.

Many pathologic processes can damage the hypothalamus and the pituitary, but tumors are the most common. Primary pituitary tumors tend to expand in a dorsal direction where the resistance is minimal, and the early signs of a pituitary tumor may be related to the involvement of the hypothalamus. To cause hypothalamic symptoms, the lesion must ordinarily involve both sides of the hypothalamus.

Since the optic pathways have a strategic position at the base of the hypothalamus they are often affected by hypothalamohypophysial tumors. A pituitary tumor, for instance, that expands in a dorsal direction is likely to encroach on the optic chiasm or one of the optic tracts, causing visual field defects. The classic symptom is a bitemporal visual field defect (bitemporal hemianopia) caused by compression of the medial fibers of the optic tracts just posterior to the chiasm. These fibers originate in the nasal retina of each eye; thus their destruction causes blindness in each temporal visual field.

Hypothalamic Syndromes

Many of the symptoms related to hypothalamic diseases can also be seen in lesions of other brain regions, especially those regions closely related to the hypothalamus, e.g., the frontal cortex, the amygdaloid body, the hippocampal formation, and various structures in the brain stem. The number of truly hypothalamic syndromes, therefore, is rather limited. The best known are diabetes insipidus and Froehlich's syndrome. Disturbances in temperature regulation is also typical of hypothalamic disorders.

Diabetes Insipidus

Lesions involving the supraoptic and paraventricular nuclei or the supraopticohypophysial tract are likely to interfere with the formation of ADH. This results in a condition known as diabetes insipidus, which is characterized by an increased production of urine (polyuria). The loss of fluid, in turn, results in an excessive thirst (polydipsia). In many cases no explanation can be found for this disease.

Dystrophia Adiposogenitalis (Froehlich's Syndrome)

Lesions of the ventromedial hypothalamus in mammals including the human result in hyperphagia and obesity. The ventromedial nucleus, there-

fore, is sometimes referred to as a "satiety center." In tumors that involve both the hypothalamus and the pituitary, the adiposity is often associated with underdevelopment of the genitalia, in which case it is called Froehlich's syndrome.

Disturbances in Temperature Regulation

Destruction of the "heat loss" center in the anterior hypothalamus may result in *hyperthermia,* which, if pronounced, may lead to the death of the patient within hours or days. Postoperative hyperthermia is sometimes seen following operations for pituitary tumors or suprasellar meningiomas. Bilateral lesions in more posterior parts of the hypothalamus may result in *hypothermia* or *poikilothermia,* a condition characterized by pronounced variations in the body temperature in response to changes in the surrounding temperature.

Many diseases are characterized by *fever,* which is caused by blood-borne substances, i.e., pyrogens. The pyrogens act on the hypothalamic thermoregulatory centers that bring about an increase in the body temperature through peripheral vasoconstriction and shivering. The constriction of the skin vessels results in a decreased skin temperature, which produces a chilly sensation. When the fever subsides, heat is released from the body by vasodilation and sweating.

Psychosomatic Disorders

People who live in "modern" highly competitive and hectic societies are apparently afflicted by psychosomatic disturbances to a greater extent than people who live in stable social environments characterized by traditions and age-dependent hierarchy rather than rapid change and competition. Environmental stress, e.g., broken families, unstable work situations, financial problems, and extreme social climbing, result in emotional arousal and neuroendocrine changes that eventually may lead to pathologic changes in the organism. Such psychosomatic disturbances are often an important factor in the development of commonly known diseases including many forms of cardiovascular disorders, asthma, peptic ulcer, and eating disorders. Although the psychosomatic diseases are not referred to as hypothalamic disorders, it is by way of the hypothalamus that the psychosomatic disturbances are executed.

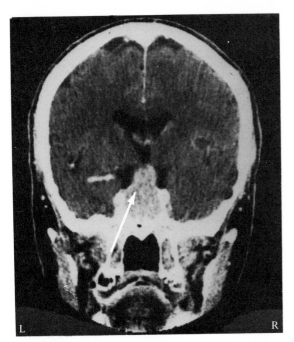

Fig. CE15. Pituitary Adenoma
The CT scan was kindly provided by Dr. V. Haughton.

CLINICAL EXAMPLE

Pituitary Adenoma

A 45-year-old male was seeking medical attention for a series of disturbing but seemingly unrelated symptoms. He had been suffering from increasingly severe headaches for a couple of years, and about a year ago he developed hypothyroidism and was treated with thyroid extract. Three months ago he realized that he was impotent, and he started to complain of visual deficits at about the same time. His appearance was that of a chronically ill man, with a shallow complexion typical of panhypopituitarism. He had decreased pubic hair and some testicular atrophy.

Neurologic examination revealed a complete bitemporal hemianopsia, but he had no other cranial nerve deficits. However, he seemed to have a general mild weakness in his musculature.

Laboratory studies showed normal thyroid hormone levels, but he had abnormally low serum testosterone. Intravenous administration of thyrotropin-releasing hormone produced only a small elevation of thyroid-stimulating hormone in the serum.

A CT scan (see figure) was obtained.

1. Where is the lesion?
2. Does the lesion account for his visual deficits?
3. How did his endocrine abnormalities arise?

Discussion

The CT scan demonstrates a mass lesion growing out of the sella turcica (arrow) and extending into the hypothalamus. Considering the clinical findings, the most likely diagnosis is a pituitary adenoma (chromophobe adenoma). The tumor, apparently, compresses the optic chiasm in the midline, thereby damaging the crossing fibers, i.e., those coming from the nasal part of the retina of each eye (Fig. 150).

The endocrine deficiencies result from destruction of the anterior lobe of the pituitary. Pituitary adenomas are slowly growing tumors, and they may reach a large size before they interfere with the well-being of the patient. Indeed, visual failure, rather than endocrine symptoms, often brings the patient to the doctor.

SUGGESTED READING

1. Haymaker, W., E. Anderson, and W. J. H. Nauta, 1969. The Hypothalamus. Charles C Thomas: Springfield, Illinois.
2. Knigge, K. M. and A. J. Silverman, 1974. Anatomy of the endocrine hypothalamus. In R. O. Greep and E. B. Astwood (eds.): Handbook of Physiology, Endocrinology. American Physiological Society, Vol. 6.
3. Martin, J. B., S. Reichlin, and G. M. Brown, 1977. Clinical Neuroendocrinology. F. A. Davis: Philadelphia.
4. Morgane, P. J. and J. Panksepp (eds.), 1979. Anatomy of the Hypothalamus. Marcel Dekker: New York.
5. Reichlin, S., R. J. Baldessarini, and J. B. Martin, 1978. The Hypothalamus. Research Publications: Association for Research in Nervous and Mental Disease, Vol. 56. Raven Press: New York.
6. Stumpf, W. E. and L. D. Grant (eds.), 1974. Anatomical Neuroendocrinology. S. Karger: Basel.

16

The Autonomic Nervous System

PERIPHERAL PARTS
  Pre- and Postganglionic Neuron
  Thoracolumbar or "Sympathetic" Division
  Craniosacral or "Parasympathetic" Division
  Afferent Visceral Fibers
  Autonomic Innervation of Some Organs

CENTRAL PARTS
  Cardiovascular and Respiratory Centers in
    Medulla Oblongata
  Hypothalamus
  Amygdaloid Body and Cerebral Cortex

CLINICAL NOTES
  Referred Pain
  Horner's Syndrome
  Autonomic Dysfunction in Spinal Cord Injuries
  Psychosomatic Disorders

SUGGESTED READING

Through its innervation of the visceral organs, the glands, and the blood vessels, the autonomic nervous system regulates the internal environment; it is largely responsible for maintaining normal bodily functions. The activities of the autonomic nervous system are, to a great extent, based on tonically active bulbar centers, intimately adjusted by reflexes from a variety of receptors in the internal organs. The autonomic activities are closely integrated with other nervous activities and with endocrine functions.

Many diseases affect the autonomic pathways, in the peripheral and the central nervous systems, and thus cause derangement of autonomic functions. Hypothalamic syndromes, in particular, are characterized by autonomic disturbances, and many emotional states, both normal and pathologic, are accompanied by autonomic nervous system activities. The autonomic system is the means for physical expression of emotion, as in the blush of embarrassment or the tachycardia of fright.

The autonomic ("vegetative" or "visceral") nervous system innervates smooth muscles, glands, and cardiac muscle. It consists of a *sympathetic* (or thoracolumbar) and a *parasympathetic* (or craniosacral) division, which usually have antagonistic effects.

The sympathetic system responds to needs requiring a mobilization of all resources, e.g., in stressful situations. It prepares the body for an emergency: the pupils dilate and heart rate, blood pressure, and cardiac output increase, favoring blood flow to skeletal muscles, myocardium, and brain. There is also an increased secretion of epinephrine and norepinephrine into the blood. At the same time, the peristaltic activity of the gastrointestinal (GI) tract is suppressed by adrenergic nerve inhibitory effects.

In contrast, the parasympathetic system reduces heart rate but stimulates the peristaltic and secretory activities of the GI tract. Autonomic activity, however, is seldom solely either sympathetic or parasympathetic; it is usually the product of a well-balanced interplay between the two parts, thereby providing an important mechanism for the maintenance of homeostasis, i.e., a condition of dynamic equilibrium in the internal environment.

Originally, the autonomic nervous system was considered to be a peripheral system with purely motor functions. However, it was soon discovered that the CNS also contains important autonomic centers, and it is now generally recognized that afferent fibers and pathways are as much part of the autonomic nervous system as they are of the somatic system. In fact, the majority of the nerve impulses in the "great visceral nerve," the vagus, are *afferents,* conveying important information about pressure, stretch, chemical environment, etc., from the visceral organs, e.g., the gastrointestinal tract, the heart, the central arteries, and the veins.

PERIPHERAL PARTS

Pre- and Postganglionic Neuron

One of the most characteristic features of the autonomic nervous system is that a significant number of the efferent neurons are located outside the CNS in *autonomic ganglia*. The efferent peripheral pathway, therefore, consists of two neurons, a *preganglionic neuron,* whose cell body is located

within the CNS, and a *postganglionic neuron,* whose cell body is located in a ganglion outside the CNS (Fig. 165). Because one preganglionic neuron usually contacts many postganglionic neurons in the peripheral ganglion, there is generally a considerable divergence of activity following stimulation of only one preganglionic neuron. This arrangement is the basis for the "mass effect" of the autonomic, especially sympathetic, system. Nevertheless, this system of divergence–convergence is highly specific, as it serves to bind together into "functional units" such parts as the vascular bed or the GI system, which for central control requires unification.

Anatomic Differences Between the Sympathetic and Parasympathetic Systems

Whereas the postganglionic sympathetic neurons are located in sympathetic ganglia at some distance from the effector organs (Fig. 166) the postganglionic parasympathetic neurons are located either in the wall (Fig. 166) of the organs they innervate (e.g., in the myenteric and mucosal plexuses of the GI tract) or in close proximity to the organs of innervation (e.g., in pulmonary, cardiac, or gastric plexuses). The parasympathetic activity, therefore, is generally more localized in its effect than the sympathetic activity.

Pharmacologic Differences Between the Sympathetic and Parasympathetic Systems

Whereas *acetylcholine* (ACh) is released at the axon terminals of the postganglionic parasympathetic fibers (cholinergic fibers), *noradrenaline* (norepinephrine) is the transmitter substance that is released from most postganglionic sympathetic fibers (adrenergic fibers). However, the sympathetic postganglionic fibers to the sweat glands and the sympathetic vasodilator fibers to the blood vessels of skeletal muscles are cholinergic, as are all preganglionic autonomic neurons.

Thoracolumbar or "Sympathetic" Division

The cell bodies of the preganglionic motor neurons of the sympathetic division (red in Fig. 167) are located in the *intermediolateral cell column* in the

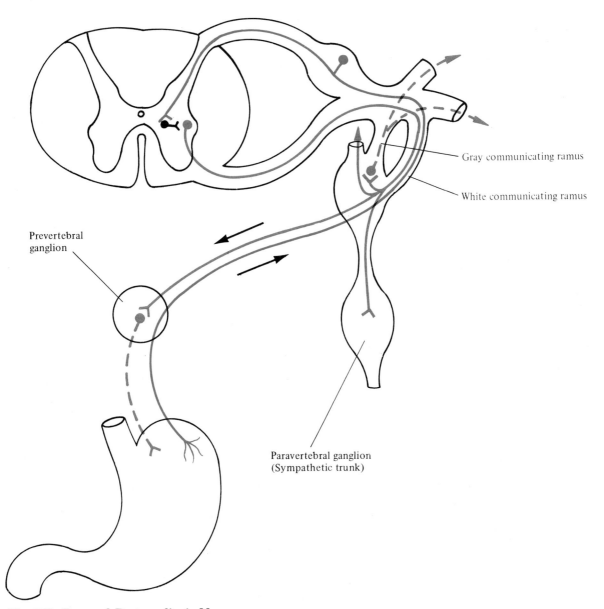

Gray communicating ramus

White communicating ramus

Prevertebral
ganglion

Paravertebral ganglion
(Sympathetic trunk)

Fig. 165. Pre- and Postganglionic Neurons
Diagram showing the arrangement of pre- and postganglionic neurons in the sympathetic autonomic system.
Preganglionic neuron, *solid red;* postganglionic neuron, *dashed red;* afferent neuron, *blue;* interneuron, *black.*

lateral horn of the spinal cord. This cell column extends from the first thoracic to the second or third lumbar segment. The preganglionic fibers exit via ventral roots T1–L2–3 and reach the *paravertebral ganglia* of the *sympathetic trunk,* which extends from the base of the skull to the coccyx on the ventrolateral side of the vertebral column. The connection between the ventral root and the sympathetic trunk is formed by the preganglionic sympathetic fibers, which are called the white *communicating rami* (Fig. 165). The color of these rami is whitish because the preganglionic fibers are myelinated.

Having reached the sympathetic trunk the preganglionic fibers can:

either   pass through the paravertebral ganglia as *splanchnic nerves* and synapse in one of the *prevertebral ganglia,* such as the *celiac ganglion,* the *superior mesenteric ganglion* or the *inferior mesenteric ganglion,*

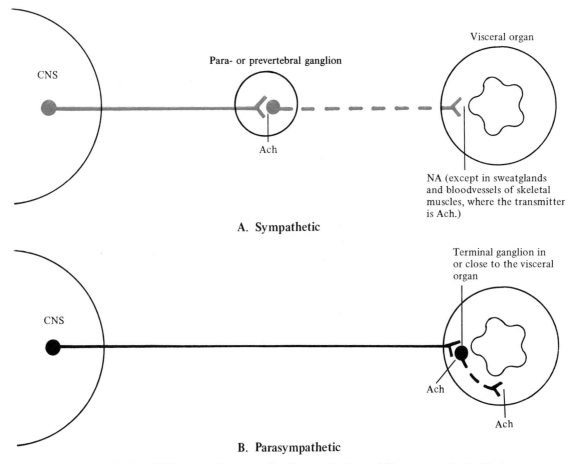

A. Sympathetic

B. Parasympathetic

Fig. 166. Major Differences Between the Sympathetic and Parasympathetic Systems

or pass up or down in the sympathetic trunk before establishing contacts with postganglionic neurons at different levels of the sympathetic trunk ganglia,

or, finally, they may establish synaptic contacts with postganglionic neurons in the paravertebral ganglion at the level of entrance.

Many of the postganglionic fibers that emerge from the different paravertebral and prevertebral ganglia join arteries and follow these, as plexuses of nerve fibers, to the different internal organs. Other postganglionic fibers return to the spinal nerves from the different levels of the sympathetic trunk as the *gray communicating rami,* so named because the majority of the postganglionic fibers

are unmyelinated.[1] In contrast with the white rami, which are present only in the thoracolumbar (T1–L2–3) part of the sympathetic trunk, the gray rami are found along the entire trunk. The postganglionic fibers that join the spinal nerves distribute to the sweat glands in the skin and to the blood vessels and the hair follicles (arrector pili muscles) in the peripheral parts of the body. These structures, incidentally, do not receive a parasympathetic innervation.

Craniosacral or "Parasympathetic" Division

The preganglionic efferent fibers in the parasympathetic division (black in Fig. 167) pass through some of the cranial nerves (the cranial part) and through the second, third, and fourth sacral nerves (the sacral part).

1. Although the terms white and gray communicating rami indicate a difference in color, it is apparently not possible to identify the two types on the basis of their color during surgery.

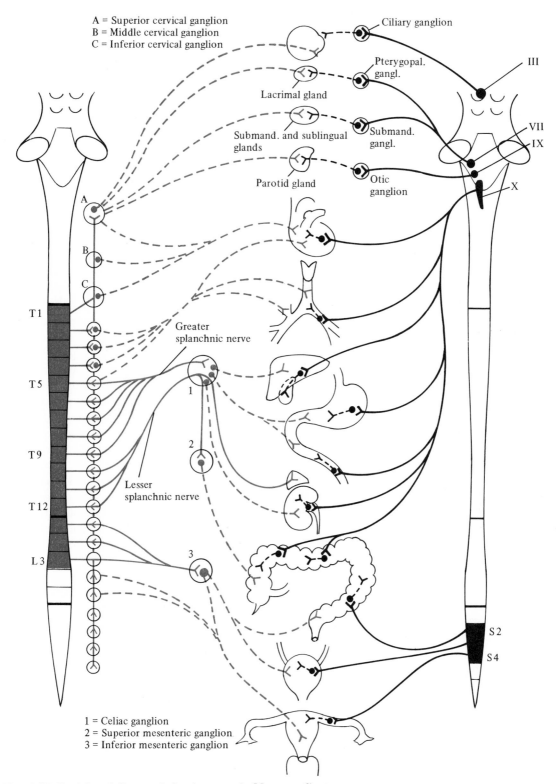

A = Superior cervical ganglion
B = Middle cervical ganglion
C = Inferior cervical ganglion

Ciliary ganglion

Pterygopal. gangl.

Lacrimal gland

III

Submand. gangl.

Submand. and sublingual glands

VII
IX

Parotid gland

Otic ganglion

X

A

B

C

T 1

Greater splanchnic nerve

T 5

1

Lesser splanchnic nerve

2

T 9

T 12

L 3

3

S 2

S 4

1 = Celiac ganglion
2 = Superior mesenteric ganglion
3 = Inferior mesenteric ganglion

Fig. 167. Peripheral Parts of the Autonomic Nervous System
Scheme of the efferent pathways of the sympathetic thoracolumbar (*red*) and parasympathetic craniosacral (*black*)
divisions of the peripheral autonomic system.

Cranial Part

The cranial part of the parasympathetic division originates in the brain stem, and the preganglionic fibers emerge along with the following four cranial nerves: the oculomotor (III), facial (VII), glossopharyngeal (IX), and vagus (X) nerves.

Oculomotor Nerve.   The parasympathetic oculomotor fibers originate in the parasympathetic nucleus (Edinger-Westphal) of the oculomotor nuclear complex. They course along in a branch of the IIIrd cranial nerve to the *ciliary ganglion,* where preganglionic fibers synapse with the postganglionic neurons that innervate the ciliary muscle and the sphincter pupillae.

Facial Nerve.   Preganglionic fibers from cells in the *superior salivatory nucleus* emerge from the skull in the nervus intermedius. Some of the fibers reach the *pterygopalatine ganglion* via the great petrosal branch and the nerve of the pterygoid canal. Other of these preganglionic axons proceed through the corda tympani and the lingual nerve to synapse in the *submandibular ganglion.* The postganglionic fibers originating in the pterygopalatine ganglion innervate the lacrimal gland and those from the submandibular ganglion terminate in the submandibular and sublingual glands.

Glossopharyngeal Nerve.   Preganglionic secretomotor fibers originate in the *inferior salivatory nucleus* and reach the *otic ganglion* through the tympanic branch of the glossopharyngeal nerve and the lesser petrosal nerve. The postganglionic fibers innervate the parotid gland.

Vagus Nerve.   The vagus nerve is the principal nerve of the parasympathetic division. It contains preganglionic parasympathetic fibers that originate in the *dorsal motor nucleus of the vagus.* The postganglionic neurons are located in ganglia that lie in the walls of the visceral organs of the thorax and the abdomen. Only a small number (10–15%) of the fibers in the vagus are efferent; the majority are afferent fibers from receptors in the different visceral organs. The visceral afferent fibers, like the autonomic afferent fibers in the facial and glossopharyngeal nerves, terminate in the *solitary nucleus.*

Sacral Part

The preganglionic fibers of the sacral part of the parasympathetic system originate in cells of the second, third, and fourth sacral segments of the spinal cord. The fibers emerge in the ventral root and later leave the sacral nerves to form the *pelvic nerves* (nervi erigentes) on each side of the rectum. Here they intermingle with sympathetic fibers. The sacral parasympathetic part innervates the descending and sigmoid colon, the rectum, the bladder, and the genitalia.

Afferent Visceral Fibers

Impulses from visceral receptors reach the CNS through afferent fibers, which follow the efferent autonomic fibers peripherally (Fig. 165). The afferent fibers, whose cell bodies are located in the spinal ganglion and in the cranial nerve ganglia of the facial (VII), the glossopharyngeal (IX), and the vagus (X) nerves, are equal in importance to the efferent fibers and greatly outnumber them. The visceral sensoric impulses play an important role in various reflexes for the coordination and adjustment of visceral functions, and only occasionally do they reach the level of consciousness.

Although our understanding of the visceral sensory system, and of its receptors and afferent pathways has increased significantly in recent years, it is still incomplete compared with our knowledge about the efferent part of the autonomic system. For instance, we know little about the type of visceral sensations that are mediated by the various ascending tracts in the spinal cord.

From a clinical point of view, the most prominent visceral sensation is pain, which is usually poorly localized and of aching quality. Visceral pain is also characterized by its capacity to induce strong autonomic responses and by its tendency to be displaced or reflected from the true source in the visceral organ to the body surface (see *Referred Pain* in Clinical Notes). The vast majority, perhaps all, of the pain fibers from the internal organs pass with the sympathetic innervation, whereas nearly all the other afferents controlling autonomic function run in the parasympathetic system.

Autonomic Innervation of Some Organs (Fig. 167)

Eye

The preganglionic sympathetic fibers to the eye, the cell bodies of which lie in the *intermediolateral cell column* in the first and second thoracic segments (ciliospinal center), proceed through the sympathetic trunk to the *superior cervical ganglion*, where they establish synaptic contacts with the postganglionic fibers. The postganglionic fibers follow the internal carotid and the ophthalmic arteries and pass uninterruptedly through the *ciliary ganglion* and the *short ciliary nerves* to end in the dilator pupillae and the superior tarsal muscle. A lesion of the sympathetic pathway to the eye results in Horner's syndrome (see Clinical Notes).

Preganglionic parasympathetic fibers, which originate in the *Edinger-Westphal nucleus* of the oculomotor nuclear complex, reach the *ciliary ganglion* through the oculomotor nerve. The postganglionic fibers pass forward in the *short ciliary nerves* and innervate the constrictor pupillae and the ciliary muscle. The parasympathetic pathway to the constrictor pupillae is an important link in the pupillary light reflex.

Heart

The preganglionic sympathetic neurons are located in the upper thoracic part of the *intermediolateral cell column* (T1–T5). They end in the three *cervical ganglia* and upper *thoracic ganglia*. The postganglionic fibers reach the heart by way of the *cardiac nerves*. Stimulation of the sympathetic fibers that innervate the pacemaker cells and cardiac muscle cells increases heart rate, transmission velocity, excitability, and the contractility of the cardiac muscle cells. This latter important effect increases both the speed and the force of the cardiac systoli.

Activation of the parasympathetic fibers, which reach the heart through the vagus, results predominantly in a reduction of the heart rate, and delays the transmission of the atrial excitation to the ventricles.

Lungs

The postganglionic sympathetic fibers, which arise from level T2–T5 of the sympathetic trunk, produce bronchodilation and vasoconstriction, whereas stimulation of the vagus results in constriction of the bronchioli and an increased glandular secretion.

Gastrointestinal Tract

The motor and secretory innervations of the GI tract are provided by the parasympathetic system, mostly through the *vagus nerves* and partly (lower colon and rectum) through the *pelvic nerves* from the sacral part of the spinal cord. The preganglionic parasympathetic fibers establish synaptic contact with the postganglionic neurons that form the *myenteric* (Auerbach's) and *mucosal* (Messner's) *plexuses* in the wall of the GI tract. Stimulation of the parasympathetic system increases peristalsis and secretion of gastric and intestinal juices, and relaxes the sphincters.

The preganglionic sympathetic fibers (from T5 to L2) pass without interruption through the *sympathetic trunk* and *splanchnic nerves* to the *prevertebral ganglia* (the celiac ganglion and the superior and inferior mesenteric ganglia). The postganglionic fibers are distributed to the GI tract as nerve plexuses around the arteries. Stimulation of the sympathetic fibers results in reduced peristalsis, decreased secretion, and contraction of the sphincters.

Adrenal Medulla

Cells of the adrenal medulla are derived from the neural crest and represent postganglionic sympathetic neurons. Accordingly, they are innervated by preganglionic sympathetic fibers, which emerge from the *lesser splanchnic nerve*. Stimulation of the adrenal medulla is followed by liberation of epinephrine and to a lesser extent norepinephrine into the bloodstream. This provides for a relatively rapid and widespread reinforcement of sympathetic activities during emergency situations and conditions of stress. The hormonal component is particularly important for the mobilization of substances such as glucose and fatty acids, from nutritional depots, while the direct nervous influence on the heart and vessels dominates the cardiovascular adjustments.

Bladder

The control of micturition is primarily a parasympathetic function. When the volume of urine in the bladder reaches a certain level, impulses from stretch receptors in the wall of the bladder pass through the *pelvic nerves* to the sacral cord, where they activate parasympathetic preganglionic neurons. Increased activity in these preganglionic fibers, which pass through the pelvic nerves to the bladder, results in contraction of the detrusor muscle. There is a concomitant inhibition of the motor neurons that innervate the external sphincter. Although the reflexes for emptying the bladder are predominantly under reflex spinal control in the newborn, they gradually become subjected to supraspinal conscious regulation.

CENTRAL PARTS

Although the integrity of the spinal cord is essential for the autonomic reflexes, several supraspinal regions are also involved in the control of autonomic functions. The brain stem reticular formation, for instance, contains important cardiovascular and respiratory centers; the cerebellum exercises a modulatory influence on autonomic functions; and in the forebrain it is, above all, the hypothalamus that is concerned with the control and modulation of autonomic functions. Other forebrain regions, especially the amygdaloid body and the cerebral cortex, also influence autonomic functions, but their activity is mediated to a considerable extent by the hypothalamus.

Cardiovascular and Respiratory Centers in Medulla Oblongata

These vital centers are represented by cranial nerve nuclei and by cell groups in the reticular formation of the medulla oblongata and lower pons. Although the respiratory reflexes are characterized by somatic rather than autonomic efferents, it is convenient to discuss the respiratory center in connection with the cardiovascular centers.

Cardiovascular Centers[2]

These centers are responsible for the integration of a series of visceral reflexes designed to keep the blood pressure reasonably well stabilized. In particular, the sympathetic centers maintain a low-frequency tonic activity. The centers receive impulses from many sensory receptors, including *pressoreceptors* (baroreceptors) in the aorta and the carotid arteries, and *"volume" receptors* in the atrial and ventricular walls. If the blood pressure increases and the vessel wall stretches, or if the heart is increasingly filled in diastole, the respective receptors increase discharge of impulses, which pass along the *glossopharyngeal* and *vagus nerves* to the *solitary nucleus* and then to the *cardiovascular centers*. The cardiovascular centers activate the parasympathetic fibers to the heart at the same time that they reduce the activity in the sympathetic fibers, thereby reducing heart rate. There is also a reduced activity in the sympathetic vasoconstrictor fibers to the arterioles, which decreases resistance to blood flow, as well as to the venous "capacitance" side, thereby favoring increased peripheral pooling of blood, and hence a reduction of venous return to the heart.

Respiratory Center

The respiratory center, whose activity is modified by impulses from the pons, is essential for the maintenance of rhythmic respiration. The center consists of aggregations of rhythmic *respiratory neurons* that include especially the *nucleus of the solitary tract* and the *nucleus ambiguus* and surrounding areas of the *reticular formation*. Although it is common to speak of a rostrally located inspiratory part and a caudally located expiratory part of the respiratory center, inspiratory and expiratory neurons to a large extent are intermingled in the respiratory center (Fig. 168). In quiet breathing only the inspiratory movement is active. The inspiratory center, which is driven by impulses from both central and peripheral chemoreceptors and various reflexes, sends impulses through re-

2. The cardiovascular centers are represented by several sets of neurons that produce effects either on the heart rate (cardioinhibitory and cardioexcitatory centers) or on the blood pressure (vasopressor and vasodepressor centers). This complex of different centers is often referred to as the vasomotor center (VMC).

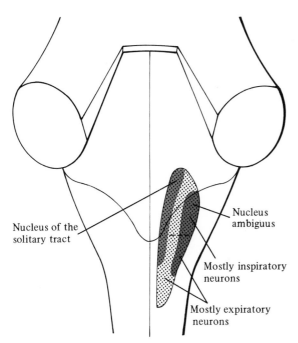

Fig. 168. Respiratory Center

The respiratory neurons are located primarily in the region of the nucleus of the solitary tract, the nucleus ambiguus and surrounding areas of the reticular formation.

ticulospinal pathways to the motor neurons that innervate the inspiratory muscles. When the inspiratory activity has reached a critical threshold, the inspiratory center is inhibited, which allows for passive expiration. The "switching off" of the inspiratory center is controlled by a neural mechanism that obtains input from several sources, including impulses through the vagus nerve from stretch receptors in the lungs (Hering-Breuer reflex), and impulses from the chest wall.

The changes in respiration that are seen in different conditions are brought about by impulses generated by chemoreceptors in the large arteries of the heart and mechanoreceptors of the lungs. There is also a mechanism for direct chemical stimulation of the respiratory center, which responds especially to an increase in the carbon dioxide content of the blood and to the pH of the extracellular fluid.

Hypothalamus

Because the functional anatomy of the hypothalamus is presented in Chapter 15, only a few com-

ments are made here regarding hypothalamic control of autonomic function. As previously indicated, the hypothalamus controls and integrates a large number of visceral functions by way of its connections with the autonomic centers in the brain stem and the spinal cord, and through its relationships with the pituitary gland. There is a certain topography in the hypothalamus in the sense that sympathetic activities can often be elicited by stimulation of the posterior hypothalamus and parasympathetic activities by stimulation of the anterior hypothalamus. However, the most prominent aspect of the hypothalamus' regulatory functions is its capacity to integrate sympathetic, parasympathetic, and somatic responses into organized patterns of activity. The regulation of body temperature (see Clinical Notes, Chapter 15) is a good example.

With the aid of modern tracer techniques, scientists recently have established the presence of direct projections from several hypothalamic regions to autonomic centers in the brain stem and the spinal cord (Fig. 169). These pathways are partly reciprocated by direct lines of communication from the solitary nucleus to the hypothalamus and the amygdaloid body. Since the solitary nucleus receives visceral afferents from both the glossopharyngeal and the vagus nerves—and apparently also from ascending pathways that originate in autonomic centers in the spinal cord—interoceptive information can be channeled directly to the hypothalamus and related forebrain structures.

Amygdaloid Body and Cerebral Cortex

It is a common experience that mental activities can influence visceral functions (e.g., goose pimples, blushing, salivation in response to strong psychic influences), and there are many experimental and clinical observations that implicate parts of the frontal and temporal lobes in the control of autonomic, as well as endocrine, functions. It should also be emphasized that the amygdaloid body, which receives highly elaborate sensory information from cortical regions in the temporal and frontal lobes, is a major modulator of hypothalamic activities.

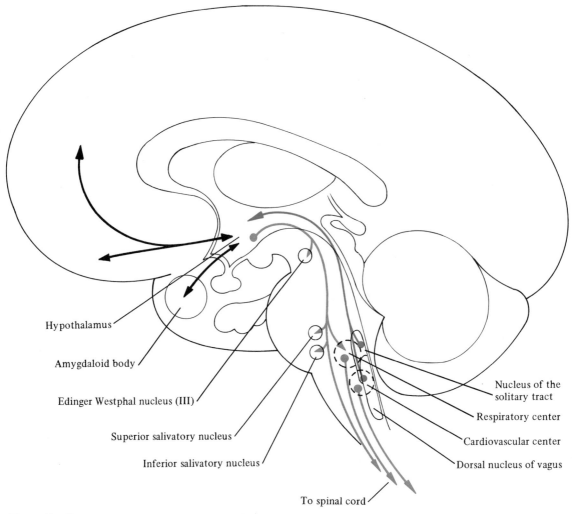

Fig. 169. Central Parts of the Autonomic Nervous System
Highly schematic figure of the most prominent central structures involved in the regulation of autonomic activities.

CLINICAL NOTES

Referred Pain

Referred pain is a clinically important although poorly understood phenomenon in which the pain is displaced or referred from its true source in a visceral organ to the surface of the body. The pain is usually referred, not to the skin overlying the affected organ, but to the skin that is innervated by the same spinal cord segment as the diseased organ (Fig. 170). For example, the pain of angina pectoris is usually felt in the upper thorax (T2–T4) or down the inside of the left arm (T1), whereas gall bladder pain is referred to thoracic dermatones (T6–T8), usually in the epigastric re-gion or dorsally underneath the right shoulder blade. Pain in the shoulder region (C3–C4) may be caused by irritation of the diaphragm.

Referred pain is a complicated phenomenon that has not been satisfactorily explained. A popular theory is that the visceral afferent fibers converge on the same pool of spinal cord neurons as the somatic afferent fibers. Because somatic pain is much more common than visceral pain, the brain becomes accustomed to interpreting the activity in a specific pool of spinal cord neurons as the result of pain stimuli in a particular skin region. When the same neural pool is stimulated by impulses from the visceral organ, the brain "misinterprets" the message as coming from the skin.

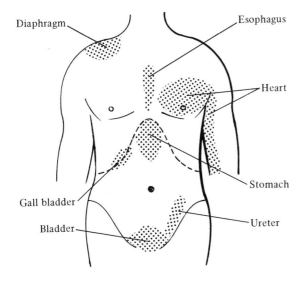

Diaphragm

Esophagus

Heart

Stomach

Gall bladder

Ureter

Bladder

Fig. 170. Referred Pain
Diagram showing cutaneous sites of reference of visceral pain commonly encountered in medical practice. It is worth emphasizing that there are significant variations from case to case.

Horner's Syndrome

Interruption of the sympathetic fibers to the eye results in *miosis* (constriction of the pupil) and *ptosis* (drooping of the eyelid) because of paralysis of the dilator pupillae and the superior tarsal muscle. There is also *anhydrosis* (loss of sweating) on the affected side of the face and neck. The eyeball also appears to lie deeper in the orbit, i.e., *enophthalmos,* but whether this is real, as a result of paralysis of the smooth muscles in the inferior orbital fissure, or only apparent because of the ptosis, is unclear.

Autonomic Dysfunction in Spinal Cord Injuries

Trauma to the spinal cord is common in highly industrialized societies and in times of war. Complete transection of the spinal cord results in paralysis and anesthesia of all body segments below the lesion. The difficult and time-consuming treatment of such patients (called paraplegics, if lower limbs and body are paralyzed; and tetraplegics, if all four limbs are involved) is often carried out in special medical centers.

The paralysis of the parasympathetic innervation to the bladder and the rectum deserves special attention. Immediately following a spinal transection autonomic functions are completely suppressed. There is retention of urine and lack of activity in the bowel. Urination and defecation must be induced by catheter and enema. As the "spinal shock" wears off after a few weeks, reflex activities resume in the bladder and the rectum, providing the lesion is rostral to the sacral parasympathetic part (S2–S4) of the spinal cord. Urination becomes automatic and precipitous, a condition known as *hypertonic* or *hyperreflexive bladder.* If the sacral segments of the spinal cord are destroyed there is no reflex control of the bladder, which will fill to capacity and overflow. This is known as *flaccid, hypotonic,* or *hyporeflexive bladder.*

Psychosomatic Disorders

Although many of the vegetative activities, e.g., secretions and motility of the GI tract, contraction of the heart, kidney function, etc., are basically automatic in nature, the autonomic control of visceral functions is closely correlated with the activity in the rest of the nervous system. This intimate relationship is clearly reflected in the organization of the central parts of the autonomic system. Except for the sympathetic and parasympathetic nuclei in the spinal cord and the brain stem, the autonomic centers in the CNS are inseparable from the rest of the nervous system

The intimate relationships between mental activities and vegetative functions are familiar to everybody. Salivation can occur by the mere thought of delicious food, embarrassment causes blushing, and sudden psychic stress can cause a dramatic change in heart rate. This intricate relationship between mental activities and visceral functions may have far-reaching consequences for a person's well-being; continuous frustration, or emergency responses that are repeated too often, will eventually lead to neuroendocrine disturbances that may result in pathologic changes in visceral organs. This psychosomatic component may be a key factor in the development of many commonly known diseases such as peptic ulcer, asthma, and hypertension, to mention a few. Since psychosomatic ailments make up a large part of the physician's practice, most clinicians will have to deal with this general pathophysiologic aspect of the autonomic nervous system.

SUGGESTED READING

1. Appenzeller, D., 1982. The Autonomic Nervous System. An Introduction to Basic and Clinical Concepts, 3rd ed. Elsevier BioMedical Press: Amsterdam.

2. Brodal, A., 1981. Neurological Anatomy in Relation to Clinical Medicine, 3rd ed. Oxford University Press: New York, Oxford, pp. 698–787.

3. DeJong, R., 1979. The Neurologic Examination. Harper and Row: Hagerstown, Maryland, pp. 491–544.

4. Henry, J. P. and P. M. Stephens, 1977. Stress, Health, and the Social Environment. A Sociobiologic Approach to Medicine. Springer-Verlag: New York, Heidelberg, Berlin.

5. Koizumi, K. and C. M. Brooks, 1980. The autonomic system and its role in controlling body functions. In V. B. Mountcastle (ed.): Medical Physiology, 14th ed. C. V. Mosby: St. Louis, Missouri, pp. 893–922.

17

Amygdaloid Body, Hippocampal Formation, and "Limbic System"

AMYGDALOID BODY
    Subdivisions
    Connections
    Functional Aspects

HIPPOCAMPAL FORMATION
    Histologic Structure
    Extrinsic Connections
    Intrinsic Connections
    Functional Considerations

"LIMBIC SYSTEM"

CLINICAL NOTES
    Psychomotor Epilepsy
    Wernicke-Korsakoff's Syndrome

SUGGESTED READING

The amygdaloid body and hippocampal formation are two large structures in the temporal lobe. They are intimately related to other areas of the cerebral cortex as well as to a number of subcortical structures in the brain and the brain stem.

As key components of the "limbic system," the amygdala and hippocampus have been implicated in emotional behavior and memory. However, to what extent and how the various "limbic system" structures are involved in these extremely complicated functions is not known. A more comprehensive knowledge of these matters would undoubtedly improve our understanding of many aspects of human behavior and make us better prepared to manage patients with psychiatric symptoms including emotional disturbances and various memory defects.

It is widely believed that certain forebrain structures form a functional system called the "limbic system" that is especially significant in affect and motivation. The two most well-known "limbic structures" are the *amygdaloid body* (amygdala) and *hippocampus,* both of which are in the temporal lobe.

Although the two structures are continuous with adjacent parts of the cerebral cortex, they have a different histologic organization. The hippocampus is a cortical structure with a somewhat simpler organization than the rest of the cerebral cortex, whereas the amygdaloid body can be divided into several subgroups, most of which are subcortical in nature. However, there are also some striking similarities between the amygdaloid body and the hippocampus, especially in regard to their connections with other parts of the brain. Both structures have extensive relationships with other cortical and subcortical structures through a multitude of extrinsic and often reciprocal connections.

AMYGDALOID BODY

Subdivisions

The amygdaloid body is a large nucleus located just in front of the inferior horn of the lateral ventricle and immediately underneath the uncus of the parahippocampal gyrus (Fig. 171). It is a heterogenous structure containing many different cellular subgroups with significant differences in cytoarchitecture, histochemical characteristics, and connections. In a simplified manner, a distinction can be made between a large *basolateral* and a small *corticomedial* nuclear group, which also contains a *central nucleus.* A large part of the amygdaloid body is occupied by the basolateral nuclear group, which has highly differentiated connections, especially with the cerebral cortex and the striatum. The small corticomedial nucleus is continuous with and closely related to the olfactory cortex whereas the medial and central nuclei, which are located in the dorsal part of the amygdaloid body, are closely related to the hypothalamus and the brain stem.

Connections

The amygdaloid body is closely related to the following structures: the cerebral cortex, striatum,

hypothalamus, brain stem, thalamus, and hippocampus.

Cerebral Cortex

The large basolateral subdivision of the amygdala receives higher order sensory information from association areas in the *frontotemporal lobes* and *insula,* whereas the smaller corticomedial part receives olfactory input from the *olfactory bulb* and the *olfactory cortex.* Since the corticoamygdaloid pathways are reciprocated by amygdalocortical pathways, the amygdaloid body is apparently in a position to modulate the incoming sensory information.

Striatum

Basolateral amygdala projects directly to most of the striatum, especially to its ventral territories including the accumbens, i.e., the *ventral striatum* (Chapter 8). The projections from the amygdala to the ventral striatum, which constitute a significant part of the ventral amygdaloid pathway, provide a direct input to the basal ganglia and the motor system.

Hypothalamus and Brain Stem

The major pathway between the amygdaloid body and the medial hypothalamus is the *stria terminalis,* which closely follows the mediodorsal aspect of the caudate nucleus as it makes a loop around the thalamus (Fig. 162). The lateral hypothalamus is connected with the amygdaloid body via the *ventral amygdaloid pathway.* Many of the projection fibers in the ventral pathway continue beyond the hypothalamus to various brain stem centers including the autonomic nuclei. Ascending projections from the brain stem to the amygdala include not only monoaminergic pathways, but also fibers carrying visceral sensory input, e.g., from the nucleus of the solitary tract. The central nucleus is a focal point for many of the hypothalamic and brain stem connections.

Thalamus

Significant projections exist between the amygdaloid body and the medial and midline thalamic

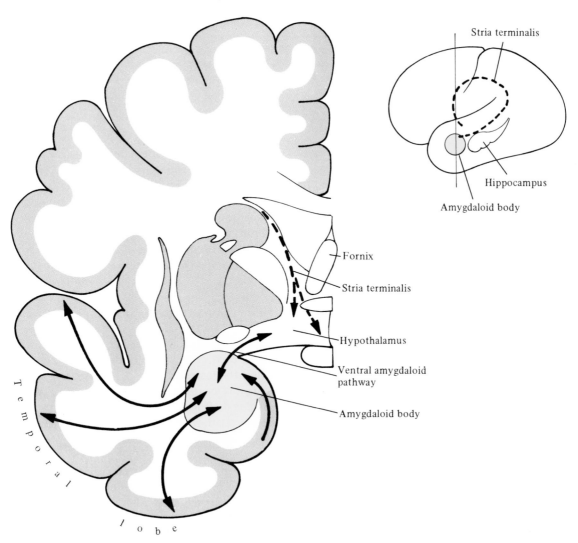

Fig. 171. Amygdaloid Body
The key figure in the *upper right corner* indicates the approximate location of the amygdaloid body in the rostral part of the temporal lobe. The approximate location of the stria terminalis has also been projected on the lateral surface of the hemisphere. A frontal section through the hemisphere rostral to the anterior tip of the temporal horn reveals that the amygdaloid body occupies a relatively large area of the temporal lobe. Some of the main connections of the amygdaloid body have been indicated with *black arrows*.

nuclei. Their functional significance is not well understood.

Functional Aspects

Bilateral destruction of the amygdaloid body and surrounding temporal neocortex results in dramatic changes referred to as the *Klüver-Bucy* syndrome, which is characterized by an increase in sexual activity, a compulsive tendency to place objects in the mouth, decreased emotionality, visual agnosia, and changes in eating behavior. On the basis of this polysymptomatic picture, the impression is easily obtained that different types of behavior, e.g., aggressive behavior, sexual behavior, and eating behavior are specifically related to amygdaloid activity. It is unlikely, however, that a specific part of the amygdaloid body or the surrounding cortical regions relates to each one of these complex behaviors.* Rather, the various

---

* Note: The visual defect in the Klüver-Bucy syndrome is in all likelihood related to involvement of temporal neocortex rather than to the amygdaloid body and its connections.

Fig. 172. Hippocampus Formation   ▷

A. The key figure in the *upper right-hand corner* indicates the approximate level for the cross section in **A.** Note that the fornix (*red*) has been transected in three places at this level.

B. Hippocampus formation and its main connections. Efferent connections (*red*) from the subiculum reach both cortical and subcortical regions. Perforant path, *blue;* intrinsic hippocampal pathways, *black*. (Modified after an original drawing by G. van Hoesen.)

symptoms are likely to be related to a more general defect, which makes it difficult to relate sensory information to past experience, or to evaluate sensory stimuli in terms of their emotional and motivational significance. It is in this context of *sensory–affective associations* that the amygdaloid connections can best be appreciated. The sensory information that is channeled through the various cortical association areas is likely to be highly relevant in behavioral terms. For the individual to respond appropriately, however, this information will have to match or interact with input reaching the amygdala from the hypothalamus and other subcortical areas known to be of importance for drive and motivation. How and where this interaction takes place is not known, but the amygdaloid body seems to be a crucial component in a functional system responsible for matching sensory and affective qualities of sensory stimuli. If this mechanism is destroyed by a lesion in or around the amygdaloid body in the temporal lobe, the response to various sensory stimuli is likely to be inappropriate, as witnessed in *Klüver-Bucy* syndrome. This is a serious handicap in the behavioral interactions with the environment.

Although the role of the amygdala in *memory* and *learning* is not well known, it should be noted that the widespread system of amygdalocortical fibers makes it possible for the amygdala to modulate and influence the activities in cortical association areas, known to be of importance for higher order sensory functions including storage of long-term memory. By virtue of its close association with the hypothalamus and other subcortical regions related to drive and motivation, the amygdaloid body is likely to provide an emotional component to the learning experience.

Experience has shown that advances in the study of anatomic pathways and interneuronal connections inspire functional inquiries; anatomic knowledge invariably puts physiologists on the right track. The amygdaloid projections to the hypothalamus no doubt reflect the importance of the amygdaloid body as a *modulator of hypothalamic activities*. It is also important to realize that the amygdaloid body is characterized by significant and direct projections both to the basal ganglia and the lower brain stem. When trying to define the role of the amygdaloid body in behavioral mechanisms, these projections deserve special attention , especially since they provide the amygdaloid body with direct lines of communication with both the *somatomotor* and *visceromotor systems*.

HIPPOCAMPAL FORMATION

The hippocampus (Ammon's horn) appears as a curved cortical structure in the floor and medial wall of the temporal horn of the lateral ventricle, where it is located in close proximity to the amygdaloid body (Fig. 172). The surface facing the ventricle is the deepest layer of a gyrus that has been folded inward in the region of the hippocampal fissure (Fig. 172A). The *dentate gyrus,* which is interlocked with the hippocampus, is a long narrow gyrus joined side-to-side to the hippocampus. The hippocampus, the dentate gyrus, and a cortical area along the other side of the hippocampus, the *subiculum,* are referred to as the hippocampal formation.

Histologic Structure

Three cortical layers are distinguished in the hippocampal formation. On the basis of architectonic differences, the cortical band of the *hippocampus proper* can be divided into three fields: CA1, CA2, and CA3. The most conspicuous cells are the pyramidal cells, which have basal dendrites directed outward toward the ventricular surface, and apical dendrites extending in a regular fashion toward the center of the structure. The myelinated axons of the pyramidal cells pass to the ventricular surface, where they form a lamina of white matter, the *alveus.*

The *dentate gyrus* is typically crenated and it can be easily recognized during the gross dissection of the human brain, where it is situated underneath

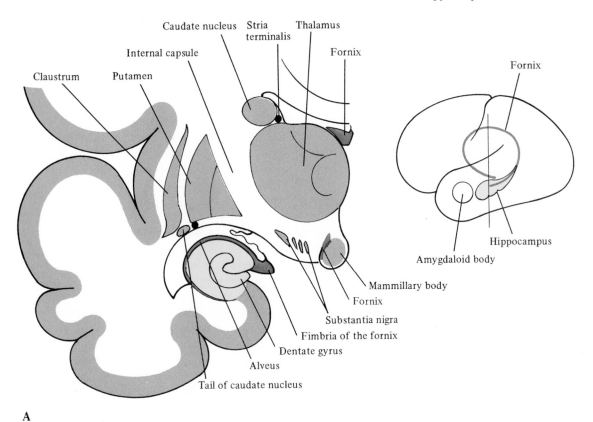

A

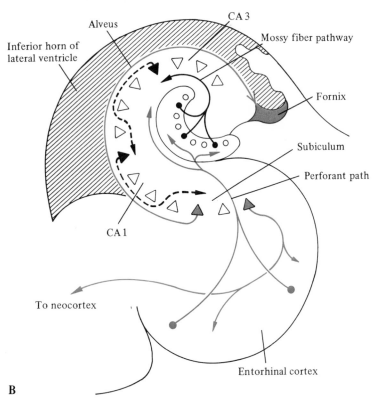

B

the fimbria of the fornix on the medial aspect of the temporal lobe. It is characterized primarily by a densely packed layer of small granular cells, which give origin to an important association pathway, the *mossy fiber system,* through which the activity in the dentate gyrus is conveyed to the cells in the hippocampal pyramidal cells (CA3).

Extrinsic Connections

The hippocampal formation, like the amygdaloid body, is intimately related to the rest of the cerebral cortex. Information from sensory cortical areas converges on the entorhinal cortex in the parahippocampal gyrus through a widespread system of anatomic pathways. The entorhinal cortex, in turn, gives origin to a massive projection system, the *perforant path,* which terminates in the hippocampus and the dentate gyrus (Fig. 172B). The entorhinal cortex, therefore, serves as an important gateway to the hippocampal formation.

The cortical input to the hippocampus is mirrored by efferent projections from the hippocampus back to the cerebral cortex. This output route from the hippocampus proceeds either directly or through subiculum to other parahippocampal areas, including the entorhinal area, and further on to association areas in all four lobes.

Another well-known efferent pathway is the *fornix,* with axons arising from pyramidal cells in primarily the subiculum. These axons proceed through the alveus to enter the fornix. The fornix is a massive fiber bundle, which can be easily identified in gross anatomic preparations of the human brain (Fig. 163B). Through the fornix, information from the hippocampal formation can reach a variety of subcortical structures, primarily the septum, the hypothalamus, and the anterior thalamic nucleus.

Intrinsic Connections

The mossy fiber pathway forms an important link in an intrinsic neuron circuit that can be schematically outlined as follows (Fig. 172B). The perforant path fibers project to the dentate gyrus, which gives origin to the mossy fiber system. This system, in turn, projects to the pyramidal cells in CA3, which sends collaterals to the CA1 pyramids. The axons of the CA1 pyramids, finally, proceed (in the alveus) to the subiculum. The latter, like the

hippocampus itself, projects to the entorhinal cortex. A significant feature in relation to this circuit is that the hippocampal formation is divided into a series of lamellae or narrow strips that are transverse to the longitudinal axis of the hippocampus. Each lamella contains intrinsic connections that project primarily to other components of that lamella. This anatomic organization has been thought to fit with a modern concept according to which the hippocampus would serve as a "cognitive map" (see below).

Functional Considerations

A list of all the functions in which the hippocampal formation is said to be involved would be almost infinite. Memory functions, motivational and attentional mechanisms, inhibitory processes, aggressive behavior, neuroendocrine activities, and many other functions have been ascribed to the hippocampus. It is becoming increasingly obvious, however, that such categorization is inadequate. Like the amygdaloid body, the hippocampus is apparently characterized by more general activities that are crucially important in a variety of behaviors.

Since bilateral removal of the medial parts of the temporal lobes, including the hippocampus, produces severe memory deficits in the human, it is generally believed that the hippocampus is of great importance for learning and memory functions. However, this opinion is by no means generally accepted. In fact, the large majority of animal experiments do not support the view that the hippocampus is specifically involved in memory mechanisms, although it is true that hippocampal lesions generally entail a tendency to affect behaviors once learned and thus cause a reduced ability for relearning. There seems to be a growing suspicion that the gross memory deficits in patients with bilateral medial temporal lesions are related as much to destruction of temporal neocortical projections in close proximity to the hippocampus as to damage to the hippocampus. Nevertheless, it should be noted that most modern theories of hippocampal function implicate memory mechanisms to a greater or lesser extent.

Although there is no generally accepted concept of hippocampal function, recent physiologic studies of the properties of single hippocampal neurons (units) indicate that the hippocampus may be critically involved in spatial orientation mechanisms that enable us to recognize and predict relationships and events in the surrounding environment. The hippocampus may serve as a "cognitive mapping system," which makes it possible for us to compare present situations with those experienced previously. Reflecting for a moment on the hippocampal connections, one is struck by the massive and well-organized afferent pathways that converge on the entorhinal area, and hence on the hippocampus formation, from different sensory regions of the cerebral cortex. Input from different sensory cortical regions would certainly be crucial for a structure that provides for flexibility in response to highly elaborate sensory information.

"LIMBIC SYSTEM"

In 1937 James Papez proposed "that the hypothalamus, the anterior thalamic nucleus, the cingulate gyrus, the hippocampus and their interconnections, constitute a harmonious mechanism which may elaborate the functions of central emotion as well as participate in emotional expressions." This was at the time a daring proposition, and it marks the beginning of the notion of the "limbic system,"[1] which has become one of the most celebrated functional anatomic systems in the brain.

From a modest beginning, the "limbic system" has grown into a multifarious system, which includes a large part of the basomedial telencephalon as well as diencephalic and mesencephalic structures believed to be of special significance for emotional and motivational aspects of behavior. Regular components of the "limbic system" include the *cingulate* and *parahippocampal gyri,* the *hippocampus,* the *septum,*[2] and the *amygdaloid body* (Fig. 173). These structures are to a considerable extent related to the *hypothalamus,* which is the main brain structure for the integration of various autonomic effects accompanying emotional expressions. The hypothalamus, therefore, is often

included in the "limbic system." Many other parts of the forebrain and the brain stem are more or less intimately associated with the above-mentioned structures. Such affiliated members of the "limbic system" include neocortical areas in the basal frontotemporal region, the olfactory cortex, ventral parts of the striatum, the anterior and medial thalami, the habenula, and parts of the medial mesencephalon. When and to what extent these parts are included in the "limbic system" concept seems to be a matter of convenience and personal preference.

The "limbic system" concept has understandably attracted the attention of especially psychologists and psychiatrists, who see an opportunity to correlate emotional behavior and disorders with specific parts of the brain. Despite its popularity, however, the "limbic system" remains an enigma to many neuroscientists, and there is no generally accepted definition of the system. Aided by modern tract-tracing methods, scientists are discovering an increasing number of interconnections between the "limbic system" and the rest of the brain. At the same time as the borders of the "limbic system" are becoming more diffuse, several parts of the system display separate functional identities. For instance, structures such as the amygdaloid body and the hippocampus have specific connections and functional significance, and it may be necessary to approach these and other "limbic" structures individually no less than in the framework of the "limbic system" concept, which invites a preconceived view in regard to their anatomic affiliations and functional significance.

The notion of the "limbic system" has no doubt served as a powerful stimulus for a variety of neuroscientific experiments. However, in spite of the fact that there has been a great deal of effort in trying to define the "limbic system," the concept continues to be one of the most elusive in modern neurology. The "limbic system" is a convenient term for many purposes, but some experts contend that it has outlived its usefulness as a scientific concept.[3]

---

1. The term "limbic" was introduced by Broca (1878), who noted that the cingulate and parahippocampal gyri, two of the main structures of the "limbic system," form a limbus or border around the diencephalon. Since the olfactory bulb and tract seemed to project to both the cingulate and the parahippocampal gyri, he referred to all these structures as "le grand lobe limbique."

2. The septal region, which is well developed in many mammals, contains the septal nuclei. In humans it consists of a dorsal cell-free part, septum pellucidum, and a ventral part, precommissural septum in the subcallosal area (Fig. 42), which contains the septal nuclei.

---

3. Rhinencephalon or "smell brain" is another commonly used, but poorly defined term. Most of the structures included in the "limbic system" have at one time or another been considered parts of the rhinencephalon. Strictly speaking, however, the term rhinencephalon should be reserved for the structures that are directly related to the sense of smell, i.e., the olfactory bulb and the retrobulbar olfactory areas (anterior olfactory nucleus, olfactory tubercle) as well as the olfactory cortex including the corticomedial amygdaloid nucleus.

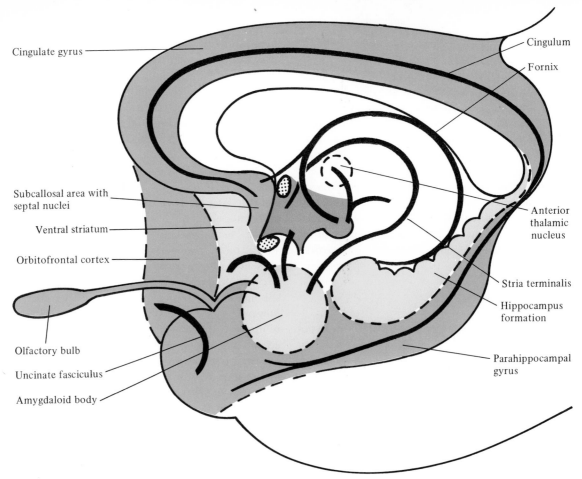

Fig. 173. Limbic System
In this highly schematic figure of the limbic system and its main connections, the orbitofrontal cortex and the rest of "le grand lobe limbique" of Broca has been colored *blue*. Some other key structures of the limbic system, e.g., hippocampus, amygdaloid body, and the ventral striatum have been indicated with *yellow color*. Hypothalamus, which is closely related to many of the above mentioned structures, has been colored *red*. Many other structures that are usually said to be affiliated with the limbic system, e.g., habenula, interpeduncular nucleus, and the limbic midbrain area, have not been indicated in the figure. (Modified after an original drawing by G. van Hoesen.)

CLINICAL NOTES

Many neurologic and psychiatric disorders are characterized by *emotional disturbances* of one type or another. Inability to control emotional expressions (uncontrollable laughter or crying, for instance) is a well-known symptom of many organic brain diseases, including vascular lesions and degenerative disorders. Such diseases generally do not respect anatomic boundaries, and their diffuse nature makes it difficult to correlate the emotional disturbances with specific brain structures.

Aggressive reactions and *rage attacks* are sometimes seen in patients with temporal lobe tumors, especially if the tumor is located in the anteromedial part of the temporal lobe. It is believed that the aggressive emotional reactions in patients with temporal lobe tumors and in temporal lobe seizures (see Chapter 19) are related primarily to the involvement of the amygdaloid body and its connections. Lesions of the amygdaloid body, i.e. *amygdalotomy,* have been used to treat patients with aggressive and violent behavior. Psychosurgery[4] however, has been heavily criticized because of the perceived threat that brain surgery might be used in a more systematic fashion to control behavior.

---

4. The history of *psychosurgery,* i.e., the treatment of mental disorders by brain operations, has been dramatic and controversial. Egas Moniz from Portugal received the Nobel Prize in 1949 for his introduction of *prefrontal lobotomy* in certain psychoses, and various types of prefrontal lobotomies were frequently applied in the early 1950s to mentally disturbed patients. The purpose of the lobotomy was to transect the

Psychomotor Epilepsy

One partial seizure with complex manifestations is psychomotor epilepsy. This is the most common type of focal epilepsy. It usually occurs as a result of a pathologic focus in the anterior part of the temporal lobe, thereby leading to another designation, *"temporal lobe epilepsy."* It is characterized by both subjective phenomena such as auditory, visual, gustatory, or olfactory hallucinations, emotional events such as fear, and stereotyped movements, usually in the form of purposeless activities such as smacking the lips or fumbling with clothes. Some patients with a pathologic focus in the anterior part of the temporal lobe also suffer from psychiatric symptoms, e.g., personality distur-bances or even severe psychoses. This has led some to describe an "epileptic personality," a term that currently is subject to much disagreement.

Wernicke-Korsakoff's Syndrome

Some persons with multinutritional deficiencies resulting from starvation or alcoholism may develop a confusional state that is particularly related to Thiamine (Vitamin B1) deficiency. Usually they suffer from ataxia, poor short-term memory, and gaze defects. Autopsy often reveals lesions of the posterior hypothalamus, medial thalamus, and dentate nuclei.

Suggested Reading

1. Anderson, P., 1975. Organization of hippocampal neurons and their interconnections. In R. L. Isaacson and K. H. Pribram (eds.): The Hippocampus, Vol. 1: Structure and Development. Plenum Press: New York, pp. 155–175.
2. Ben-Ari Y. (ed.), 1981. The Amygdaloid Complex. Elsevier/North-Holland Biomedical Press: Amsterdam.
3. Hall, E., 1975. The anatomy of the limbic system. In G. J. Mogenson and F. R. Calaresu (eds.): Neural Integration of Physiological Mechanisms and Behavior. University of Toronto Press: Toronto, pp. 68–94.
4. Isaacson, R. L., 1982. The Limbic System, 2nd ed. Plenum Press: New York.
5. MacLean, P. D., 1978. Challenges of the Papez heritage. In: Limbic Mechanisms. The Continuing Evolution of the Limbic System Concept. Plenum Press: New York, pp. 1–15.
6. O'Keefe, J. and L. Nadel, 1978. The Hippocampus as a Cognitive Map. Oxford University Press: Oxford, England.
7. Swanson, L. W., 1979. The hippocampus. Trends in Neuroscience 2: 9–12.
8. Valenstein, E. S., 1973. Brain Control. John Wiley: New York.
9. Van Hoesen, G. W., 1982. The parahippocampal gyrus: New observations regarding its cortical connections in the monkey. Trends in Neuroscience 5, 10: pp. 345–350.

frontothalamic projection fibers. The introduction of antipsychotic drugs, as well as the undesirable side effects following the operations, led to a rapid decline in psychosurgery during the second half of the 1950s.

Since some patients cannot be helped by pharmacologic agents or by other conservative treatments, psychosurgery can occasionally offer welcome relief from suffering. However, the field of psychosurgery has changed character as a result of advances in our understanding of the brain, and the development of new stereotaxic operative procedures. The aim of modern psychosurgical methods is to sever specific fiber bundles or to destroy certain nuclear groups as in amygdalotomy. *Cingulotomy* is another form of psychosurgery, which is sometimes used to treat intractable pain.

Psychosurgery should be performed only on patients who suffer from severe psychotic disorders or intractable pain, and where all other therapy has failed. A noted psychiatric neurosurgeon has formulated the guideline: "The brains of our patients are so disturbed that they only produce suffering."

18
Thalamus

THALAMIC NUCLEI AND THALAMOCORTICAL
CONNECTIONS
    Anterior Nuclear Group
    Medial Nuclear Group
    Ventrolateral Nuclear Group
    Lateral and Medial Geniculate Bodies

THALAMIC FUNCTIONS
    Sensory Relay Nuclei
    Pulvinar and Associative Functions
    Thalamus and the Motor System
    Anterior Thalamic Nucleus and Papez's Circuit
    Reticular Nucleus and Intralaminar Nuclei

CLINICAL NOTES
    Thalamic Syndrome

SUGGESTED READING

The thalamus and the cerebral cortex are closely related through an extensive system of reciprocal connections. Both structures, however, have distinct characteristic functional–anatomic attributes, and it is therefore convenient to treat them in separate chapters.

Thalamus is the gateway to the cerebral cortex, but it is more than just a collection of relay stations; it is a supreme integration center for sensory and motor activities. Impulses arriving through the various sensory pathways are processed in specific parts of the thalamus before they are transmitted to the cerebral cortex. Some thalamic nuclei, which serve as integration centers for impulses from the basal ganglia and the cerebellum, project to the motor cortex. Other parts of the thalamus are associated with "limbic system" structures known to be of special importance for emotional and motivational mechanisms.

THALAMIC NUCLEI AND THALAMOCORTICAL CONNECTIONS

Anterior Nuclear Group

The *anterior nucleus* (A) consists of three subdivisions. It receives a significant part of its input from the mammillary body through the mammillothalamic tract, and it is connected with the cingulate gyrus on the medial side of the hemisphere (Fig. 174). The pathway from the mammillary body to the cingulate gyrus via the anterior nucleus is part of Papez's circuit (see below).

Medial Nuclear Group

The main nucleus in this group, the *mediodorsal nucleus* (MD), projects in an orderly fashion to extensive parts of the frontal lobe, i.e., the prefrontal cortex including the orbitofrontal cortex. MD, in turn, receives corticothalamic projections from the prefrontal cortex, but it also receives input from other parts of thalamus as well as from a variety of subcortical structures including the amygdaloid body, the ventral pallidum, and the midbrain reticular formation.

Ventrolateral Nuclear Group

Ventral Group

This group includes the *ventral anterior* (VA) and *ventral lateral* (VL) nuclei as well as the *ventral posterior* (VP) nucleus. The VA–VL complex receives input from the basal ganglia and cerebellum and is closely related to the motor and premotor cortex (areas 4, 6, and 8) in the frontal lobe. The ventral posterior nucleus (VP), which is often referred to as the ventrobasal complex, is the main somatosensory region of the thalamus. Its two parts, the *ventral posterolateral* (VPL) and the *ventral posteromedial* (VPM) nuclei, serve as relay nuclei in the somatosensory pathways and project primarily to the somatosensory cortex (areas 3, 1, and 2) in the postcentral gyrus.

Lateral (Dorsal) Group

This group contains three nuclei, the *lateral dorsal nucleus* (LD), the *lateral posterior nucleus* (LP),

and the *pulvinar* (P). They are connected reciprocally with extensive areas in the parietal, occipital, and temporal lobes.

Lateral and Medial Geniculate Bodies

The *lateral geniculate body* (LG) receives fibers from both eyes through the optic tract, and it projects through the optic radiation primarily to the striate cortex (area 17) in the region of the calcarine sulcus and to a lesser extent to the surrounding areas 18 and 19 in the occipital lobe.

The *medial geniculate body* (MG) is a relay nucleus in the auditory pathway. It receives fibers from the two inferior colliculi, and it projects via the auditory radiation to the auditory cortex (areas 41 and 42) in the superior temporal gyrus.

THALAMIC FUNCTIONS

Because the thalamocortical projection fibers, the *thalamic radiation,* reach practically all areas of the cerebral cortex, thalamus is likely to play a key role in most forebrain functions. The cortical areas that receive input from the thalamus project back to the thalamic nuclei, from where they receive their input. This widespread system of reciprocal connections indicates a close cooperation between the thalamus and the cerebral cortex in whatever functions they are involved.

The caudal half of the thalamus is in general related to the ascending sensory pathways and to the parieto-occipitotemporal cortex whereas the rostral half of the thalamus is characterized foremost by its relationships to motor and limbic system activities as witnessed by its connections with the cerebellum, basal ganglia, hypothalamus, and amygdaloid body as well as various cortical areas in the frontal and limbic lobes.

Sensory Relay Nuclei

The sensory relay nuclei, VPL–VPM (somatosensory system), LG (visual system), and MG (auditory system) are part of the ventral tier of thalamic nuclei. They are located in the caudal half of the thalamus, and since they serve as relay stations in the main sensory pathways to the cerebral cortex, they are discussed in relation to the ascending sensory pathways (Chapter 6), the visual pathways

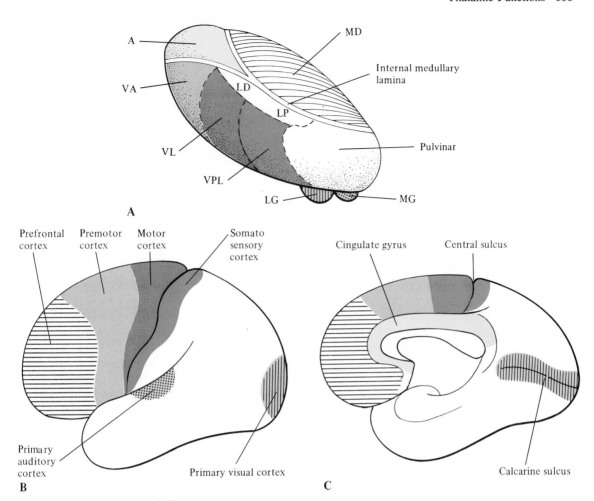

Fig. 174. Thalamocortical Connections
A. Dorsolateral view of the thalamus showing the main subdivisions.
B. Lateral surface of the cerebral hemisphere showing the main projection areas of the various thalamic nuclei.
C. Medial surface of the cerebral hemisphere.

(Chapter 13), and the auditory pathways (Chapter 12). Although it is customary to refer to these nuclei as sensory relays, it is important to remember that they receive significant input, not only from the sensory pathways, but also from the cerebral cortex and from other thalamic nuclei. A considerable amount of integration is likely to take place in these as well as in other thalamic nuclei.

Pulvinar and Associative Functions

Pulvinar is remarkable for its large size and its multifarious relations with the cerebral cortex and many subcortical structures. Its functions are not well-known, but its widespread reciprocal relationships with the parieto-occipitotemporal association

cortex and visual association areas indicate that it collaborates closely with the cerebral cortex in many important cognitive functions including complex visual and language functions.

Thalamus and the Motor System

The VA and the VL nuclei are important components of the motor system in the sense that they transfer basal ganglia and cerebellar activities to the motor cortex (Chapter 8). However, like all other thalamic relay nuclei, the VA–VL complex is more than a simple relay for transmission of impulses to the cerebral cortex. Its various subnuclei receive a complicated pattern of inputs, not only from the globus pallidus and the dentate nucleus, but also from other parts of the basal ganglia, the reticular formation, and the cerebral cortex, as well as from nearby thalamic nuclei. Therefore, the impulses from the basal ganglia and the cerebellum interact in the VA–VL complex with information from other sources before they are transmitted in a modified form to the motor cortex and its descending corticospinal and corticoreticulospinal pathways.

The projections from the MD to the prefrontal cortex form an integral part of a more widespread thalamofrontal projection system that originates in continuous cell columns that stretch through both the MD and the VA–VL complex. It seems as if this anatomic continuity that characterizes the thalamocortical projections of the MD and the VA–VL complex is matched by a functional continuity. As discussed above, the VA–VL complex forms part of a classic pallidothalamocortical loop, which is known to be of great significance for control of motor functions, and evidence obtained by modern tract-tracing methods indicates that MD represents an integral part of the motor system by virtue of its relationship to the ventral part of the basal ganglia, i.e., the ventral striatopallidal system. This system seems to be especially designed for the processing of limbic system input. Without attempting to define the function of MD in more precise terms, it seems that MD has a special role in integrating emotionally and motivationally powerful stimuli before they finally influence the effector mechanisms of the frontal cortex.

Anterior Thalamic Nucleus and Papez's Circuit

About 50 years ago, the American neuroanatomist James Papez suggested that the anterior thalamic nucleus and its projections to the cingulate gyrus belong to a circuit that constitutes an important part of the structural basis of emotion. The circuit leads from the hippocampus to the mammillary body via fornix, and then to the anterior thalamic nucleus by way of the mammillothalamic tract. Thalamocortical projections connect the anterior thalamic nucleus with the cingulate gyrus, from where the impulses finally reach the hippocampus via several intervening structures including the cingulum bundle. It should be noted that the circuit is by no means closed. Indeed, its main components, the cingulate gyrus and hippocampus, are characterized by widespread corticocortical and subcortical relations besides those identified as part of Papez's circuit. Papez's original idea regarding the anatomic basis of emotion has had a great impact on the many branches of neuroscience trying to elucidate the relationship between brain and behavior (Chapter 17).

Reticular Nucleus and Intralaminar Nuclei

The *reticular nucleus* surrounds the thalamus like a shield and it is traversed by practically all fibers interconnecting the thalamus and the cerebral cortex. These fibers establish synaptic contacts with the neurons in the reticular nucleus, and since the reticular neurons send axons to other thalamic nuclei and to the midbrain reticular formation, the reticular nucleus of the thalamus is in a position to integrate corticothalamic and thalamocortical activity and transmit information back to the thalamus and the midbrain.

The *intralaminar nuclei* and some related *midline nuclei* are characterized by significant projections to the striatum, and they are therefore likely to be important in the control of movements. The intralaminar nuclei also project diffusely to widespread areas of the cerebral cortex, and these pathways form part of the anatomic substrate for the ascending activating system (see Chapter 10).

CLINICAL NOTES

Thalamic Syndrome

Tumors and especially vascular lesions related to the middle and posterior cerebral artery may involve thalamus to some extent. A typical condition is the *thalamic pain syndrome* (of Dejerine-Roussy), which is caused by destruction of the sensory relay nuclei in the posterior half of thalamus. It is most often caused by occlusion of the thalamogeniculate branches of the posterior cerebral artery. In addition to injury of the internal capsule with transitory hemiparesis and homonymous hemianopsia, there is usually loss of deep sensation and impairment of superficial sensation on the opposite side of the body. Position sense is affected more frequently than other sensory functions. An agonizing concomitant of this syndrome is a "burning" or "knife-like" pain, which usually appears after several weeks or months, when the other sensory functions begin to return.

SUGGESTED READING

1. Brodal, A., 1981. Neurological Anatomy in Relation to Clinical Medicine. Oxford University Press: New York, Oxford, pp. 94–107.

2. Macchi, G., et al. (eds.), 1983. Somatosensory Integration in the Thalamus. Elsevier/North Holland: Amsterdam.

3. Poggio, G. F. and V. B. Mountcastle, 1980. Functional organization of thalamus and cortex. In V. B. Mountcastle (ed.): Medical Physiology, 14th ed., Vol. 1. C. V. Mosby: St. Louis, Missouri, pp. 271–276.

4. Rose, J. E. and C. N. Woolsey, 1949. Organization of the mammalian thalamus and its relationship to the cerebral cortex. Electroencephalogr. Clin. Neurophysiol. 7: 391–404.

19

Cerebral Cortex

STRUCTURE OF THE CEREBRAL CORTEX
   Cortical Layers
   Brodmann's Map
   Cortical Columns

CORTICAL CONNECTIONS
   Projection Fibers
   Association Fibers
   Commissural Fibers

CORTICAL FUNCTIONS
   Cross-Control and Cerebral Specialization
   Cortical Localization
   Frontal Lobe
   Parietal Lobe
   Occipital Lobe
   Temporal Lobe

CLINICAL NOTES
   Frontal Lobe Syndrome
   Parietal Lobe Syndrome
   Occipital Lobe Syndrome
   Temporal Lobe Syndrome
   Epilepsy
   Language Disorders

CLINICAL EXAMPLE
   Epilepsy

SUGGESTED READING

The cerebral cortex is intimately related to most major structures in the brain and spinal cord, and it has reached an enormous degree of development in the human brain. In general, the organization of the cerebral cortex is characterized by a mixture of laminar and vertical (columnar) features. Its intrinsic organization is extremely complicated, and only recently have some of its local circuit connections been elucidated.

Sensory impulses impinge on cerebral cortex, where they are analyzed and related to previous experience, and ultimately transformed into action, if needed. Indeed, a variety of both cortico-cortical and corticosubcortical neuron circuits are being exploited in the process of preparing for an appropriate response to the information received. The cerebral cortex is also instrumental in the elaboration of various types of mental activities including memory, learning, intelligence, and language abilities.

STRUCTURE OF THE CEREBRAL CORTEX

Cortical Layers

The cerebral cortex is a 2–4 mm thick and highly convoluted sheath of gray substance. About half of its surface is hidden in the depth of the various sulci and fissures. The nerve cell bodies of the cerebral cortex are disposed in more or less well-defined layers as shown by Nissl stains. Although the arrangement of these layers varies in different parts of the cortex, it is usually possible to distinguish six different layers (Fig. 175).[1]

I. The *molecular layer* is a fiber-rich superficial layer with few cell bodies but with many axonal branches and apical dendrites from pyramidal cells with cell bodies in deeper layers.

II and III. The *external granular* and *external pyramidal layers* contain mostly small and medium-sized pyramidal cells. Each pyramidal cell has an apical dendrite, which extends toward the surface of the cortex, and several basal dendrites that arborize at the base of the cell body. The axons of the pyramidal cells in these two layers project to deeper cortical layers, or to other cortical areas in the same or the opposite hemisphere. Layer III pyramidal cells also project to subcortical structures.

IV. The *internal granular layer* is primarily composed of densely packed small stellate (star-shaped) cells. The dendritic trees of these cells are quite variable, and the axons ramify extensively in the same or nearby layers. Layer IV also contains a large number of horizontally directed myelinated fibers (the outer band of Baillarger) from various thalamic relay nuclei.

V. The *internal pyramidal layer* is composed of medium-sized and large pyramidal cells, and it contains the giant pyramidal cells of Betz in the motor cortex. The pyramidal cells of layer V give rise to many of the corticofugal fibers to the striatum, brain stem, and spinal cord.

VI. The *multiform layer* contains a variety of small and medium-sized stellate and pyramidal cells. This layer also gives rise to corticofugal projection fibers.

---

1. Since the olfactory cortex and hippocampus are characterized by three layers, they are together referred to as *allocortex* ("other cortex") as opposed to the six-layered *neocortex* or *isocortex.*

Brodmann's Map

The cerebral cortex is heterogenous, and it can be divided into different areas on the basis of variations in relative thickness and cell density of the different layers, as well as in the size, shape, and arrangements of cells. The best known of these cytoarchitectural maps is the one published by the German histologist Brodmann in 1909 (Fig. 176). He identified about 50 different regions, and the hope was that the different cytoarchitectural areas could be related to specific functions. This, however, has been possible only to a limited extent, primarily in regard to primary motor and sensory areas. Nevertheless, Brodmann's numbers are of great interest, and many of them are used by clinicians and scientists for reference purposes.

Granular and Agranular Cortex

The cortical areas that receive the primary sensory pathways are characterized by strongly developed granular layers II and IV for the reception of afferent impulses. Pyramidal layers III and V, by contrast, are less developed. This type of cortex, i.e., *granular cortex,* is found especially in the striate area (area 17), the auditory cortex (areas 41 and 42), and in the somatosensory cortex (areas 3, 1, and 2). Other areas, e.g., the motor cortex (areas 4 and 6), the frontal eye field (area 8), and part of Broca's speech area (area 44), all of which give rise to prominent corticobulbar and corticospinal projections, have well-developed pyramidal layers, whereas the granular layers are less distinct. This type of cortex is referred to as *agranular cortex.* The granular and agranular types can be said to represent the prototypes of sensory and motor cortices, but they are only two extremes in a continuum of structural types.

Cortical Columns

Whereas the cortical layers represent a longitudinal arrangement, other histologic features reflect a vertical (perpendicular to the surface) organization. Axons as well as apical dendrites, either solitary or in bundles, tend to have a vertical orientation (Fig. 175). Even the nerve cells seem to be arranged in vertical columns, and detailed Golgi

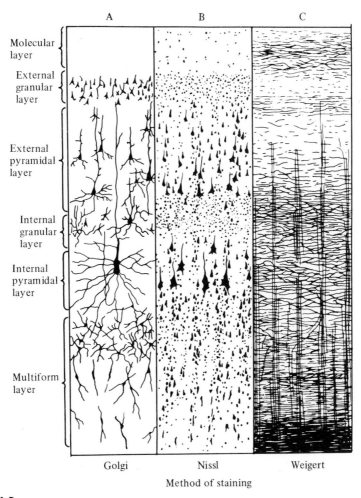

Fig. 175. Cortical Layers
Diagram showing the layers of the cerebral cortex. **A.** Golgi method. **B.** Nissl stain. **C.** Weigert myelin stain.
(After Brodmann.)

studies of interneuronal connections suggest the existence of considerable communication in a vertical direction, i.e., between nearby cells in different layers. Physiologic studies, likewise, have indicated the presence of a vertical organization in the form of cell columns, in which all cells in a given column respond to the same stimulus. Columnar cortical organization, therefore, is conceived of as a basic principle of great functional importance.

A *functional column* is about 300 μm wide and consists of hundreds to thousands of neurons, which are heavily interconnected in a direction perpendicular to the cortical surface. These functional units are activated by specific stimuli. For instance, some columns in the somatosensory cor-

tex are activated by touch, others by position of a joint, etc. Since all neurons within a single column have the same receptive field, a vertical column in the somatosensory cortex represents an elementary functional unit, which is both place- and modality-specific. Functional columns in the visual cortex are illustrated in Fig. 154.

Although the discovery of functional columns was greeted with great enthusiasm, we are still far from knowing the true nature of cortical columns and how different columns interact with each other. The intrinsic circuitry of the cerebral cortex is extremely complicated, and a multitude of interneurons, collateral pathways, and synaptic relationships provide an almost unlimited number of possibilities for impulse transmission.

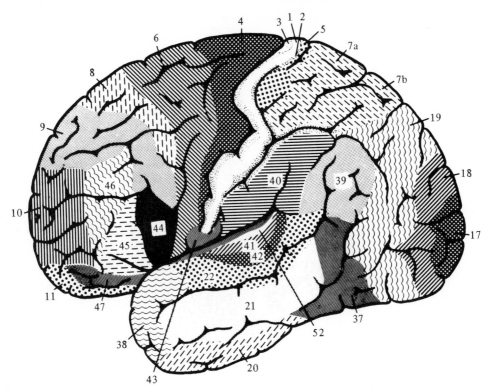

Fig. 176. Brodmann's Map
From Bindman, L. and O. Lippold, 1981. The Neurophysiology of the Cerebral Cortex. With permission of University of Texas Press, Austin.)

CORTICAL CONNECTIONS

Projection Fibers

The multitude of cortical projection fibers is astounding, and it reflects the fact that the cerebral cortex influences practically every functional system in the brain and the spinal cord. Most subcortical structures receive *corticofugal projections.* Examples of corticofugal pathways were discussed in previous chapters, e.g., corticostriatal and corticothalamic pathways (see Chapters 8 and 18), or cortical projections to the amygdaloid body and the hippocampus (see Chapter 17). Many of the corticofugal projections, e.g., the corticospinal, the corticoreticular, and the corticopontine pathways (see Chapters 7 and 9) pass through the internal capsule.

The *corticopetal projections* are no less impressive. Foremost among these are the various thalamocortical projections from all the ascending sensory pathways (chapters 6, 12, and 13). A recently discovered cholinergic corticopetal system originates in the basal nucleus of Meynert (see Chapter

8) and monoaminergic pathways from the locus ceruleus and the raphe nuclei in the brain stem reach widespread areas of the cerebral cortex (see Chapter 10). The amygdaloid body and the hippocampus are also characterized by a widespread system of corticopetal connections (see Chapter 13).

Association Fibers

Blunt dissection of the major fiber systems reveals a number of significant association pathways, including short *arcuate fibers* as well as long bundles such as the *cingulum,* the *arcuate fasciculus,* the *superior and inferior occipitofrontal fasciculus,* and the *uncinate fasciculus.* Gross anatomic dissections, however, cannot reveal the specific connections of the various fiber bundles, but this has been done with modern tract-tracing methods, and the results obtained indicate that the associative connections are extremely complex, but precisely organized.

Association fibers from primary sensory areas

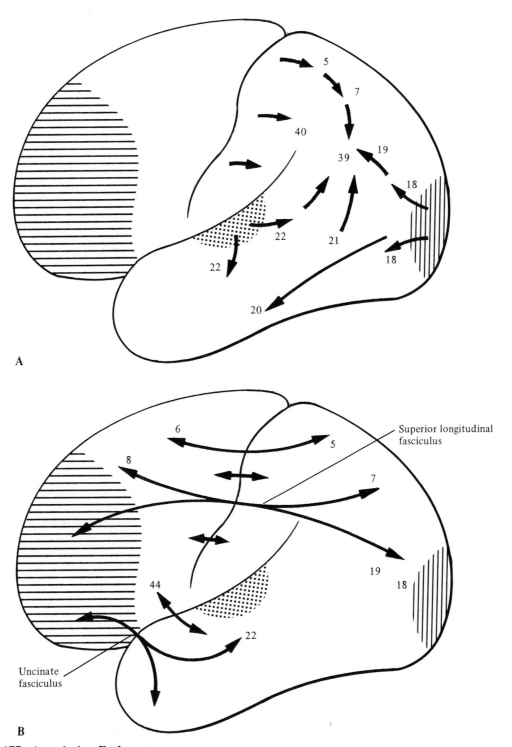

Fig. 177. Association Pathways
A. Highly schematic figure showing sequential processing of sensory information. Although the figure indicates unidirectional connections most of the corticocortical connections are in fact bidirectional as shown in **B.**
B. Some examples of short and long association fibers, which provide the anatomical substrate for very specific interactions between different cortical areas.

to nearby association areas provide the substrate for a type of sequential or serial processing of information (Fig. 177A). Further, impulses from the different sensory systems converge on a multimodal parietotemporal region occupied approximately by the angulare and supramarginal gyri (areas 39 and 40). Integration of various types of sensory information is of special importance for complex functions including linguistic abilities (see Cortical Functions).

Sensory impulses have ample opportunity to affect the motor cortex before they reach the multimodal region in the parietotemporal junction area. For instance, abundant short reciprocal fibers connect the primary somatosensory cortex in the postcentral gyrus with the motor cortex in the precentral gyrus (Fig. 177B). Other association fibers interconnect sensory association area (areas 5, 18–19, and 22) with the premotor cortex (areas 6 and 8). Long association fibers, finally, converge on the prefrontal cortex from several sensory processing areas (see below).

Association Cortex

It is customary to divide the cerebral cortex into motor, sensory, and association areas. Association cortex is represented by a vast territory in the frontal lobe, i.e., the prefrontal cortex, and by extensive parietotemporal areas intercalated between the somatosensory, visual, and auditory cortices. The term association cortex indicates that these regions are involved in associative functions, e.g., in the analysis and elaboration of sensory information, in the integration of different sensory modalities, and in the planning of motor actions.

It was previously believed that higher integrative functions were dependent primarily on cortical association pathways. It has become evident, however, that the association areas, like the primary sensory areas, are connected with thalamic cell groups, some of which may even be related to specific sensory and motor systems. The distinction between projection areas and association areas, therefore, is not so clear as previously thought. Nevertheless, the concept of association areas as a substrate for associative cortical functions is still useful, even if it falls short of explaining the mechanisms of higher brain functions. Both corticocortical and corticosubcortical neuronal circuits are likely to be involved in mental activities.

Commissural Fibers

The overwhelming majority of the over 300 million commissural fibers is contained in a massive fiber bundle, the *corpus callosum.*. Commissural fibers between the two temporal lobes pass, not only through the corpus callosum but also through the *anterior commissure.* The commissural connections are not uniformly distributed across the cerebral hemisphere; some areas, e.g., the hand and foot areas in the somatosensory and motor cortices and part of visual area 17, do not receive commissural fibers. The commissural fibers transmit information and learning from one hemisphere to the other.

CORTICAL FUNCTIONS

The dramatic development of the cerebral cortex is generally considered to be the key to man's superiority over other animals. The pioneer American neuroanatomist C. Judson Herrick, for instance, referred to the cerebral cortex as "the organ of civilization." Since cortical functions, such as language, cannot be studied by the ablation method in experimental animals, our knowledge of the localization of speech function is based primarily on patients with cortical lesions. It is also possible to study the responses in conscious patients, whose cortex is being stimulated during brain operation. Further, some modern radiographic techniques provide a dynamic picture of cerebral blood flow (Fig. 178) or metabolic rate, both of which are sensitive indicators of brain activity.

Cross-Control and Cerebral Specialization

A more or less complete crossover characterizes the long somatosensory fiber systems as well as the descending corticospinal pathways, and the crossover takes place in the large sensory (lemniscal) and motor (pyramidal) decussations in the lower part of the medulla oblongata. This means that sensory impulses from one side of the body impinge primarily on the cortical sensory areas in the opposite hemisphere, and that the cortical motor areas in one hemisphere control the movements of the opposite arm and leg. This type of cross-control makes some sense if one realizes that visual stimuli from a threatening object in the right

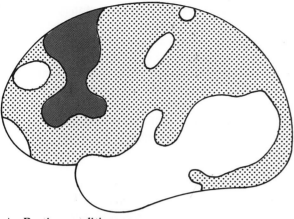

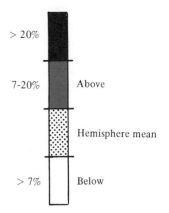

> 20%

7-20%   Above

Hemisphere mean

> 7%   Below

A. Resting condition

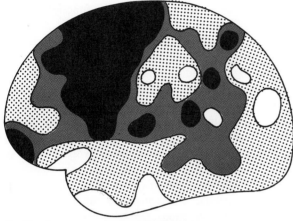

B. Hand movements conceived

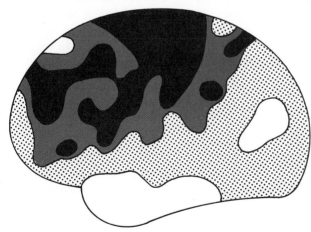

C. Hand movements performed

Fig. 178. Cerebral Blood Flow During Hand Movement

Cerebral blood flow distribution in resting condition (A), during motor ideation (B) and during actual movement of the right hand (C). Note the increased blood flow in the supplementary motor area when the hand movement was conceived (B) and in motor cortex when the movement was carried out (C). Relative flows are plotted in accordance with the scale to the right. The figures represent means of 6 studies. (The *black* and *white* diagrams were transcribed from original color photographs, which were kindly provided by Dr. D. Ingvar.)

visual field reaches the left cerebral hemisphere, which, in turn, controls the motor responses on the right side of the body, i.e., on the side of the threatening object.

Many of the more complex brain functions are allocated to one of the cerebral hemispheres. Hemisphere specialization is not unique to the human brain, but it has been observed mostly in man. The ability to perform fine manipulative hand movements is one example. Most people are right-handed, which indicates that the left motor cortex is usually more resourceful than the motor areas on the right side in regard to hand skills. Language abilities and mathematical skills, likewise, are located mainly in the left hemisphere, whereas the right cerebral cortex is usually dominant in regard to musical skills, the recognition of complex visual patterns, and emotions.

The reason for hemisphere specialization is not clear, but scientists have speculated that higher brain functions involve so many millions of neurons that a duplication of the mechanism in both hemispheres would be wasteful. Besides, it might be incompatible with an orderly behavior.

Cortical Localization

Some general aspects of function must be mentioned before we discuss cortical localization. The classification of functions as motor, sensory, secretory, etc. is convenient, but ambiguous. Almost any type of functional event represents a composite of several elementary processes that take place simultaneously in many parts of the brain, and a specific function cannot usually be localized to a particular structure in the brain. Our tendency to dichotomize between motor and sensory illustrates the difficulties. A movement does not occur without some type of external stimulus or internal expectation, and it is difficult, if not impossible, to determine where "sensory" becomes "motor" in a neuronal chain. Functional centers are in reality integration centers; they are represented by groups of neurons that integrate various functional aspects, e.g., motor and sensory. The cortical motor and sensory areas are typical examples; neither is purely motor nor purely sensory. Although the primary somatosensory cortex (areas 3, 1, and 2) in the postcentral gyrus is foremost a receptive area for somatosensory impulses, it is also to some extent related to motor functions, which is re-

flected by the fact that some of the pyramidal tract fibers originate in the area. It is therefore common to refer to the primary somatosensory cortex as sensorimotor I (SmI). The primary motor cortex (area 4) in the precentral gyrus is for similar reasons referred to as motorsensory I (MsI).

A functional center does not exist in isolation from the rest of the nervous system. For the sake of simplicity, a functional "center" can be conceived of as a "distribution center," in the sense that it is connected to many other parts of the nervous system. It derives its importance from the fact that it represents an essential part of a neuronal circuit, or a series of circuits, that are of special importance for the function in question. If the center is damaged, the function is impaired to a lesser or greater extent.

It is difficult to say to what extent cortical localization of function can be correlated with histologic boundaries. As previously indicated, Brodmann's cytoarchitectural areas can be related to specific functions only to some extent. Nevertheless, since structure and function are closely related, it is likely to be proven someday that the various cortical subdivisions, which can be defined on the basis of specific histologic structure and distinct patterns of connections, subserve different functional mechanisms or different aspects of a specific function.

Although the cortical functions will be discussed in relation to various lobes, it should be noted that the macroscopic boundary by which hemispheric lobes and gyri are defined do not necessarily indicate functional boundaries.

Frontal Lobe

Motor Areas

A large part of the frontal cortex in front of the central sulcus is related to the control of movements, primarily on the opposite side of the body (see Chapter 7). These motor areas include *primary motor cortex* (Brodmann's area 4), *premotor cortex* (area 6), *frontal eyefield* (area 8), and *motor speech area* of Broca (areas 44 and 45).

A *supplementary motor area* is located in the upper part of area 6, primarily on the medial side of the hemisphere. It contains a bilateral representation of the whole body and is involved in complex motor phenomena. Merely thinking of performing a movement increases the blood flow in the supplementary motor area, which indicates that this part of the cortex is related to planning or programming of movements (Fig. 178).

Prefrontal Cortex

The prefrontal cortex is located in front of the motor areas. It increased dramatically through phylogenetic development, and its importance is reflected by the fact that it represents about a quarter of the entire cerebral cortex in the human brain. The functions of the prefrontal cortex are still to a large extent shrouded in mystery; they are subtle and psychologic in nature, and therefore difficult to study. Some insight into this problem, however, has been gained from studying patients with frontal lobe damage, e.g., war injuries, or by observing the effect of limited psychosurgical operations on the prefrontal cortex.

The New England railroad worker Phineas Gage is the most famous "lobotomized" patient in the history of medicine. According to a report published in a medical journal more than a century ago, this unfortunate man was struck by a thick iron bar that penetrated his forehead. Miraculously, the man survived and was able to walk with help to see a doctor. The crowbar had inflicted massive damage to his left frontal lobe, which resulted in a striking deterioration of his personality. Quoting from the medical journal: "Gage lived for twelve years afterwards; but whereas before the injury he had been a most efficient and capable foreman in charge of laborers, afterwards he was unfit to be given such work. He became fitful and irreverent, indulged at times in the grossest profanity, and showed little respect for his fellow man. He was impatient of restraint or advice, at times obstinate, yet capricious and vacillating. A child in his intellectual capacity and manifestations, he had the animal passions of a strong man."

The famous crowbar case proves that the frontal lobe is crucially involved in organizing and controlling our behavior. However, it is not known how the prefrontal cortex accomplishes this task, but the effect is evident in both intellectual and emotional aspects of behavior.

Some insight into these difficult problems can be gained from an analysis of the multitude of connections that exist between the prefrontal cor-

tex and the rest of the CNS. Prominent are the long association pathways, which converge on the prefrontal cortex from many other parts of the cerebral cortex. The transcortical pathways apparently provide the prefrontal cortex with information from areas related to sensory processing and perceptual experience. Other pathways are closely related to affective and emotional spheres, and to the biologic needs of the body. For instance, a variety of subcortical structures including the striatum, thalamus, and amygdaloid body, as well as various cell groups in the basal forebrain and brain stem, are directly connected with the prefrontal cortex. Although it is difficult to comprehend the function and relative significance of all these different pathways, it should be mentioned that several of the structures that are related with the prefrontal cortex belong to the "limbic system," which is believed to be of special importance for various motivational and emotional aspects of behavior (see Chapter 17).

In summary, it is apparent that the prefrontal cortex controls many aspects of our personality; it is of crucial importance for a series of mental faculties, e.g., initiative and concentration, judgment and foresight, and it subserves important functions in the emotional sphere, reflected in concern and sometimes anxiety for ourselves and the surroundings. The prefrontal cortex is a crucial component of a system that makes it possible for us to perceive the consequences of our actions. The prefrontal cortex is eminently suited for these tasks; through a multitude of connections with practically every major cortical and subcortical region in the brain, it is constantly being informed about events within and outside the body, and it adjoins and partly overlaps the motor areas, which are immediately responsible for the motor acts through which our behavior is expressed.

Parietal Lobe

Somatosensory Projection Areas

The main or *first somatosensory area* (SmI) for reception of tactile and proprioceptive impulses is located in the postcentral gyrus. It is represented by three parallel strips (areas 3, 1, and 2), which extend throughout the longitudinal extent of the postcentral gyrus (see Chapter 6). The different cytoarchitectonic areas have been shown to contain their own specific representation of the body. A *second somatosensory area* (SmII) is located along the superior lip of the lateral fissure adjacent to the insula. Both the first and the second sensory areas receive input from the same thalamic relay nucleus, i.e., the ventral posterior nucleus (VP). However, the somatotopic organization is more precise in SmI than in SmII.

Posterior Parietal Association Cortex

This rather extensive region includes the *superior parietal lobule* (areas 5 and 7) and the *inferior parietal lobule* (supramarginal and angular gyri). The posterior parietal area is generally considered to be a sensory association area for higher order sensory processing and for the integration of various types of sensory information. How and to what extent the superior parietal lobule is involved in sensory discrimination is not yet clear. Sensations of *touch* and *pressure* are clearly the domain of the somatosensory cortex in postcentral gyrus. *Stereognosis* and *two-point discrimination,* likewise, are closely related to the postcentral gyrus.

The *supramarginal* (area 40) and *angular* (area 39) *gyri,* seems to be a region of convergence for different types of sensory information. For instance, the interrelationship of visual and auditory stimuli is of special importance for language functions, and the inferior parietal lobule, most often in the left hemisphere, is therefore considered to be part of the *posterior language area* (see Clinical Notes).

The integration of various somatosensory and visual stimuli is important for the formation of the "body image," i.e., the awareness of the body, and the ability to correlate the position of the various parts of the body to each other and to the environment. A patient with a parietal lesion may not be aware of the contralateral half of the body. This and other forms of sensory neglect are characteristic of the parietal lobe syndrome (see Clinical Notes).

A highly developed and precisely organized system of association fibers, the superior longitudinal fasciculus, connects the parietal association cortex with the motor and premotor areas (Fig. 177B). Therefore, although the posterior parietal cortex is generally considered to subserve sensory rather than motor functions, its activities can nevertheless be of immediate consequence in motor expression.

Occipital Lobe

The occipital lobe is primarily related to visual functions. The primary visual cortex, the *striate area* (area 17), is the main receiving area of the optic radiation (Chapter 13). Each striate area, which is located primarily in the calcarine fissure on the medial surface of the hemisphere, receives visuotopically organized impulses from the ipsilateral halves of the two retinae. The contralateral visual field, therefore, is represented by a retinotopic map in the striate area. Several other retinotopically organized areas are located in the surrounding *parastriate* and *peristriate cortices* (areas 18 and 19). They are believed to be concerned with specific aspects of the visual image, including steroscopic feature and color vision.

Temporal Lobe

The temporal lobe contains receiving areas for two of the sensory systems, i.e., the auditory and the olfactory systems. Auditory cortex is located on the lateral side in the region of the lateral fissure, whereas the olfactory cortex is located in the region of the uncus of the parahippocampal gyrus on the medial side of the temporal lobe (see Chapter 14). The posterior part of the temporal lobe, as well as nearby parietal and occipital areas, are of special importance for language functions.

Most of the *auditory cortex* (areas 41 and 42) is located on the dorsal surface of the superior temporal gyrus, and it is therefore to a large extent hidden in the lateral fissure (Fig. 146). The auditory cortex is tonotopically organized, i.e., it is characterized by a spatial representation of tonal frequencies. Area 22 immediately surrounding the auditory cortex is also related to auditory functions and its posterior part, which is included in Wernicke's language area, is essential for the comprehension of spoken language (see Clinical Notes). Like the auditory cortex, area 22 is primarily located on the dorsal surface of the temporal lobe in a region referred to as *planum temporale.* The planum is usually larger on the left side, and this asymmetry is apparently related to the fact that the left hemisphere has specialized in language functions.

To be able to recognize faces is of crucial importance in many of our daily activities, and clinical–

anatomic studies indicate that extensive areas on the underside of the temporal and occipital lobes, apparently including parts of both the parahippocampal and fusiform gyri, are of special importance for *face recognition.*

Memory, Learning, and Neuronal Plasticity

There seems to be a close relationship between the temporal lobe and *memory functions,* but little is known about the mechanisms involved. However, some of the cortical areas in the temporal lobe serve as important gateways for information from widespread areas of the neocortex to two of the most prominent limbic system structures, i.e., the amygdaloid body and the hippocampus formation (see Chapter 17). The efficiency with which memory traces are being formed is known to be closely linked to emotional and motivational factors that are related to the limbic system. Since some of the neocortical areas in the temporal lobe are important mediators of neocorticolimbic interactions, the temporal neocortex would certainly be in a position to play a crucial role in the storage of new information. To assume that memory functions are localized only to the temporal lobes, however, is no doubt an oversimplification. Whatever the nature of memory traces may be, many parts of the brain are likely to be involved.

Although different aspects of memory have been studied intensively in recent years, little is yet known about the specific mechanisms involved in storage and retrieval of information in the brain. It is becoming increasingly obvious, however, that neuronal connections can be modified in response to experience and environmental stimuli. In other words, the nervous system is characterized by a high degree of plasticity. This is especially evident in the developing brain, in which the formation of specific synaptic relationships and neuronal circuits is crucially dependent on proper environmental stimulation. This, no doubt, has far-reaching implications for all aspects of human development and its relationship to behavior and mental health, especially since the definitive dendritic and axonal branching patterns and synaptic relationships are not established until long after birth.

But plastic changes and remodeling of neuronal pathways are apparently not restricted to the developing brain. Some of the success with which a person recovers from a brain lesion may depend on a reorganization of synaptic connections, possibly including the formation of new axonal branches, i.e., *collateral sprouting.* It is likely that the normal process of memory and learning has a similar basis. The neuronal plasticity does not necessarily have to involve anatomic changes in interneuronal connections; it may be restricted to subtle changes in synaptic configuration or simply biochemical alterations without obvious structural concomitants.

Many parts of the brain are probably involved in the storage and retrieval of information, but it seems that the cerebral cortex plays a key role in many aspects of memory functions in the human brain. The temporal lobe seems to be especially important for the acquisition of new memories.

CLINICAL NOTES

The cerebral cortex is involved in a variety of different functions, and cortical lesions are characterized by great diversity of symptoms and signs. Motor and sensory abnormalities are common, as are disturbances in language function and mental and emotional state.

Frontal Lobe Syndrome

Lesions of the motor areas cause spastic paralysis of the contralateral side of the body. If the lesion encroaches on Broca's area in the dominant hemisphere, it is likely also to affect speech (see below).

The term "frontal lobe syndrome" is often used to denote a prefrontal lesion. The effects of such a lesion are to some extent dependent on the site of the lesion and on the patient's premorbid personality. The clinical picture, therefore, can vary considerably from patient to patient. Severe bilateral lesions always have a noticeable effect on personality; the patient cannot concentrate and is easily distracted. A general lack of initiative, foresight, and perspective is also common. If a patient with a frontal lobe lesion were to play chess, he or she would probably not be able to think of more than one move at a time. Another characteristic symptom is apathy, i.e., a severe emotional indifference, especially if the lesion involves the medial or orbital frontal cortex.

Parietal Lobe Syndrome

Lesions in the parietal lobe result in cortical sensory syndromes. Impaired somatic sensation and loss of discriminative sensory functions on the opposite side of the body usually appear as a result of circumscribed lesions in the postcentral gyrus.

Lesions involving the posterior parietal association cortex are characterized by more complex sensory defects. The most striking symptoms are neglect of sensory stimuli and disturbance of spatial relationships. For instance, a patient with a posterior parietal lesion, especially on the right side, may not be aware of the contralateral half of the body. The absence of awareness of illness, e.g., hemiplegia, is called *anosognosia*. Severe bilateral lesions may result in a general lack of spatial perception and topographic sense; the patient is unable to draw a simple diagram or describe how to get from his home to work

The lack of understanding of the significance of sensory stimuli is referred to as *agnosia*.[2] The definition implies that a higher order perceptual disturbance can be clearly identified in the absence of a defect in the primary sensation or in intellectual capacity. Considering the complexity of the thalamocortical and corticocortical connections, and of the physiologic mechanisms involved in sensory processing, it is questionable if such a clear distinction can ever be made between primary sensory defects and higher order perceptual disturbances in patients with cortical lesions.

Tactile agnosia means inability to recognize objects by touch. It is related to, but different from, *astereognosis*, which is a loss of the ability to judge the form of an object by touch. Agnosias occur not only in parietal lesions but also in disease of the occipital or temporal cortices. *Visual agnosia* is a failure to interpret visual images, and *auditory agnosia* is a failure to recognize what is heard (see below). Disorders of the execution of learned movement that cannot be accounted for either by weakness, ataxia, or sensory loss is termed *apraxia*. Apraxias involving both sides of the body are most often seen in left parietal lobe lesions that interrupt the association pathways between the parietotemporal junction area and the premotor areas in the frontal lobe. A lesion that interrupts the callosal fibers between the motor areas in the left and the right frontal lobes usually causes apraxia in the left limbs only. The term apraxia is not used if the failure to carry out a command is due to a severe deficit of comprehension, e.g., in a patient suffering from sensory aphasia (see below).

Occipital Lobe Syndrome

The occipital lobe is essential for the reception and recognition of visual stimuli, and a lesion in this part of the brain results in characteristic visual defects, which depend on the site of the lesion. A unilateral lesion causes *homonymous defects,* i.e., visual defects related to the corresponding halves of the two retinae, whereas a bilateral lesion results in *cortical blindness.* It is important to remember that the pupillary light reflex does not involve occipital pathways and is preserved in occipital lobe lesions. A patient suffering from *visual agnosia* cannot recognize or identify an object in spite of the fact that vision and mental capacities are intact. The object, however, can be recognized immediately by palpation. Visual agnosia, like all forms of agnosias, rarely occurs in isolation. Inability to recognize faces is called *prosopagnosia,* and this rare disorder can be seen following bilateral lesions on the undersides of the occipital lobes.

Temporal Lobe Syndrome

Visual Defects: Meyer's Loop

The ventral fibers in the optic radiation, which are related to the lower part of the retina, detour into the temporal lobe before proceeding to the visual cortex. A temporal lobe lesion that interrupts this loop (Meyer's loop) produces a *contralateral upper homonymous visual defect* (Fig. 156).

Cortical Deafness and Auditory Agnosia

Unilateral lesions in the auditory cortex do not produce significant deafness because of significant crossover at many points along the central auditory connections. Bilateral lesions, however, do

---

2. The Greek word for "knowledge" is gnosis, and *gnosia* refers to the ability to recognize the form and nature of persons and things. This faculty depends on a comparison of present sensory input with past experience.

cause deafness, but such lesions are extremely rare. *Auditory agnosia* (psychic deafness) is an inability to recognize what is heard despite the fact that the auditory projection system to the auditory cortex is intact. The responsible lesion is often located in the auditory association cortex (area 22) in the superior temporal gyrus. *Auditory–verbal agnosia* (word deafness: inability to recognize spoken words) is an important element in Wernicke's aphasia (see below).

Memory Disturbances

Although memory functions and learning cannot be localized to a single structure in the brain, the temporal lobes seem to be of special significance for memory functions. For instance, stimulation of the lateral temporal association cortex in awake patients undergoing brain surgery has aroused complex memories of auditory and visual images. Further, temporal lobe lesions have a general tendency to produce memory deficits, especially of recent memory. The memory deficits may not be obvious following unilateral lesions, but bilateral temporal lobe ablations, which have occasionally been performed in patients suffering from severe epilepsy, have resulted in profound disturbances in memory and learning.

Memory and learning deficits are important symptoms in several clinical disorders. In *Alzheimer's disease* (Chapter 8), forgetfulness is often the first and primary symptom of a mental deterioration.

Concussions (see Clinical Notes, Chapter 3) have a profound effect on the memory mechanisms, and the disturbance in memory, *amnesia*, is of great clinical relevance. A patient who has suffered a concussion usually cannot remember events that occurred immediately before the accident. This is called *retrograde amnesia* and may only involve the events that took place a couple of seconds before the accident. Similarly, the patient has no recollection of the period following the accident, i.e., *anterograde* or *post-traumatic amnesia*. The duration of amnesia is an important index of the severity of the concussion.

Korsakoff's psychosis is a clinical syndrome characterized primarily by severe memory disturbances. The ability to form new memories is lost, and since little or nothing can be remembered, the patient is in a hopeless state of confusion. Persons with poor food intake resulting from chronic abuse of alcohol may develop a severe Vitamin B_1 (thiamine) deficiency that may lead to Korsakoff syndrome.

Epilepsy

Epilepsy ("falling sickness") is a common disorder, characterized by paroxysmal attacks of brain dysfunction, often with alteration of consciousness. Epileptic seizures are the result of disorderly discharge of cerebral neurons triggered by some type of pathology in the brain. In many cases no original disease can be found, but the possibility of an underlying structural or metabolic disease should always be investigated. For instance, a pathologic focus in the form of scar tissue may well exist, even if the original trauma or disease passed unnoticed. Epilepsy may be the very first symptom of a neurologic disease such as infection, malformation, brain tumor, etc.

There are two groups of convulsive seizures: *partial* and *generalized*. Although seizure activity may start in any part of the brain, cortical seizures have attracted special attention because of the characteristic symptomatology. They give rise to partial (focal) epilepsies whose symptoms vary depending on the site of the irritative focus. Lesions in the region of the central sulcus, for instance, give rise to motor or sensory symptoms, and focal fits of occipital origin are characterized by visual symptoms. A focus in the primary motor cortex may result in an abnormal excitation that spreads across the sensorimotor cortex in a sequence determined by its functional–anatomic organization; this is a *Jacksonian*[3] *fit*. This partial motor seizure starts as jerking (clonic) movements in one part of the body, e.g., a finger, and spreads to other regions on the same side in a sequential fashion corresponding to the somatotopic organization of the motor cortex (Fig. 115B).

Hallucinations (false perceptions) are often preliminary symptoms of a partial epileptic seizure. Temporal lobe lesions may cause hallucinations involving hearing, smell, taste, or vision, whereas

---

3. The famous British neurologist Hughlings Jackson, who lived in the 19th century, suggested that epilepsy resulted from an abnormal discharge of neurons. On the basis of careful clinical examinations, he also predicted that the various parts of the body must be represented in a somatotopic fashion in the cerebral cortex.

posterior parietal and occipital injuries usually cause visual hallucinations. The subjective psychic experience may be followed by a period of unresponsiveness possibly characterized by automatic motor acts; the patient may smack his lips, make swallowing movements, or fumble with his clothes. Such convulsions are called *partial seizures with complex manifestations.* An older term was *psychomotor epilepsy.*[4] A special type of psychomotor attack is referred to as the *"uncinate fit"* (see Clinical Notes, Chapter 14).

Some seizures are generalized from the start. Others begin as a focal epilepsy and then develop into a *generalized motor seizure* ("grand mal") with loss of consciousness and clonic contractions of all the muscles in the body, a frightening experience when seen for the first time. The violent muscle contractions produce a rigid distortion of the body, breathing is impaired, and the skin turns blue from lack of oxygen. The tongue and cheek may be bitten and bloody saliva drool from the mouth. Most convulsions, partial or generalized, stop spontaneously within 1–3 min. Longer attacks require intervention and intravenous medication.

Language Disorders

The importance of language, i.e., the comprehension and communication of ideas and feelings, can hardly be overestimated. Language is the very essence of social intercourse, and a severe language disorder, *aphasia,* is devastating to the patient.

Language functions are localized to the left hemisphere (Fig. 179) in more than 95% of the population, and it is convenient to distinguish between two major cortical language areas. The *expressive speech area* (Broca's area) is concerned primarily with motor aspects of speech. Another more extensive region in the parieto-occipitotemporal junction, the *receptive speech area,* is of great importance for comprehension of spoken and written language.

A lesion in *Broca's area,*[5] which is located in the inferior frontal gyrus (areas 44 and 45), results

in *motor or nonfluent aphasia,* i.e., Broca's aphasia. Although the muscles of articulations may not be paralyzed, the patient can speak only with great difficulty. A patient with Broca's aphasia usually has a right-sided hemiplegia as well, because of involvement of the left precentral gyrus.

Another type of language disorder, i.e., *sensory aphasia,* appears when the lesion is located in the posterior part of the superior temporal gyrus (area 22) and in the angular and supramarginal gyri (areas 39 and 40). A sensory aphasia is characterized by disturbances in the comprehension of the spoken language, *word deafness,* and in difficulties in reading, *alexia,* and writing, *agraphia.* Some call this type of aphasia *fluent aphasia* or *Wernicke's aphasia,* in honor of Carl Wernicke from Poland, who made extensive studies on aphasic patients in the 19th century and thereby laid the groundwork for our present understanding.

Although it is customary to speak of an expressive and a receptive language area it is important to recognize that such a functional subdivision is a gross simplification. Language functions are very complicated, and clinical–pathologic studies have shown that language disorders are hardly ever purely motor or purely sensory. A patient with Broca's motor aphasia, for instance, also has some difficulty in grammar and in comprehending language. The language areas are closely interconnected with each other (via the arcuate fasciculus) as well as with many other parts of the brain, including the thalamus, and more widespread areas of the cerebral hemisphere are likely to be involved in complex language functions.

CLINICAL EXAMPLE

Epilepsy

A 47-year-old left-handed male presented with a 15-year history of seizures.

Twenty years earlier, while in military service, he was struck by shrapnel that entered the right frontal region. He was rendered unconscious for about an hour, and when he returned to consciousness he had a left hemiparesis and expressive speech difficulty. His wound was debrided and thereafter he made a good recovery, clearing his hemiparesis and aphasia. He took anticonvulsant medication prophylactically for about 2 years. After discharge from the service, he became a car dealer.

---

4. Since this type of seizure is commonly seen in patients with lesions in the temporal lobe, it is often referred to as temporal lobe epilepsy. However, the attack can probably be related also to other parts of the brain, especially the frontal lobe.

5. The French anthropologist and anatomist Paul Broca discovered as early as in 1861 that a lesion in the inferior frontal gyrus on the left side could have a disastrous effect on a person's ability to speak.

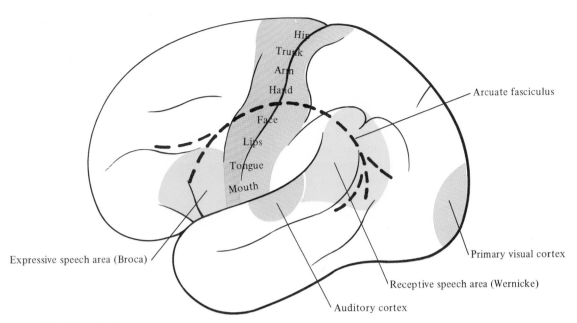

Fig. 179. Speech Areas
The expressive and receptive speech areas have been indicated by yellow color in this diagram of the lateral surface of the left cerebral hemisphere. Note that the expressive speech area of Broca is located immediately in front of the motor area for mouth, tongue and lips. (Modified from Geschwind, N. 1979. Specializations of the human brain. Scientific American, 241:3, 158–171.)

Five years later, while enjoying a cup of coffee, he suddenly experienced jerking, beginning in the thumb and forefinger of the left hand. He dropped the cup, and as he watched the convulsive movements spread to involve the forearm and shoulder, his head drew to the left, and he was unable to speak though he tried to call out. After about 2 min, his seizure ceased and he was left with weakness of the left arm for a further 10–15 min and he regained the power of speech within the same time.

Following this, he had similar episodes at approximately 2–3-week intervals, and some of the attacks progressed to loss of consciousness and urinary incontinence. Each time, however, the attack commenced in the thumb and index finger of the left hand and spread to the face and occasionally to the leg before consciousness was lost. Occasionally he was able to abort an attack by grasping his forearm just above the wrist.

On examination, he was a cooperative person who showed a mild left lower facial weakness and slight diminution of power in the long finger extensors and wrist extensors of the left hand. Rapid alternating movements were less well performed on the left than on the right, and the stretch reflexes were hyperactive in the left upper extremities as compared with the right. The remainder of the

neurologic examination was entirely normal, though tests of speech function revealed an occasional paraphasic speech error and an occasional word substitution on reading.

Skull X-rays revealed a frontal skull defect resulting from the posttraumatic surgical procedure. The EEG (electroencephalogram) showed right frontal electrographic seizure activity during sleep.

1. What type of seizure does the patient suffer from?
2. Why do the seizures often start in the thumb and forefingers?
3. Why did the patient have a mild aphasia?

Discussion

This is a partial seizure of posttraumatic origin. The term Jacksonian seizure is applied to simple partial seizures of either motor or sensory variety when in their propagation across the cerebral cortex, they reveal a motor or sensory march (compare Fig. 115 B). Because of the organization of the cerebral cortex of man with the majority of the surface expression of the cortex involved with the thumb, forefinger, mouth, and tongue function, these areas are predominantly involved in irritative cortical phenomena. At any time, the seizure may become secondarily generalized by propagating to centrencephalic structures and thus to both hemispheres simultaneously.

Following such a seizure, a postictal or Todd's paralysis is common and this again may be caused by inhibition or by neuronal exhaustion on the basis of increased metabolic activity or clearing in the seizure focus. The patient's speech disturbance indicates that his language areas are located in the right hemisphere, which is dominant for speech in about 50% of left-handed people. The speech deficit, like the paralysis, is transitory.

Patients may frequently abort the spread of an epileptic march by grasping the extremity above where the seizure phenomenon is occurring. The reason for this is not clear but it may have to do with evocation of inhibitory neurotransmitters.

Patients with posttraumatic epilepsy can usually be treated successfully with anticonvulsant medication, and only rarely do such patients require neurosurgical therapy with excision of the epileptic focus.

SUGGESTED READING

1. Bindman, L. and O. Lippold, 1981. The Neurophysiology of the Cerebral Cortex. University of Texas Press: Austin, pp. 3–60.

2. Brodal, A., 1981. Neurological Anatomy in Relation to Clinical Medicine, 3rd ed. Oxford University Press: New York, pp. 788–848.

3. Dreifuss, F. E. and S. I. Lee, 1981. Epilepsy, Case Studies. Medical Examination Publishing Co.: Garden City, New York.

4. Geschwind, N., 1979. Specializations of the human brain. Scientific American 241(3): 158–168.

5. Geschwind, N., 1980. Some special functions of the human brain. Dominance, language, apraxia, memory and attention. In V. B. Mountcastle (ed.): Medical Physiology, 14th ed., Vol. 1. C. V. Mosby: St. Louis, Missouri, pp. 647–665.

6. Lassen, N. A., D. H. Ingvar, and E. Skinhöj, 1978. Brain function and blood flow. Scientific American 239(4): 62–71.

7. Poggio, G. F. and V. B. Mountcastle, 1980. Functional organization of thalamus and cortex. In V. B. Mountcastle (ed.): Medical Physiology, 14th ed., Vol. 1. C. V. Mosby: St. Louis, Missouri, pp. 276–298.

20
Neuronal Transmitters and Modulators

ACETYLCHOLINE

NEUROPEPTIDES
  Substance P
  Opioid Peptides: Endorphins and Enkephalins
  Other Peptides

AMINO ACIDS
  γ-Aminobutyric Acid
  Glycine
  Glutamate and Aspartate

SUGGESTED READING

Some of the most exciting discoveries in recent years concern the chemical nature of neuronal systems. About 30 different substances are known or suspected transmitters, and many more are likely to be discovered. The various substances can be identified within neuronal cell bodies and axon terminals by the aid of fluorescence histochemical and immunocytochemical techniques, and it has been shown that each of the transmitters has a specific pattern of location in the brain.

With the development of the Golgi method in the latter half of the last century a new era in the tracing of neuronal pathways began, and the mapping of interneuronal connections has been a classic pursuit ever since. Indeed, the tracing of neuronal circuits and synaptic relationships has intensified considerably during the last decades as a result of the development of increasingly more sensitive neuroanatomic tract-tracing methods. A momentous event occurred in the early 1960s with the development of the Falck-Hillarp fluorescence histochemical method for the demonstration of biogenic amines. By the aid of this method it became possible to identify and characterize neurons and pathways, not only in regard to their morphology, but also on the basis of their neurotransmitter content. The subsequent introduction of the immunocytochemical techniques for the identification of neurotransmitter-synthesizing enzymes and peptides has virtually revolutionized the study of neuronal systems and pathways. Many chemically distinct pathways have been identified, and the diversity of chemically coded systems in the brain is remarkable; about 30 different substances have been recognized either as putative neurotransmitters or as modulators of interneuronal communication, and many more will undoubtedly be discovered.

Acetylcholine (ACh) was the first neurotransmitter to be identified more than 50 years ago, but the lack of a specific method for localizing ACh in neurons and terminals hampered the study of cholinergic pathways for many years. The monoaminergic pathways, on the other hand, have been intensively studied since the introduction of the histofluorescence method 20 years ago, and the various monoamine systems, which are discussed in Chapter 10, belong to the best known transmitter systems in the CNS. In recent years a number of neuropeptides and amino acids have been added to the list of known or suspected transmitters.

Transmitters and modulators produce their effect by interacting with *receptors,* i.e., uniquely shaped macromolecules located on the surface of the receiving cell. The transmitter will bind only to the receptor that fits its shape as a key fits a lock. A number of receptors have been isolated and characterized in regard to their specificity for a particular transmitter or modulator. Cholinergic, adrenergic, and opiate receptors are well-known examples.

ACETYLCHOLINE

ACh is the main neurotransmitter in the peripheral nervous system. It is used as a transmitter at the neuromuscular junction and in autonomic ganglia. The postganglionic parasympathetic fibers to the sweat glands are also cholinergic. But ACh is an important transmitter also in the CNS, and one of the most prominent cholinergic systems arises in the basal nucleus of Meynert (Fig. 117), which is located close to the basal surface in the region of the anterior perforated space. The large neurons in this nucleus and in nearby regions of the basal forebrain project to widespread regions of the cerebral cortex. One hypothesis that has attracted much attention in recent years is that the symptoms of *Alzheimer's disease* are due, at least in part, to massive degeneration of these cholinergic cells. Another cholinergic system is related to the striatum, where many of the interneurons are ACh as their transmitter. Loss of striatal cholinergic interneurons seems to be one of the main features in *Huntington's disease* (see Clinical Notes, Chapter 8).

The breakdown of ACh is facilitated by *acetylcholinsterase* (AChE), which can be localized by the aid of histochemical methods. AChE, however, is found not only in cholinergic pathways but also in noncholinergic neurons and it is therefore not a perfect marker for ACh utilizing neurons. With the development of antibodies against *choline acetyltransferase* (ChAT), the enzyme that catalyzes the synthesis of ACh, it has recently become possible to trace cholinergic pathways by the aid of immunocytochemical methods. This will greatly facilitate a full characterization of cholinergic systems.

NEUROPEPTIDES

Peptides, i.e., short chains of amino acids, have been found to play important roles in neurotransmission mechanisms. Substance P (SP) was the first peptide to be discovered in the brain in 1931. Other peptides were first identified as pituitary hormones, e.g., ACTH and vasopressin, or as hypothalamic releasing hormones, e.g., thyrotropic-releasing hormone (TRH). Several gastrointestinal peptides, e.g., SP, vasoactive intestinal polypeptide (VIP), and cholecystokinin (CCK), are also present in the brain. More than 15 different peptides have been identified as neuroactive peptides and some of the most exciting discoveries concern a group of endogenous peptides with opioid activity, referred to as endorphins, including the enkephalins (ENK). Most of the peptides are present in many regions of the CNS, especially in the hypothalamus and amygdaloid body. Cerebellum, thalamus, and the cerebral cortex contain only a few peptides.

Substance P

Substance P (P for preparation) was the first neuroactive peptide to be discovered in 1931 and it has a wide distribution both in the central and peripheral nervous system. It probably serves many functions, although little is known about its physiology. Many of the primary sensory neurons in the dorsal root ganglia contain SP, which is believed to be specifically concerned with the transmission of pain impulses in the dorsal horn of the spinal cord (see Clinical Notes, Chapter 6).

Many of the fiber systems related to the hypothalamus and the amygdaloid body contain SP, but little is known concerning its functional significance. One of the highest concentrations of SP is found in the substantia nigra, where it seems to be directly involved in the regulation of the nigrostriatal dopamine system. Many of the SP fibers in the substantia nigra are likely to arise in the striatum and globus pallidus, and it is of interest to note that patients with *Huntington's disease* have a marked decrease of the SP content in substantia nigra, presumably because of a loss of striatal neurons.

Opioid Peptides: Endorphins and Enkephalins

All endogenous peptides with opioid activity are referred to as endorphins. In 1975 two endorphins were identified in the brain and they were named enkephalins (from the Greek word: "in the head"). Both enkephalins are pentapeptides, and they are identical except for the terminal amino acid, which is either methionine (met-ENK) or leucine (leu-ENK). The enkephalins, which are widely distributed both in the central and peripheral nervous systems, have recently attracted much attention

for their apparent role as transmitters in an endogenous pain-inhibiting system, which is believed to originate in the brain stem and project to the spinal cord where it supposedly interferes with transmission of pain impulses (see Clinical Notes, Chapter 6). Procedures for healing chronic pain, e.g., *acupuncture* and *brain stimulation,* may well derive their effect by stimulating the endogenous pain-inhibiting system.

Although the analgesic effects of the enkephalins have created understandable excitement, there are many enkephalin systems in the brain and they are likely to be involved in a multitude of functions. Many of the interneuronal systems, e.g., in the olfactory bulb, neocortex, and cerebellum, are enkephalinergic, and the enkephalins seem to play an important role in neuroendocrine regulation. They are also involved in basal ganglia functions, as witnessed by the fact that one of the most prominent enkephalin systems in the brain originates in the striatum and terminates in the globus pallidus.

Other Peptides

Some of the most well-known peptides, e.g., *ACTH, oxytocin, vasopressin, somatostatin* (growth hormone-release inhibiting hormone), *thyrotropic-releasing hormone* (TRH), and *luteinizing hormone-releasing hormone* (LH-RH) were first identified as hormones secreted by the pituitary gland or by hypothalamic cells. Although these substances are involved in neuroendocrine functions, they are apparently related also to other activities. ACTH-containing fibers, for instance, are found in many extrahypothalamic areas including the thalamus, amygdaloid body, and brain stem and it is believed to play an important role in motivational mechanisms as well as in memory and learning. Somatostatin, likewise, has a wide distribution in the brain and spinal cord, and it seems to have a generally inhibitory effect on synapses.

Other peptides, e.g., VIP and CCK, were initially identified in the gastrointestinal system and believed to be gut hormones. Both substances, however, have been discovered in many parts of the brain, especially in the forebrain and cerebral cortex, where they are believed to be involved in a number of activities related to cortical functions, neuroendocrine effects, and control of cerebral blood flow.

AMINO ACIDS

γ-Aminobutyric Acid

γAminobutyric acid (GABA) is the most common inhibitory transmitter in the CNS and it is believed that about one-third of all synapses in the brain are GABAergic. Neurons containing GABA can be identified by staining them with antibodies against glutamic acid decarboxylase (GAD), the enzyme that catalyzes the biosynthesis of GABA. Most local-circuit neurons seem to be GABAergic, the most well-known examples being the stellate and basket cells in the cerebral and cerebellar cortices (Fig. 122). There are also several inhibitory GABAergic projection systems in the brain. One of the most prominent is the Purkinje cell projection to the deep cerebellar nuclei. Some of the major projection systems of the basal ganglia are also GABAergic and inhibitory, including projections from the striatum to globus pallidus, and from these structures to the substantia nigra. The symptoms in patients with *Huntington's disease* seem to be due in part to loss of GABAergic interneurons in the basal ganglia.

Glycine

Glycine is another inhibitory transmitter, which is found especially in the spinal cord, and it is believed that the interneurons in the ventral horn use glycine as their transmitter.

Glutamate and Aspartate

These two amino acids occur in high concentration in many parts of the brain and they are believed to be the main excitatory transmitters in the CNS. Examples of glutamate or aspartate systems are the corticostriatal pathway, the parallel fiber system in cerebellum, and several of the hippocampal pathways, including the perforant path and the mossy fiber system.

SUGGESTED READING

1. Bloom, F. E., 1980. Neurohumoral Transmission and the Central Nervous System. In: Goodman and Gilman's The Pharmacological Basis of Therapeutics. MacMillan: New York, pp. 235–257.
2. Bloom, F. E., 1981. Neuropeptides. Scientific American 245(4): 148–169.
3. Cooper, J. R., F. E. Bloom, and R. H. Roth, 1982. The Biochemical Basis of Neuropharmacology, 4th ed. Oxford University Press: New York.
4. Emson, P.C. (ed.), 1983. Chemical Neuroanatomy. Raven Press: New York.
5. Iversen, L. L., 1979. The chemistry of the brain. Scientific American 241(3): 118–129.

21
Cerebrovascular System

CEREBRAL BLOOD FLOW
  Regulation
  Fainting and Syncope

STROKE
  Cerebral Thrombosis and Hemorrhage
  Collateral Circulation
  Stroke Therapy

VASCULAR ANATOMY AND NEUROVASCULAR SYNDROMES
  Internal Carotid System
  Vertebral–Basilar System

NORMAL ANGIOGRAMS

CLINICAL EXAMPLES
  Middle Cerebral Artery Territory Infarct
  Internal Carotid Artery Occlusion
  Anterior Spinal Artery Syndrome

SUGGESTED READING

Cerebrovascular disease (stroke) is one of the most common of all disorders and a major cause of disability and death. Continuous and vigorous research, however, is gradually improving our abilities to diagnose and prevent strokes, and an increasing number of stroke victims are being successfully treated by a competent medical staff.

As in most diseases of the nervous system, the clinical features of stroke are to a large extent dependent on the anatomic localization of the pathologic process, and the examination of a stroke patient is likely to become an exercise in futility unless one has a basic understanding of the main arteries and their distribution. Fortunately, it is relatively easy to acquire such knowledge.

The frequency of cerebrovascular disorders makes the cerebrovascular system one of the most important subjects in clinical neurology. Pathologic changes in brain arteries alone are responsible for almost 50% of all neurologic disorders in a general hospital, and patients with strokes resulting from an occlusion or a hemorrhage in one of the cerebral arteries are frequent encounters in general practice. Since the various features of a stroke syndrome cannot be understood without a basic knowledge of the course and distribution of the major arteries, the morphology of the cerebral vessels is a subject of the highest priority in any neuroscience course for medical students. Blood vessels and vascular disorders related to the meninges are discussed in Chapter 3.

The cerebrovascular system can be visualized radiographically by injecting a contrast medium into the carotid or vertebral arteries. Roentgenograms obtained in this manner are termed angiograms. To be able to interpret the angiograms and to appreciate various abnormalities of the cerebrovascular system, its normal anatomic appearance must be known. The anatomy of the cerebrovascular system is a matter of genuine concern for most experts of the CNS, regardless of whether they are interested in its clinical–pathologic aspects or more basic physiologic problems of blood flow.

CEREBRAL BLOOD FLOW

Regulation

Although the brain represents only 2% of the body weight, it receives about 15% of the cardiac output. It cannot effectively store either oxygen or glucose, and is critically dependent on a continuous blood supply. Signs of brain dysfunction appear if the supply of blood is discontinued for only 8–10 sec, and irreversible neuronal damage occurs if the arrest is extended for 3–5 min.

Although the cerebral vessels are supplied with autonomic nerves, neurogenic control is apparently of minor importance under normal conditions. Instead, the cerebral blood flow appears to be regulated locally by metabolic factors such as H^+, K^+, and adenosine. This local control of blood flow permits a discrete distribution in response to regional variations in activity. For example, arithmetic, volitional hand movement (Fig. 178),

or alteration in visualized light is associated with increased blood flow in specific areas of the brain. In addition, the brain has the capacity to maintain relatively constant blood flow despite large changes in systemic blood pressure. This phenomenon, which is known as *autoregulation,* also appears to be under metabolic control. However, when mean arterial pressure decreases to less than 50–70 mm Hg, autoregulation fails and blood flow decreases.

Cerebral blood flow changes with altered levels of oxygen (Pa_{O_2}) and carbon dioxide (Pa_{CO_2}) in the arterial blood. When Pa_{O_2} is decreased to 50 mm Hg (hypoxia), cerebral blood flow is increased two-fold. Changes in Pa_{CO_2} have an even more dramatic effect, with hypercarbia causing an increase and hypocarbia a decrease in blood flow.

Fainting and Syncope

A sudden reduction in blood flow or an inadequate amount of oxygen in the blood may result in *faintness,* characterized by a feeling of weakness and dizziness. If the deficiencies in the cerebral blood flow are more pronounced, the patient may suffer a more or less complete loss of consciousness, i.e., *syncope.* Episodic attacks of faintness and syncope are common, and can be caused by a number of conditions, including cardiac disease, defective vasovagal reflexes, or by strong emotions.

STROKE

A cerebrovascular disease that results in a sudden appearance of neurologic deficits is referred to as *stroke* or *cerebrovascular accident (CVA).* These terms include both blockade of a cerebral artery (or vein) or hemorrhage from an artery (or vein). If the patient suddenly becomes unconscious, the term *apoplexia* is often used. *Transient ischemic attacks (TIAs)* are often forerunners of a major stroke.

Cerebral Thrombosis and Hemorrhage

Arterial strokes are much more common than venous strokes. The immediate cause of a CVA is usually an occlusion of a vessel by a thrombus (blood clot or cholesterol deposit) or bleeding from a ruptured vessel, which results in destruction of nervous tissue. Atherosclerosis and hypertension are the main contributing factors to cerebrovascular accidents. Bleeding that spreads through the subarachnoid space rather than within the brain tissue is called a *subarachnoid hemorrhage* (SAH). It is often the result of a ruptured aneurysm or trauma. Less frequently, SAH is caused by a rupture of an *arteriovenous malformation* (*AVM*).

Collateral Circulation

Although the location and the size of the pathologic process to a large extent determine the symptoms of a CVA, the effect on the brain tissue of a gradually developing occlusion is also dependent on the available anastomotic channels and the possibility for collateral circulation. The clinical importance of the *circle of Willis* (Fig. 35) should be emphasized in this context. A thrombosus in the internal carotid artery is likely to cause a massive cerebral infarct resulting in the death of the patient but it may also go unnoticed if there is an efficient collateral circulation in the cirlce of Willis.

Anastomotic channels between the external carotid and the internal carotid systems in the region of the ophthalmic artery may be of great functional importance in the case of a carotid artery thrombosis. Collateral circulation through superficial pial anastomoses between the major arteries of the cerebrum (anterior, middle, and posterior cerebral arteries) can also be quite effective. Similar anastomoses exist in the cerebellum between the superior cerebellar, anterior inferior cerebellar, and posterior inferior cerebellar arteries. The perforating arteries to the deep structures of the cerebrum, cerebellum, and brain stem, however, are in effect "end arteries," and occlusions of these arteries usually have severe effects.

Stroke Therapy

Stroke therapy is aimed at restoring circulation and preventing further strokes. A special form of therapy is endarterectomy, surgical removal of an obstruction usually in the carotid artery at the level of the bifurcation. Although similar operations on the upper intracranial parts of the vertebral artery, where most atherosclerotic plaques in the vertebral–basilar system are located, have traditionally been considered too difficult, great progress has recently been made in vascular microsurgery, and there is hope that atherosclerotic plaques in the vertebral arteries, and maybe even in some of the other large arteries on the base of the brain, can be successfully removed in the near future. Partial occlusion of internal carotid or vertebral–basilar systems can often be arrested by anticoagulation.

VASCULAR ANATOMY AND NEUROVASCULAR SYNDROMES

The brain is supplied with blood through four large trunks, the paired internal carotid arteries and vertebral arteries, which approach the ventral brain surface where they unite to form the *circle of Willis* (Figs. 180 and 32).

Each internal carotid artery enters the skull through the carotid canal, and at the level of the optic chiasm bifurcates to form the anterior cerebral and the middle cerebral arteries. The *internal carotid system* and its two main branches, the anterior and middle cerebral arteries, supply approximately the rostral two-thirds of the brain including the main parts of the basal ganglia and the internal capsule (Fig. 181). Cerebrovascular lesions in the territory of the internal carotid artery are characterized by contralateral signs: hemiplegia, hemianesthesia, and hemianopia. If the deficits are on the right side of the body there is usually aphasia as well, as a result of infarction in the distribution of the left middle cerebral artery (see Clinical Examples).

The two vertebral arteries, which enter the skull through the foramen magnum, unite at the pontomedullary junction to form the basilar artery (Fig. 32 in dissection guide). The basilar artery divides into the two posterior cerebral arteries at the pontomesencephalic junction. The *vertebral–basilar system* supplies the cerebellum, the brain stem, most of the thalamus, and the posterior parts of the hemispheres. Lesions in this system may result in cerebellar ataxia, various brain stem syndromes, and, in case of involvement of the posterior cerebral artery, a homonymous hemianopia.

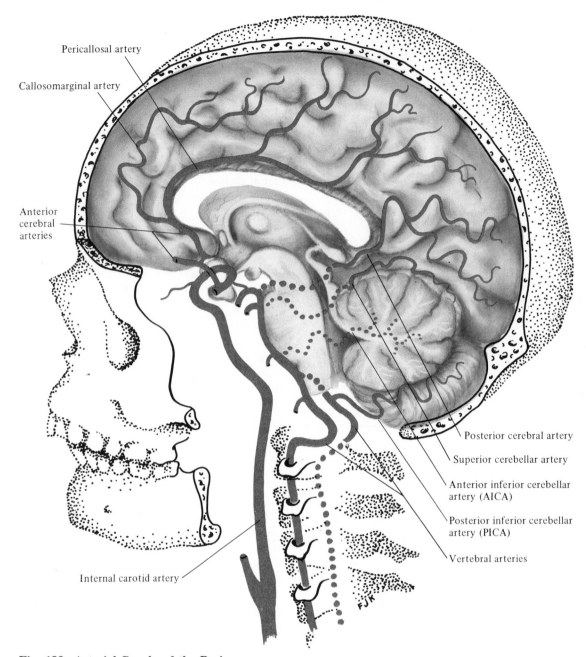

Pericallosal artery

Callosomarginal artery

Anterior cerebral arteries

Internal carotid artery

Posterior cerebral artery

Superior cerebellar artery

Anterior inferior cerebellar artery (AICA)

Posterior inferior cerebellar artery (PICA)

Vertebral arteries

Fig. 180. Arterial Supply of the Brain
Semidiagrammatic figure showing the two major arteries, the internal carotid artery and the vertebral artery, carrying blood to the brain. The left hemisphere has been removed in order to show the distribution of the anterior and posterior cerebral arteries on the medial side of the hemisphere. The three main cerebellar arteries are also illustrated.

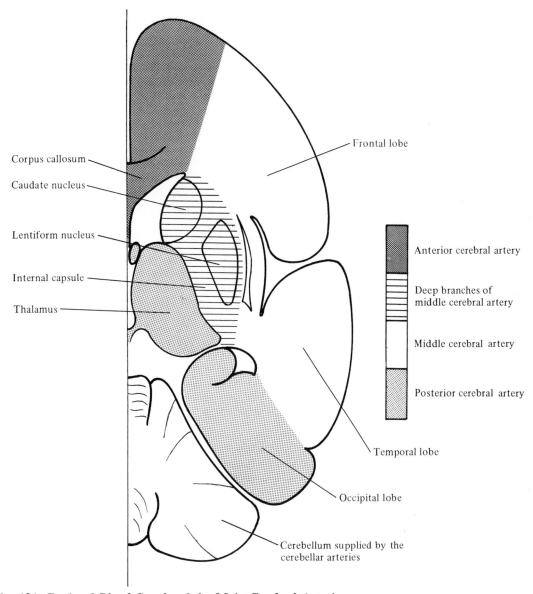

Fig. 181. Regional Blood Supply of the Main Cerebral Arteries
Diagram of the cerebral hemisphere showing the territories of the main cerebral vessels in a nearly horizontal section corresponding approximately to the CT scan shown in Fig. 77 in the Dissection guide. (Modified from C. M. Fisher, 1975. The Anatomy and Pathology of the Cerebral Vasculature. In: Modern Concepts of Cerebrovascular Disease [Ed. J. S. Meyer]. Spectrum Publications, Inc., New York, Toronto, London, Sidney.)

Internal Carotid System

Internal Carotid Artery

This artery arises from the common carotid artery in the neck and passes through the carotid canal of the petrous bone. It then turns medially and proceeds through the cavernous sinus. In doing

so, it curves in a S-like shape, forming the carotid siphon (Fig. 187B). The intracranial portion of the internal carotid artery bifurcates into the middle and the anterior cerebral artery lateral to the optic chiasm. Before it divides, however, it gives rise to the following branches:

1. Inferior and superior hypophysial arteries

2. Ophthalmic artery
3. Posterior communicating artery
4. Anterior choroidal artery.

Vascular Syndrome. Atheromatous plaques often form at bifurcations, and the region of the carotid bifurcation is a common site of internal carotid occlusion. The clinical picture of carotid artery thrombosis varies according to the compensatory capacity of the circle of Willis. Carotid thrombosis can be completely silent or it can cause massive destruction of those parts of the ipsilateral hemisphere that are supplied by the middle and anterior cerebral arteries (Fig. 181). Most often the territory of the middle cerebral artery is affected, giving rise to contralateral weakness and sensory loss, most pronounced in the face and arms. The speech areas are usually involved if the lesion is on the left side. Involvement of the anterior cerebral artery usually gives rise to sensorimotor deficits in the contralateral foot and leg.

Many of the strokes related to the internal carotid artery are preceded by transient ischemic attacks (TIAs). These TIAs, like more permanent strokes, manifest themselves in many forms depending on the artery that is temporarily occluded: monocular blindness (ophthalmic artery), hand weakness (middle cerebral artery), and speech and hand disorders (middle cerebral artery of dominant hemisphere). Since sclerotic plagues in the internal carotid artery can often be removed surgically, or thrombosis treated medically, it is important to be aware of these warning attacks before the brain is permanently damaged.

Middle Cerebral Artery

This is the major branch of the internal carotid artery. It proceeds laterally toward the lateral fissure between the frontal and temporal lobes (Fig. 35 in dissection guide). It lies below the anterior perforated space on its way to the lateral fissure. A series of 7–10 branches, the *striate arteries,* arise at right angles from the proximal segment of the middle cerebral artery and perforate this space. The medial group of the striate arteries is joined by the *recurrent artery of Heubner* from the anterior cerebral artery. The striate arteries supply the main part of the striatum, including the fundus striati, the globus pallidus, and the internal capsule.

When the middle cerebral artery reaches the lateral fissure at the level of the limen insulae it divides into several cortical branches on the surface of the insula. Most of these branches exhibit a tortuous course on the surface of the insula before they pass out of the lateral fissure to distribute to most of the cortex and underlying white matter on the lateral side of the hemisphere (Fig. 182).

Vascular Syndrome. The middle cerebral artery and its branches supply the main part of the cerebral hemisphere, including not only the basal ganglia and a major part of the internal capsule, but also important motor centers in the frontal lobe and somatosensory centers in the parietal lobe. The speech areas are also supplied by this artery, usually on the left side. A neurovascular syndrome resulting from occlusion of the stem of the middle cerebral artery, therefore, includes contralateral hemiplegia and hemianesthesia, homonymous heminopia, as well as global aphasia in most patients with left-sided lesions.

Of all cerebral arteries, the middle cerebral artery is the one most often affected by a cerebrovascular accident. The large majority of *cerebral embolisms* (detached blood clot, often from the heart), affect the middle cerebral artery, and the site of occlusion depends on the size of the embolus (see Middle Cerebral Artery Infarction in Clinical Examples). Most of the emboli are small and usually reach far peripherally into some of the cortical branches, thereby producing only part of the full-fledged middle cerebral artery syndrome. The embolic stroke is characterized by an abrupt onset.

The striate arteries are a common site of cerebral hemorrhages that usually include the basal ganglia and the internal capsule. A typical hemorrhagic stroke has a sudden onset, develops gradually during several hours, and is often fatal. Better control of hypertension has apparently brought about a gratifying reduction of hemorrhagic strokes in many countries.

Anterior Cerebral Artery

The anterior cerebral artery is smaller than the middle cerebral artery. The proximal trunk gives rise to perforating branches to the striatum and the anterior hypothalamus. It then proceeds to the interhemispheric fissure, where it communicates with the opposite anterior cerebral artery

Motor cortex   Somatosensory cortex

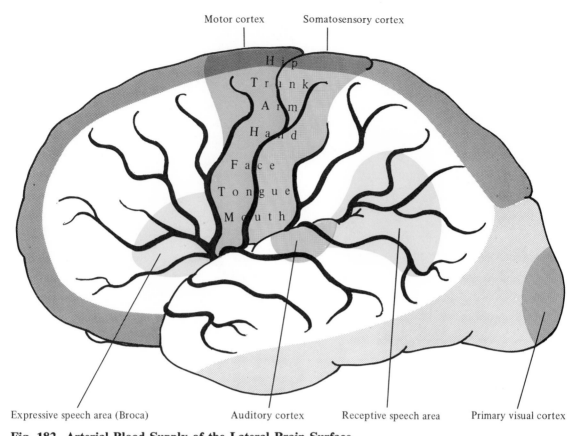

Expressive speech area (Broca)   Auditory cortex   Receptive speech area   Primary visual cortex

Fig. 182. Arterial Blood Supply of the Lateral Brain Surface
Diagram showing the territories of the main cerebral vessels and the branches of the middle cerebral artery and the main area of cerebral localization on the lateral surface of the left hemisphere. (*Dark gray* = territory of anterior cerebral artery; *light gray* = territory of posterior cerebral artery.)

through the anterior communicating artery (Fig. 35 in dissection guide). The distal trunk beyond the anterior communicating artery proceeds to the medial side of the frontal lobe toward the genu of the corpus callosum, where it divides into a *callosomarginal* and a *pericallosal trunk* (Fig. 183). Their branches supply most of the corpus callosum as well as the medial surfaces of the frontal and parietal lobes, including the leg area in the paracentral lobule.

Vascular Syndrome.   The anterior cerebral artery syndrome is characterized primarily by paralysis of the contralateral leg and foot. Behavioral disturbances, e.g., mental confusion and slowness, may also be apparent.

Vertebral–Basilar System

Vertebral Artery

The two vertebral arteries, which carry about one-third of the blood to the brain, represent the first branches of the subclavian arteries. They ascend through the transverse foramina of the cervical vertebrae before entering the skull through the foramen magnum. The arteries give off segmental branches both to the intraspinal circulation and to the neck muscles throughout their extracranial course. The muscular branches may be able to serve as anastomotic channels between the external carotid system and the vertebral–basilar system. The vertebral arteries supply the medulla oblongata with small bulbar branches and they give off two larger branches, the *anterior spinal artery* and the *posterior inferior cerebellar artery* (*PICA*) (Fig. 32). PICA is one of the most variable arteries in the vertebral–basilar system. Although it often

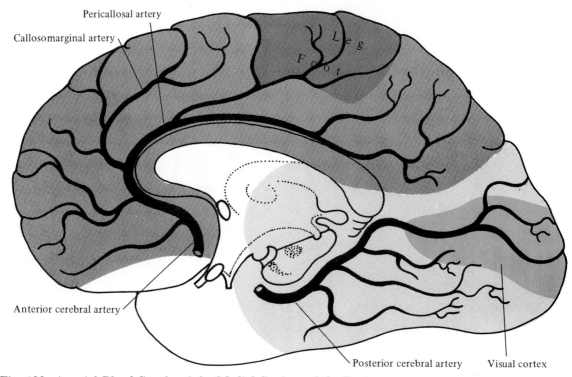

Pericallosal artery

Callosomarginal artery

Anterior cerebral artery

Posterior cerebral artery   Visual cortex

Fig. 183. Arterial Blood Supply of the Medial Surface of the Brain
Diagram of the medial aspect of the brain showing the territories of the main cerebral vessels and the cortical branches of the anterior and posterior cerebral arteries and their relations to the main areas of cerebral localization.

comes from the vertebral artery and makes a contorted loop on the side of the medulla before it reaches the inferior surface of the cerebellum, it may also have a common origin with the anterior inferior cerebellar artery from the basilar artery.

Vascular Syndromes. The two vertebral arteries are seldom of equal size, and if the larger artery is occluded, the smaller artery may not always be able to compensate for the deficiency. This can be devastating, especially if the collateral circulation is insufficient. The signs following occlusion of the vertebral artery are also characterized by variability. A well-known syndrome, the *lateral medullary syndrome of Wallenberg,* is caused by an infarct in the lateral part of the medulla oblongata (Fig. 184). It is characterized by contralateral impairment of pain and temperature in the trunk and extremities (spinothalamic tract), ipsilateral impairment of pain and temperature on the face (descending tract and nucleus of V), ipsilateral Horner's syndrome of miosis, ptosis, and decreased sweating (descending sympathetic fibers), dysphagia and dysarthria (nucleus ambiguus), vertigo, nausea, and nystagmus (vestibular nuclei), and sometimes ipsilateral limb ataxia (inferior cerebel-

lar peduncle). Although the lateral medullary syndrome is most often caused by an occlusion of the vertebral artery, it can also be caused by a lesion in PICA or the anterior inferior cerebellar artery.

Occlusion of the vertebral artery can sometimes result in a *medial medullary syndrome* with ipsilateral paralysis of the tongue (XII), contralateral paralysis of arm and leg (corticospinal tract), and contralateral impairment of touch and position sense (medial lemniscus).

The Basilar Artery

The basilar artery is formed by the union of the two vertebral arteries at the pontomedullary junction. It gives rise to the *anterior inferior cerebellar arteries,* the *internal auditory arteries,* the *pontine arteries,* and the *superior cerebellar arteries* before it bifurcates into the two *posterior cerebral arteries* at the upper border of pons.

Vascular Syndromes. Since the brain stem contains a large number of structures including the cranial nerve nuclei and long fiber tracts, it is obvi-

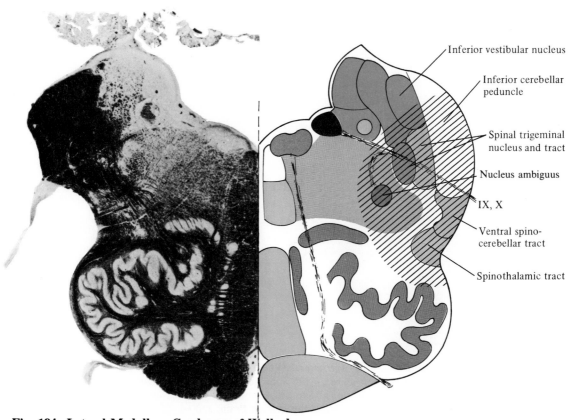

Fig. 184. Lateral Medullary Syndrome of Wallenberg
Cross-section through the rostral medulla oblongata. The crosshatched area shows the extent of the lesion (compare Fig. 127. The myelin stained left half of the medulla is reprinted from DeArmond, S. J., M. M. Fusco, and M. M. Dewey, 1976. Structure of the Human Brain, 2nd ed. With permission of Oxford University Press).

ous that vascular insufficiency of the basilar artery or one of its many branches may present a variety of different symptoms depending on the site of the occlusion, as well as the efficiency of the collateral circulation.

A total occlusion of the basilar artery may occur suddenly or following transient ischemic attacks. The full-fledged *basilar artery syndrome* includes disturbance of consciousness, often coma (reticular formation), tetraplegia (corticospinal tracts), impaired sensation (long somatosensory pathways), impaired vision or blindness (visual cortex), disorders of eye movements, facial paralysis and nystagmus (cranial nerve nuclei and their interconnection), and cerebellar ataxia (cerebellar peduncles and cerebellar hemispheres). Death usually follows within a few days.

More restricted syndromes occur if the vascular lesion is related to some of the branches from the basilar artery. Occlusion of paramedian arteries involves the corticospinal tract, the medial lemniscus, and the nuclei of cranial nerves III, IV, and VI. Infarcts related to the circumferential arteries

usually include parts of cerebellar peduncles and the cerebellum, the spinothalamic tract, and the nuclei of cranial nerves V, VII, and VIII. The following syndromes may serve as examples:

Medial pontine syndrome. Depending on the dorsal and lateral extent of the lesion, the medial pontine syndrome can include some or all of the following symptoms (compare Fig. 128 in Chapter 10): contralateral paralysis of arm and leg (corticospinal tract), homolateral paralysis of the face (VII), contralateral impairment of touch and position sense (medial lemiscus), and inward deviation of the homolateral eye (VI). There may also be paralysis of conjugate gaze to the side of the lesion (see "Gaze Center" for Horizontal Eye Movements, Chapter 11). If the lesion is located somewhat more rostral in pons, the VIth and VIIth cranial nerves may escape involvement.

Lateral pontine syndrome (anterior inferior cerebellar artery): The lateral pontine syndrome often includes impairment of pain and temperature on contralateral side of the body (spinothalamic tract), impaired facial sensation on the homolateral

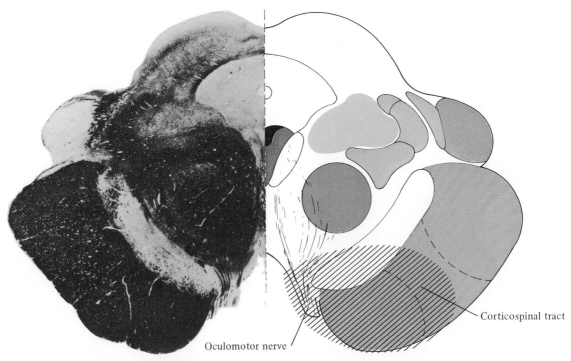

Oculomotor nerve

Corticospinal tract

Fig. 185. Mediobasal Mesencephalic Syndrome of Weber
Cross-section through the mesencephalon showing the approximate extent of a lesion giving rise to Weber's syndrome (compare Fig. 129. The myelin stained left half of the section is reprinted from DeArmond, S. J., M. M. Fusco, and M. M. Dewey, 1976. Structure of the Human Brain, 2nd ed. With permission of Oxford University Press).

side (V), vertigo, nystagmus and deafness on the homolateral side (VIII), homolateral facial paralysis (VII), paralysis of conjugate gaze to the side of the lesion (VI), and cerebellar ataxia on the homolateral side (middle cerebellar peduncle and cerebellar hemisphere).

Mediobasal mesencephalic syndrome of Weber (Fig. 185) includes contralateral paralysis of arm and leg (corticospinal tract) and ipsilateral paralysis of the oculomotor nerve, i.e., homolateral ophthalmoplegia with ptosis, dilation of pupil, absent light reflex, and outward deviation of the eye (III). Although Weber's syndrome is often due to an aneurysm in the posterior part of the circle of Willis (see Clinical Examples, Chapter 11), it can also result from involvement of the paramedian thalamoperforating branches of the basilar or posterior cerebral artery, in which case the red nucleus and its cerebellar connections may be involved, giving rise to crossed tremor and cerebellar ataxia.

Posterior Cerebral Artery

Thalamoperforating branches from the proximal part of this artery enter the posterior perforate substance to reach the medial part of the mesencephalon, the hypothalamus, and the thalamus. Distal to the *posterior communicating* artery, other perforating branches, the *thalamogeniculate arteries,* enter the cerebral peduncle to reach thalamus and the geniculate bodies. The posterior cerebral artery also gives rise to several *posterior choroidal arteries,* which enter the choroid plexus, where they form anastomoses with the anterior choroidal artery (Fig. 34 in dissection guide). The *cortical branches* finally supply the medial sides of the temporal and occipital lobes including the visual cortex (Figs. 183 and 186).

Vascular Syndrome. An occlusion of the proximal trunk of the posterior cerebral artery damages both the thalamus and the occipital lobe. The involvement of the visual cortex in the occipital lobe results in homonymous hemianopia, whereas the thalamic involvement causes a *"thalamic syndrome,"* which consists of hemiparesis, impair-

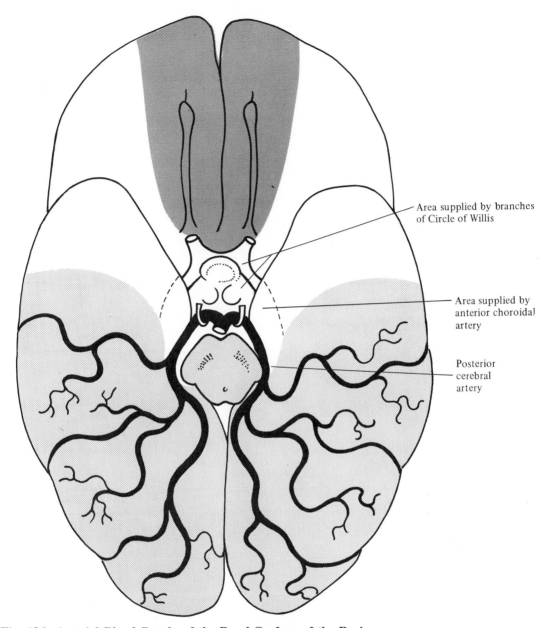

Area supplied by branches
of Circle of Willis

Area supplied by
anterior choroidal
artery

Posterior
cerebral
artery

Fig. 186. Arterial Blood Supply of the Basal Surface of the Brain
Diagram of the ventral brain surface showing the territories of the main cerebral vessels as well as the branches
of the posterior cerebral artery. (*Dark gray* = territory of anterior cerebral artery; *white* = territory of the
middle cerebral artery.)

ment of superficial and deep sensation, spontaneous and agonizing pain, and choreatheoid
movements, ataxia, or tremor, all on the side of
the lesion.

Normal Angiograms

Cerebral angiography is a relatively safe and very
valuable procedure for the diagnosis of various
pathological processes in the brain, especially tu-

mors, abscesses, and cerebrovascular disorders. It
is usually performed by catheterizing the femoral
artery. Following cannulation of one of the large
arteries in the neck, a contrast medium can be
injected into the appropriate cerebral vessels. Normal routine angiograms are illustrated in Fig. 187.

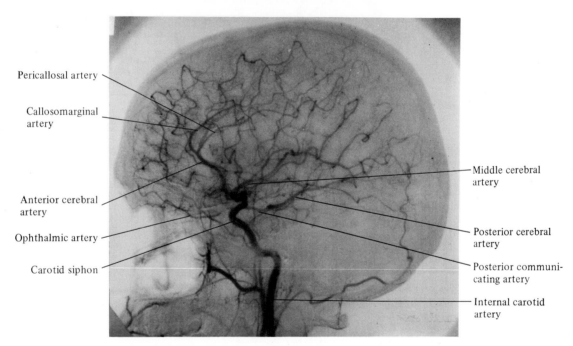

A. Internal carotid artery and its branches in frontal projection

B. Internal carotid artery and its branches in lateral projection

Fig. 187. Normal Angiograms

A. Internal carotid artery and its branches in frontal projection.
B. Internal carotid artery and its branches in lateral projection. Note that the posterior communicating artery and the main stem of the posterior cerebral artery have also been filled.

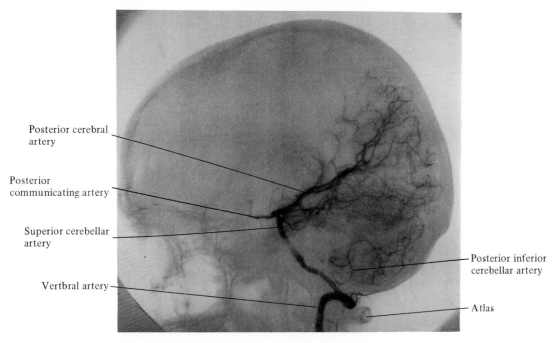

Posterior cerebral artery

Posterior communicating artery

Superior cerebellar artery

Vertbral artery

Posterior inferior cerebellar artery

Atlas

C. Vertebral and basilar arteries and their branches in lateral projection

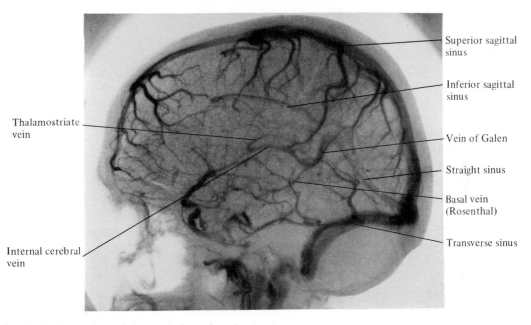

Thalamostriate vein

Internal cerebral vein

Superior sagittal sinus

Inferior sagittal sinus

Vein of Galen

Straight sinus

Basal vein (Rosenthal)

Transverse sinus

D. Cerebral veins and dural sinuses in lateral projection

C. Vertebral and basilar arteries and their branches in lateral projection.
D. Cerebral veins and dural sinuses in lateral projection. (**A–D,** Micrograph courtesy of L. Morris. The angiograms were obtained by the subtraction method, which gives an excellent visualization of vessel detail.)

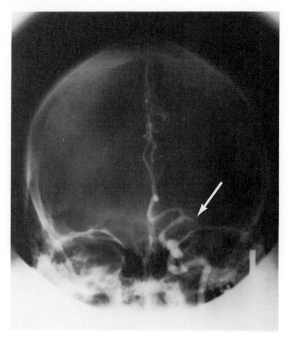

A (left). Middle Cerebral Artery Occlusion (Frontal Projection)

B (above). Middle Cerebral Artery Occlusion (Lateral Projection)

Fig. CE21A and B.
The angiograms were kindly provided by Dr. L. Morris.

CLINICAL EXAMPLES

Middle Cerebral Artery Territory Infarct

A 68-year-old left-handed female with coronary artery disease was admitted with crushing chest pain. Electrocardiogram showed an acute anterior myocardial infarction and she was admitted to the Coronary Care Unit.

She improved over the next 3 days but then, suddenly, developed more chest pain and a cardiogram showed extension of her myocardial infarct. Her condition deteriorated quickly with the development of ventricular fibrillation but, fortunately, she was converted back to normal sinus rhythm with electric counter shock.

After recovery from the counter shock, she was able to speak and had no difficulty understanding spoken and written language. It was noted, however, that she had a right homonymous hemianopsia. Her right lower facial muscles were very weak, but she could wrinkle her brow well on the right side. Her tongue deviated slightly to the right when protruded. She had a right hemiparesis with moderate weakness in the arm, but only mild weakness in the leg. She also had impaired stereognosis and graphesthesia in her right upper extremity but could still recognize pain in her right arm, al-

though she had difficulty localizing the site of the stimulus.

An emergency arteriogram was performed. The angiograms from that study (Figs. A and B) were obtained after selective catheterization of the left internal carotid artery and injection of X-ray dye.

1. What vessel is occluded?
2. Is the lesion demonstrated on the arteriograms appropriate to her neurologic deficits?
3. Why are the weakness and sensory deficits more pronounced in the arm than in the leg?
4. Why is only the lower part of her face on the right side paralyzed?
5. Why was she not aphasic?

Discussion

The patient developed sudden neurologic deficits in the wake of an acute myocardial infarction and cardiac arrhythmia. Since the arteriogram demonstrates occlusion of the left middle cerebral artery (arrow), it is likely that her heart condition resulted in the development of an embolus, which entered the general circulation and lodged itself in the middle cerebral artery. Note the absence of the middle cerebral artery and most of its branches in both the frontal and lateral projections (Figs. A and B).

The area of the left hemisphere supplied by the middle cerebral artery includes the motor and sensory areas controlling face, upper extremity, and trunk on the right side of the body (Fig. 182). The optic radiation in the left hemisphere is also involved. Motor cortex subserving leg movement is supplied by the anterior cerebral artery (Fig. 183) and is preserved in middle cerebral artery occlusions. Furthermore, since the lower limb is less affected than the upper limb, the corticofugal and corticopetal fibers connected with the cortical leg area must be largely intact. In other words, the occlusion of the middle cerebral artery has not deprived the internal capsule of all its blood supply.

The subdivisions of the facial nuclei controlling upper facial muscles receive bilateral corticobulbar innervation in most individuals (Fig. 139). Therefore, upper facial muscle function is usually preserved in unilateral cortical infarctions.

The motor and sensory language areas, which are supplied by the middle cerebral artery are usually located in the left hemisphere (Fig. 179), especially in right-handed people. This patient is left-handed, however, and the right hemisphere is dominant for language in about 50% of left-handed people. Since the patient did not become aphasic her right hemisphere is apparently dominant in regard to language.

Internal Cartoid Artery Occlusion

A middle-aged right-handed male was well until the evening of admission when he suddenly found himself unable to speak. Nor could he walk because of profound right-sided weakness.

On examination, he was alert but could not speak and was unable to understand requests. He had a right homonymous hemianopsia, and he could not look to the right. Lateral gaze to the left, however, was normal. There was weakness of the right lower facial muscles, and a profound right-sided hemiparesis involving arm and leg equally. Muscle tone and stretch reflexes were reduced on the right. Within half an hour he slowly began to get drowsier and he was comatose within 3 h.

An arteriogram (Fig. C), which was obtained after injection of dye into the left common carotid

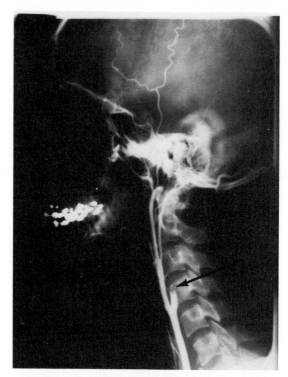

Fig. CE21C. Internal Carotid Artery Occlusion
The angiogram was kindly provided by Dr. L. Morris.

artery, shows complete occlusion of the left internal carotid artery 2 cm distal to its origin (arrow).

1. Why was the patient aphasic?
2. Why did he have a right homonymous hemianopsia?
3. Why was the hemiparesis of equal degree in his arm and leg?
4. Why was he unable to look voluntarily to the right?
5. Why did he gradually become comatose?

Discussion

Sudden occlusion of the internal carotid artery usually occurs as a result of extensive atherosclerosis. The occlusion is usually followed by rapid infarction of brain tissue. The size of the infarction is a function of the amount of collateral circulation that can be provided from the left posterior cerebral artery and from flow across the circle of Willis from the vertebral basilar system or the internal carotid artery of the opposite side (see Figs. 32 and 179).

The aphasia arose because of infarction of cortical language areas in the left hemisphere (Fig. 179).

The right homonymous hemianopsia most likely appeared because of damage to the left optic radiation, which is normally supplied by the middle cerebral artery. Equal weakness in arm and leg suggests that the infarct included the distribution areas of both the middle cerebral artery (arm and face) and the anterior cerebral artery (leg) (see Figs. 180 and 181). Infarction of the left frontal eye field, which is supplied by rostral branches of the middle cerebral artery, caused inability to voluntarily gaze to the right.

Symptoms following occlusion of the internal carotid artery are characterized by great variability, which is a product of the availability of collateral circulation. The clinical picture often resembles that of a middle cerebral artery occlusion (see above), especially if the anterior communicating artery is able to provide blood supply to the anterior cerebral artery on the affected side. In this patient there was little sign of collateral circulation, and the occlusion caused a massive infarct involving the anterior two-thirds of the hemisphere. The large size of the infarct and concomitant hemispheral swelling made the patient comatose and he died a few days later.

Anterior Spinal Artery Syndrome

A 70-year-old man with known hypertension and atherosclerosis was awakened in the middle of the night with excruciating upper abdominal pain that radiated into his back. Within minutes his legs became paralyzed and numb.

On examination his blood pressure was 200/120. A loud bruit was heard over his abdominal aorta and his femoral pulses were reduced in intensity. Cranial nerves and upper extremity functions were normal, but there was flaccid paraplegia of the lower extremities with reduced muscle tone and absent stretch reflexes. Pain and temperature sensations were completely lost below the level of T8 bilaterally, whereas vibration and position sense were intact. An emergency abdominal aortogram demonstrated a dissecting aneurysm of his upper abdominal aorta, and the *radicular artery of Adamkiewicz* was apparently occluded.

His blood pressure was carefully lowered and he underwent successful emergency repair of his aneurysm. Examination 10 days later showed some

power in his legs, but his right leg was much weaker than the left. Muscle tone and stretch reflexes were now increased in both legs and he had bilateral Babinski's signs. Touch, position, and vibratory sensations in his legs remained intact. He could also feel pain and temperature in his right leg, but not in the left leg or lower trunk below the level of the T10 dermatone.

1. Where is the initial lesion in the CNS?
2. Why were touch, position, and vibratory sensations in his legs preserved?
3. Why were his upper extremity motor and sensory functions preserved?
4. As he recovered, his deficits became asymmetric in the sense that his right leg was weaker than his left leg but certain sensory functions were more impaired in his left side compared to his right side. How do you explain this discrepancy?

Discussion

The patient suffered from an acutely dissecting aneurysm of his aorta with occlusion of the artery of Adamkiewicz (radicular artery of the lumbar enlargement), which is the major supplier of blood to the anterior spinal artery in the lower thoracic and lumbosacral part of the spinal cord. This resulted in infarction of the anterior two-thirds of the spinal cord below the midthoracic level. The posterior one-third of the spinal cord, which is supplied from intracranial and multiple extracranial branches is usually much less affected by sudden occlusion of any single vessel.

Touch, position, and vibratory sensations in the lower extremities were preserved because the posterior columns and dorsolateral fasciculi, which are nourished by the posterior spinal arteries, had not been damaged (see Fig. 105). His upper extremity functions were preserved because the part of the anterior spinal artery that supplies the cervical and upper thoracic region receives blood from the vertebral arteries or from branches of the subclavian arteries. Motor paralysis and dissociated sensory loss below the level of the lesion are typical for an anterior spinal artery syndrome.

As spinal cord infarctions resolve, asymmetrical deficits commonly arise. In this case the spinothalamic and corticospinal tracts appear to be more damaged on the right than on the left side.

SUGGESTED READING

1. Adams, R. D. and M. Victor, 1981. Principles of Neurology, 2nd ed. McGraw-Hill: New York, pp. 529–593.

2. Brodal, A., 1973. Self-observations and neuro-anatomical considerations after a stroke. Brain 96:675–694.

3. Escourolle, R. and J. Poirier, 1978. Manual of Basic Neuropathology, 2nd ed. W. B. Saunders: Philadelphia, pp. 67–104.

4. Fisher, C. M., 1975. The anatomy and pathology of the cerebral vasculature. In J. S. Meyer (ed.): Modern Concepts of Cerebrovascular Disease. Spectrum Publications: New York, pp. 1–41.

5. Osborn, A. G., 1980. Introduction to Cerebral Angiography, Harper and Row, Hagerstown, Maryland.

6. Wilson, McC. 1972. The Anatomic Foundation of Neuroradiology of the Brain. Little, Brown: Boston.

Epilogue

Zwar ist's mit der Gedankenfabrik
Wie mit einem Weber-Meisterstück,
Wo ein Tritt tausend Fäden regt,
Die Schifflein herüber hinüber schiessen,
Die Fäden ungesehen fliessen,
Ein Schlag tausend Verbindungen schlägt.

'Tis with the workshop of men's brain
As with a piece of tapestry:
One treadle guides a thousand skeins.
You shoot the shuttle to and fro,
You do not see the thin threads grow,
But a thousand are knit at a single blow.[1]

It is difficult to imagine a structure that matches the brain in complexity. Yet, its form and function can be appreciated without studying the detailed anatomy of every region. It is necessary, however, to have some insight into the functional anatomy of the human brain and spinal cord in order to meet the challenges presented by a patient with a brain lesion. Such basic knowledge can usually be obtained within the framework of the neuroscience course provided enough time is set aside for a systematic study of the topographic anatomy of the nervous system. It may be a cliché to say that form and function go hand in hand, but it is worth emphasizing that any attempt to understand the signs and symptoms in a patient with a neurologic disorder becomes an exercise in futility if the brain is conceived of as a Black Hole.

The last few decades have witnessed new and exciting reasons for cultivating the anatomy of the nervous system. There has been a phenomenal surge in the neurosciences, and some of the most impressive advances concern the chemical nature of nervous system activity. The list of transmitters and modulators in the CNS continues to grow. With a detailed knowledge of these chemicals, their function and location, there is reason to believe that we will be able to identify specific defects in nervous and mental disorders. This is likely to lead to the development of specific drugs that would allow a "magic bullet" approach, treating only the disordered portion of the brain. Indeed, recent progress in the understanding of the brain has resulted in improved treatment for several neurologic disorders, e.g., Parkinson's disease, a chronic movement disorder that affects hundreds of thousands of people in the world every year. Some of the most debilitating mental illnesses such as dementia, schizophrenia, and affective psychoses have to some extent been correlated with specific structural changes or biochemical disturbances in the brain. This is a good beginning, and an increasing number of neuroscientific programs are now being pursued with great expectations. The triumph of a breakthrough in the understanding and treatment of some of the crippling brain disorders would, for many, match the excitement of a successful space voyage. But it will take extraordinary efforts to make this dream come true. One of the first priorities must be to correlate the various chemicals with a detailed analysis of brain anatomy, and these studies are already underway in many laboratories. The results obtained can only be understood and exploited by those who have a reasonable knowledge of the anatomy of the CNS.

It would be an unfortunate oversight not to mention some of the spectacular advances that have taken place in the field of noninvasive imaging methods for medical diagnosis in recent years. *X-ray computed tomography* (CT scan) is now available in most medical centers and several of

---

1. Goethe, J. W. Faust, First Part. Translated by G. M. Cookson. Routledge and Sons: London, 1927. E. P. Dutton: New York.

the clinical examples in this book have been presented with appropriate CT scans. *Nuclear magnetic resonance* (NMR) and *positron emission tomography* (PET) techniques, which have been under development for several years, will undoubtedly perpetuate the revolution in neurologic, neurosurgical, and psychiatric diagnosis generated by the CT scan. These new methods are based on the identification and localization of chemical substances within the body, and they reveal the anatomy of the brain and spinal cord to the extent to which there are chemical differences between the structures of the CNS.

The image formation in the PET technique is based on the γ-radiation resulting from the annihilation of positrons emitted by isotopes introduced into the body by injection or inhalation. Radionuclides such as ^{11}C, ^{15}O, and ^{13}N are suitable for the labeling of metabolic substances, making it possible to obtain a dynamic picture of various life processes including the brain's energy consumption or the cerebral blood flow. With possibilities to label neurotransmitters and to measure receptor concentrations the PET technique has understandably created much excitement among those interested in the functional anatomy of the CNS. Ideally the isotopes used should have short half-lives, which generally requires a cyclotron for isotope production. This makes the procedure very costly and at least for the time being less suitable for routine diagnosis.

NMR scanning exploits the penetration of magnetic fields through the body and measures their interaction with the nuclei of atoms present in the tissue, e.g., hydrogen and phosphorus atoms. As illustrated in Fig. A, NMR provides an excellent discrimination between white and gray matter, and the infarct (arrow) can be accurately located in the basal ganglia. NMR investigations of cellular metabolism may in the future be able to provide valuable information regarding many pathologic conditions including ischemia and hypoxia. NMR does not involve any radioactivity. The image formation is based on the naturally occurring properties of particular atomic nuclei, and the radio frequency energies utilized in NMR observations do not seem to have any adverse biological effects. The NMR method, therefore, has some distinct advantages compared with the traditional radiologic techniques and the PET technique, which employ ionizing radiation.

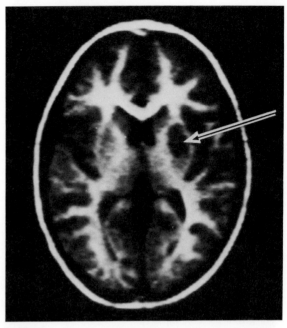

Fig. A.
NMR image of a horizontal section through the human brain showing an infarction in the basal ganglia. The infarct seems to involve primarily the lentiform nucleus and the anterior limb of the internal capsule at this level. (The micrograph was kindly provided by Dr. L. Crooks, University of California, San Francisco.)

These few examples of recent advances in basic and clinical neurosciences do indicate that the anatomy of the CNS is becoming increasingly more important. Not only the scientist who aspires to new discoveries, but also the medical practitioner, who utilizes recent advancements, must understand the basic structure of the human brain and spinal cord. This volume provides some of the foundation for both of these vital activities or professions.

Appendix

Figures 189–203 are reproduced from Medical Research Council, Memorandum No. 45, Aids to the Examination of the Peripheral Nervous System. With permission of Her Majesty's Stationary Office, London.

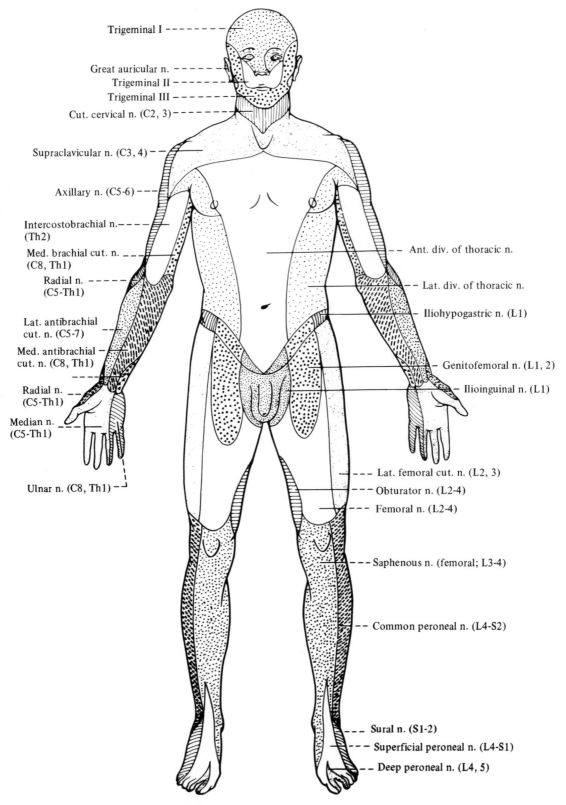

Trigeminal I

Great auricular n.
Trigeminal II
Trigeminal III
Cut. cervical n. (C2, 3)

Supraclavicular n. (C3, 4)

Axillary n. (C5-6)

Intercostobrachial n.
(Th2)
Med. brachial cut. n.
(C8, Th1)
Radial n.
(C5-Th1)

Lat. antibrachial
cut. n. (C5-7)

Med. antibrachial
cut. n. (C8, Th1)

Radial n.
(C5-Th1)
Median n.
(C5-Th1)

Ulnar n. (C8, Th1)

Ant. div. of thoracic n.

Lat. div. of thoracic n.

Iliohypogastric n. (L1)

Genitofemoral n. (L1, 2)

Ilioinguinal n. (L1)

Lat. femoral cut. n. (L2, 3)
Obturator n. (L2-4)
Femoral n. (L2-4)

Saphenous n. (femoral; L3-4)

Common peroneal n. (L4-S2)

Sural n. (S1-2)
Superficial peroneal n. (L4-S1)
Deep peroneal n. (L4, 5)

Fig. 188. The Cutaneous Distribution of the Peripheral Nerves
A. On the anterior aspect of the body.

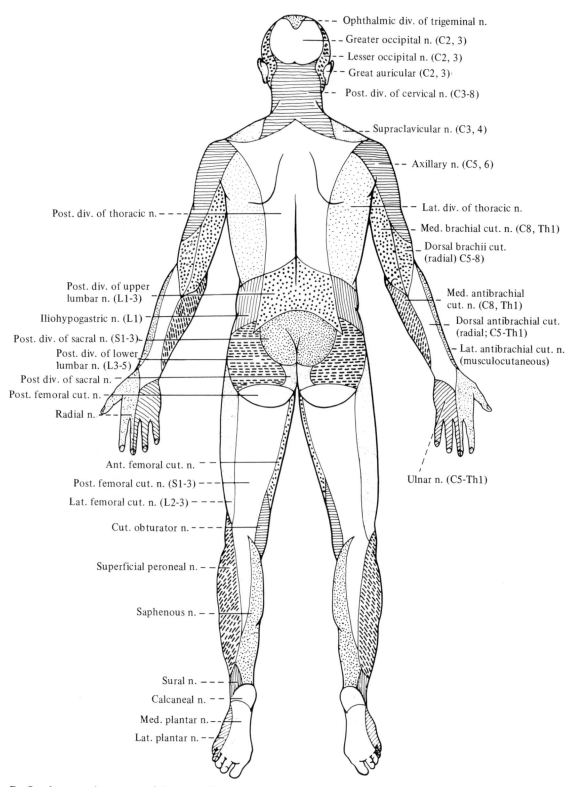

Ophthalmic div. of trigeminal n.

Greater occipital n. (C2, 3)

Lesser occipital n. (C2, 3)

Great auricular (C2, 3)

Post. div. of cervical n. (C3-8)

Supraclavicular n. (C3, 4)

Axillary n. (C5, 6)

Lat. div. of thoracic n.

Med. brachial cut. n. (C8, Th1)

Dorsal brachii cut. (radial) C5-8)

Med. antibrachial cut. n. (C8, Th1)

Dorsal antibrachial cut. (radial; C5-Th1)

Lat. antibrachial cut. n. (musculocutaneous)

Ulnar n. (C5-Th1)

Post. div. of thoracic n.

Post. div. of upper lumbar n. (L1-3)

Iliohypogastric n. (L1)

Post. div. of sacral n. (S1-3)

Post. div. of lower lumbar n. (L3-5)

Post div. of sacral n.

Post. femoral cut. n.

Radial n.

Ant. femoral cut. n.

Post. femoral cut. n. (S1-3)

Lat. femoral cut. n. (L2-3)

Cut. obturator n.

Superficial peroneal n.

Saphenous n.

Sural n.

Calcaneal n.

Med. plantar n.

Lat. plantar n.

B. On the posterior aspect of the body (From R. de Jong, 1979. The Neurologic Examination. With permission of Harper and Row, Hagerstown.)

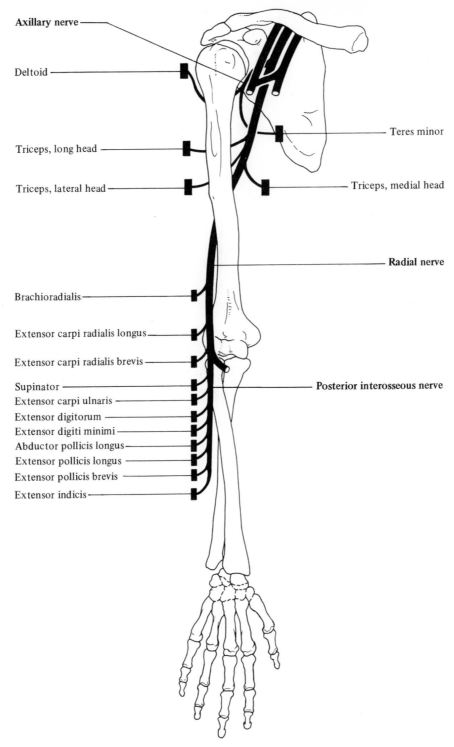

Fig. 189.
Diagram of the axillary and radial nerves and the muscles which they supply. (Modified from Pitres and Testut.)

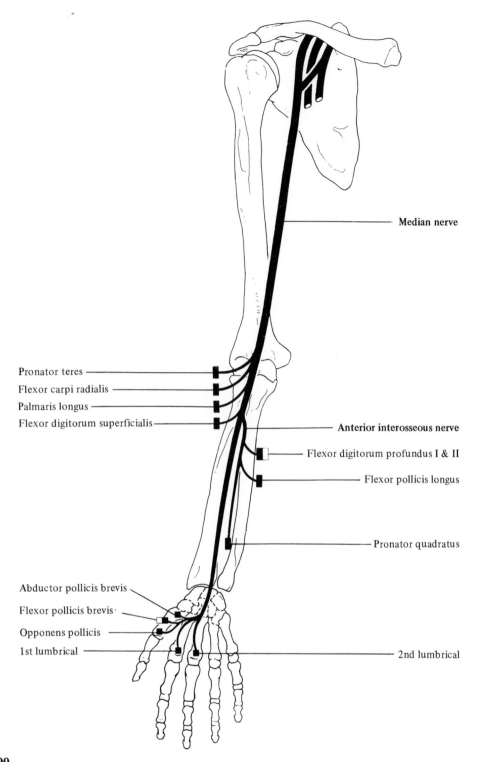

Fig. 190.
Diagram of the median nerve and the muscles which it supplies. (Modified from Pitres and Testut.) Note: the white rectangle signifies that the muscle indicated receives a part of its nerve supply from another peripheral nerve.

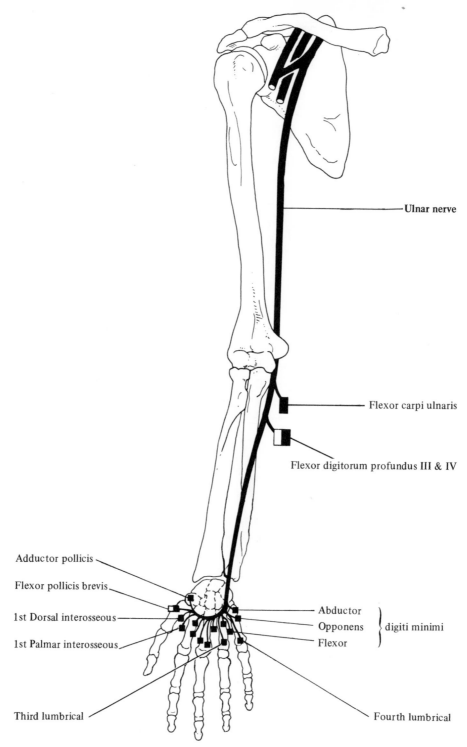

Ulnar nerve

Flexor carpi ulnaris

Flexor digitorum profundus III & IV

Adductor pollicis

Flexor pollicis brevis

1st Dorsal interosseous

1st Palmar interosseous

Abductor
Opponens } digiti minimi
Flexor

Third lumbrical

Fourth lumbrical

Fig. 191.
Diagram of the ulnar nerve and the muscles which it supplies. (Modified from Pitres and Testut.)

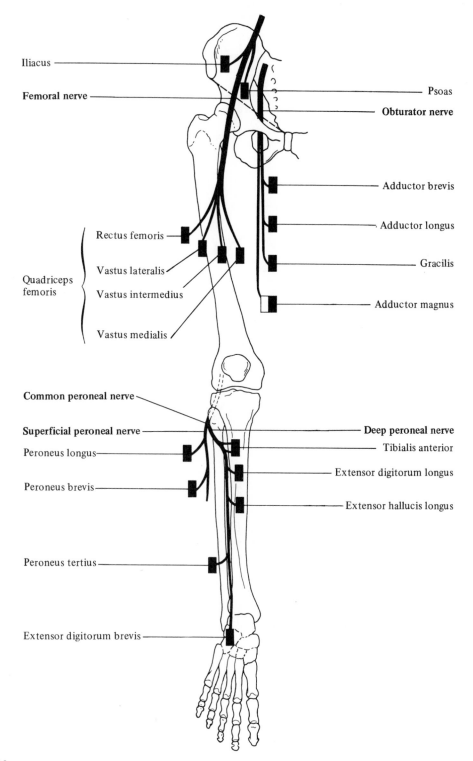

Iliacus

Femoral nerve

Psoas

Obturator nerve

Adductor brevis

Adductor longus

Rectus femoris

Gracilis

Quadriceps
femoris

Vastus lateralis

Vastus intermedius

Adductor magnus

Vastus medialis

Common peroneal nerve

Superficial peroneal nerve

Deep peroneal nerve

Peroneus longus

Tibialis anterior

Extensor digitorum longus

Peroneus brevis

Extensor hallucis longus

Peroneus tertius

Extensor digitorum brevis

Fig. 192.
Diagram of the nerves on the anterior aspect of the lower limb, and the muscles which they supply. (Modified from Pitres and Testut.)

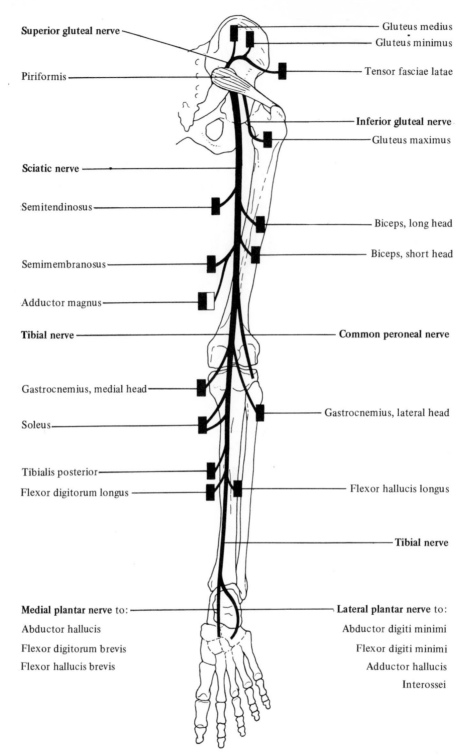

Superior gluteal nerve
Piriformis
Sciatic nerve
Semitendinosus
Semimembranosus
Adductor magnus
Tibial nerve
Gastrocnemius, medial head
Soleus
Tibialis posterior
Flexor digitorum longus
Medial plantar nerve to:
Abductor hallucis
Flexor digitorum brevis
Flexor hallucis brevis

Gluteus medius
Gluteus minimus
Tensor fasciae latae
Inferior gluteal nerve
Gluteus maximus
Biceps, long head
Biceps, short head
Common peroneal nerve
Gastrocnemius, lateral head
Flexor hallucis longus
Tibial nerve
Lateral plantar nerve to:
Abductor digiti minimi
Flexor digiti minimi
Adductor hallucis
Interossei

Fig. 193.
Diagram of the nerves on the posterior aspect of the lower limb, and the muscles which they supply. (Modified from Pitres and Testut.)

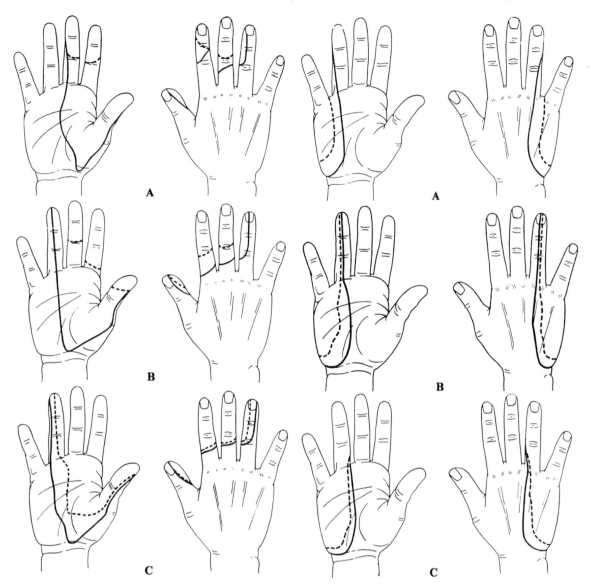

Fig. 194.
The approximate areas within which sensory changes may be found in lesions of the median nerve. **A** small area, **B** average area, and **C** large area. Light touch, continuous line; pin-prick, dotted line. Immediately after complete division of the median nerve, the insensitive area on the palm of the hand may be somewhat larger than is shown. (Modified from Head and Sherren (1905) *Brain:* 28, 116.)

Fig. 195.
The approximate areas within which sensory changes may be found in lesions of the ulnar nerve. **A** small area, **B** average area, and **C** large area. Light touch, continuous line; pin-prick, dotted line. Immediately after complete division of the ulnar nerve, the insensitive area on the palm of the hand may be somewhat larger than is shown. (Modified from Head and Sherren.)

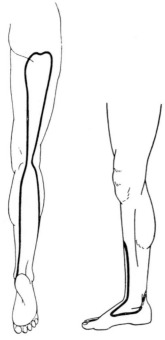

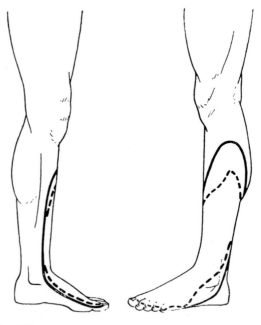

Fig. 196.
The approximate area within which sensory changes may be found in lesions of both the sciatic and the posterior cutaneous nerve of the thigh.

Fig. 197.
The approximate area within which sensory changes may be found in lesions of the common peroneal nerve above the origin of the superficial peroneal nerve. Light touch, continuous line; pin-prick, dotted line. (Modified from M.R.C. Special Report No. 54, 1920.)

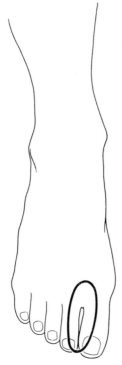

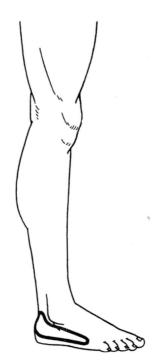

Fig. 198.
The approximate area within which sensory changes may be found in lesions of the deep peroneal nerve.

Fig. 199.
The approximate area within which sensory changes may be found in lesions of the sural nerve.

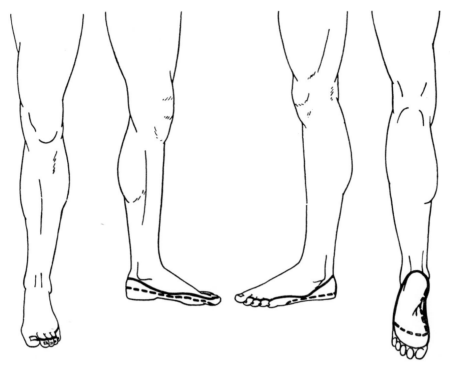

Fig. 200.
The approximate area within which sensory changes may be found in lesions of the tibial nerve. Light touch, continuous line; pin-prick, dotted line. (Modified from M.R.C. Special Report No. 54, 1920.)

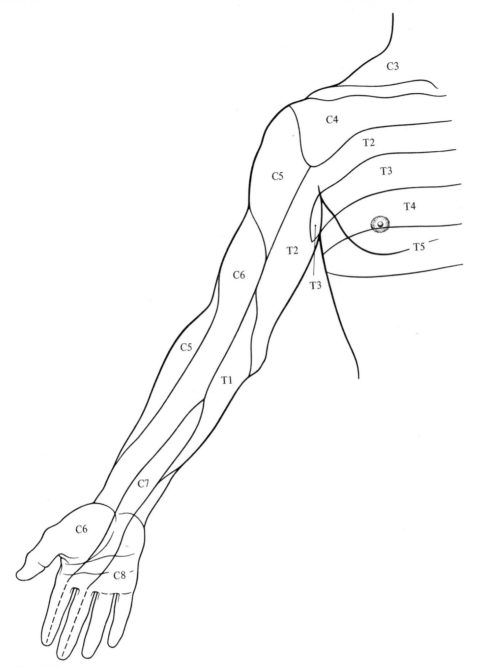

Fig. 201.
Approximate distribution of dermatomes on the anterior aspect of the upper limb.

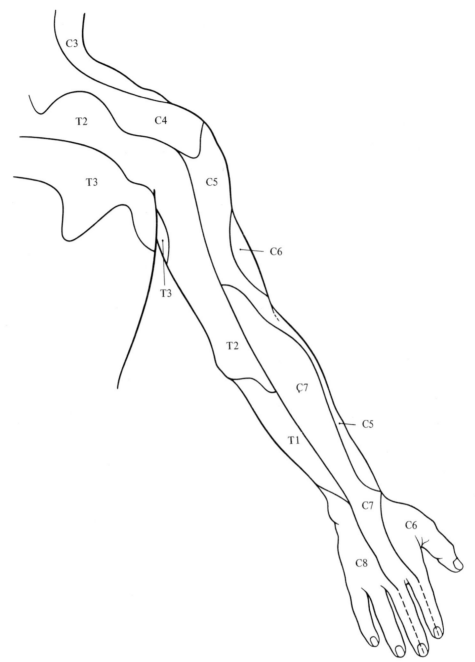

Fig. 202.
Approximate distribution of dermatomes on the posterior aspect of the upper limb.

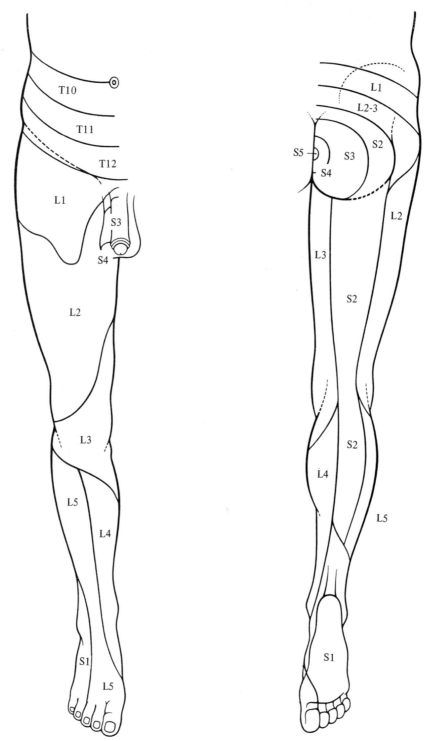

Fig. 203.
Approximate distribution of dermatomes on the lower limb.

Index

Acceleration
  linear, 247
  rotational, 247
Accumbens, 112
Acetylcholine, as neurotransmitter, 354
ACTH, 355
Acupuncture, 180
Adenohypophysis
  development of, 21
  relation to hypothalamus, 304
Adenoma, pituitary, 307
Adrenal medulla, autonomic innervation of, 315
Aggressive reactions, 328
Agnosia, 348
  auditory, 348, 349
  auditory-verbal, 349
  tactile, 348
  visual, 284, 348
Agraphesthesia, 179
Alcohol consumption in pregnancy, affecting fetus, 34
Allocortex, 338
Alveus, 324
Alzheimer's disease, 201, 349, 354
Amino acids, as transmitters in CNS, 355
γ-Aminobutyric acid, 208, 214, 355
Amnesia, 349
  anterograde or posttraumatic, 349
  retrograde, 349
Ampullae, in semicircular canals, 247
Amygdala, 29, 92–93, 114, 322–324, 327
  and autonomic function, 317
  basolateral part of, 322
  connections of, 322–323
  corticomedial part of, 322
  functional aspects of, 323–324
Amygdalotomy, 328
Anencephaly, 35
Anesthesia, 161
Aneurysm, of internal carotid artery, 285–286

Angiography, cerebral, 59–60, 358, 367
Angle, cerebellopontine, 97
  tumors in, 64, 257–258
Anhydrosis, in Horner's syndrome, 319
Anosmia, 293
Anosognosia, 348
Ansa
  hypoglossi, 254
  lenticularis, 113, 203
Aperture
  lateral, of Luschka, 27, 44, 61, 65, 97
  median, of Magendie, 27, 44, 65, 97
Aphasia, 350
  Broca's, 350
  motor or nonfluent, 350
  sensory or fluent, 350
  Wernicke's, 350
Apparatus, Golgi, 128
Apraxia, 348
Aqueduct, cerebral, 7, 27, 65
  development of, 18
Arachnoid granulations, 44
Arachnoidea
  of brain, 40, 53
  of spinal cord, 44
Area(s)
  association, 342
    auditory, 268
    posterior parietal, 346
  Broca's motor speech, 69, 121, 344
    lesions in, 350
  Brodmann's, 338, 340
  motor, 69, 119, 120, 187, 344–345
    supplementary, 189, 192, 344
  parastriate, 277, 346
  peristriate, 277, 346
  postrema, 253
  somatosensory, 69, 119, 169, 175–176, 345–346
    first, 345
    second, 346

speech
  motor, 69, 121, 344, 350
  sensory, 71, 119, 346, 350
  striate, 346
  subcallosal, 73
  vestibular, 104
Artery
  auditory, internal, 54, 364
  basilar, 54–55, 123, 364–366
  callosomarginal, 57, 65
  carotid, internal, 54, 56, 359, 361–362
    aneurysm of, 285–286
    occlusion of, 371–372
  central, of retina, 21
  cerebellar
    anterior inferior, 54, 364
    posterior inferior, 54, 363–364
    superior, 55, 364
  cerebral
    angiography of, 59–60, 358, 367
    anterior, 54, 56, 122, 123, 362–363
    middle, 54, 56, 123, 362
      infarction of, 370–371
    posterior, 55–56, 123, 364, 366–367
      cortical branches of, 366
      thalamoperforating branches of, 366
  choroidal
    anterior, 56, 58, 86
    posterior, 56, 58, 366
  communicating
    anterior, 56
    posterior, 56, 366
  hypophysial, 56
  labyrinthine, 54
  ophthalmic, 56
  pericallosal, 57, 65
  pontine, 54, 364
  recurrent, of Heubner, 56, 362
  spinal, anterior, 54, 363
    lesions in, 177–178, 372
  striate, 56, 362
  thalamogeniculate, 366
  vertebral, 54, 363–364

Arteriovenous malformation, rupture of, 359
Aspartate, 355
Astereognosis, 179, 348
Astrocytes
  fibrous, 141
  protoplasmic, 141
Astroglia, 141
Ataxia
  cerebellar, 222–223
  Friedreich's, 162, 178
Atrophy, 161
  optic, 282
Audiometers, 270
Auditory system, 261–270
  temporal lobe in, 346
Auricle, 262
Autonomic nervous system, 4, 309–319
  afferent visceral fibers in, 310–314
  amygdaloid body affecting, 317
  central parts of, 316–317
  cerebral cortex affecting, 317
  hypothalamus affecting, 304–305, 317
  organs innervated by, 315–316
  parasympathetic or craniosacral division of, 312–314
  peripheral parts of, 310–316
  in spinal cord injuries, 319
  sympathetic or thoracolumbar division of, 310–312
Autoradiography, in neuroanatomic tract-tracing, 143–145
Autoregulation of cerebral blood flow, 358
Axis, optic, 272
Axon, 4, 128, 132–136
  collateral sprouting of, 149, 347
  initial segment of, 132
  myelinated, 136
  terminals or boutons of, 4, 136
  transection of
    anterograde or Wallerian degeneration from, 143
    retrograde reaction from, 128, 143
  transport in
    fast, 136
    slow, 136

Barrier, blood-brain, 150
Basal ganglia, 6, 199–209
Basis pedunculi cerebri, 104, 107, 115, 117, 122, 228
Behavior, prefrontal cortex affecting, 328, 345
Bell's palsy, 245, 254–255
Bladder
  autonomic innervation of, 316
  hypertonic or hyperreflexive, 319
  hypotonic or hyporeflexive, 319

Blind spot of retina, 274
Blindness, causes of, 280
Blood-brain barrier, 150
Blood flow, cerebral, 358
Body
  amygdaloid, 29, 92–93, 114, 322–324, 327. See also Amygdala
  of caudate nucleus, 91
  of corpus callosum, 68
  of fornix, 68, 113
  geniculate
    lateral, 61, 91, 276, 332
    medial, 91, 115, 268, 332
  mammillary, 21, 61, 114, 116, 296, 299
    fiber connections of, 302
  Nissl, 128
  pineal, 68, 89
  trapezoid, 266
Bouton, 4, 136
Bouton en passant, 136
Brachium, 6
  conjunctivum, 99
  of inferior colliculus, 228
  of superior colliculus, 106
  pontis, 99
Brain
  development of, 11–30
  dissection of, 51–123
  subdivisions of, 6–7
Brain stem, 7, 65, 104–110, 225–228
  hemorrhage in, 256
  lesions of, 176
  vascular syndromes of, 364–367
Brown-Séquard syndrome, 178
Buds, taste, 243
Bulb, olfactory, 62, 288
  layers of, 291
  relation to amygdala, 291, 322
Bundle
  forebrain, medial, 300
  olivocochlear, 266, 269

Calcar avis, 86
Canal
  auditory, external, 262
  central, of spinal cord, 11, 65, 110
  facial, 243
  semicircular, 246
Capsule
  external, 30, 79, 91, 93
  extreme, 30, 91–92
  internal, 29, 76, 79, 93–95, 113, 117
    anterior limb of, 93, 121
    genu of, 30
    infarct in, 196–197
    lesions in, 95, 193
    posterior limb of, 95, 121, 175
    retrolenticular part of, 30, 95
    sublenticular part of, 30, 95
    topography of, 29

CAT scans of brain, 54, 119–123
Cataract, 280
Cauda equina, 11, 152
Cavity, tympanic, 262
Cell body, 128
Cells
  basket, 212
  Betz, 187
  of cerebellar cortex, 212
  granular
    in cerebellar cortex, 212
    in olfactory bulb, 291
  hair
    in cochlear duct, 266
    in semicircular canals, 247
  nerve. See Neurons
  neuroglial, 141–142
  periglomerular, in olfactory bulb, 291
  pigment, retinal, 272
  Purkinje, 16, 132, 212
  pyramidal, 132
    giant, 187
  retinal, 272–274
  stellate, 132
    of cerebellar cortex, 212
Centers
  cardiovascular, in medulla oblongata, 316
  functional, 344
  gaze, 238
  hypothalamic, 303
  oculomotor, cerebellum related to, 222
  respiratory, in medulla oblongata, 316–317
  semioval, 86, 119
  vomiting, 253
Centrum medianum, 115
Cerebellopontine angle tumor, 64, 257–258
Cerebellum, 7, 61, 65, 97–104, 211–224
  afferent connections of, 217–219
  connections with vestibular nuclei, 249
  cortex of, 212–217
  development of, 15
  efferent connections of, 220
  functions of, 222
  localization of lesions in, 223
  metastases to, 223–224
  nuclei in, 219–220
  peduncles of, 99–100. See also Peduncles, cerebellar
Cerebrospinal fluid, 27, 43–44, 53
  excessive. See Hydrocephalus
  lumbar puncture for, 47–48
Cerebrovascular system, 357–372
  anatomy of, 359–367
  angiography of, 59–60, 358, 367
  blood flow regulation in, 358

collateral circulation in, 359
in strokes, 95, 358–359
syndromes of, 359–367
  anterior cerebral artery, 363
  anterior spinal artery, 372
  basilar artery, 364–366
  internal carotid artery, 362,
    371–372
  middle cerebral artery, 362,
    370–371
  posterior cerebral artery, 366–
    367
  vertebral artery, 364
in transient ischemic attacks, 362
Chemical substances, teratogenic effects of, 34
Chiasm, optic, 21, 61, 68, 116, 276,
  296
  lesions of, 284
Cholinergic systems, 354
  ascending, in hypothalamus, 303
Chorda tympani, 243
Chorea, Huntington's, 208–209
Chromatolysis, 128, 143
Chromosomal abnormalities, and
  neurologic disorders, 30–34
Cilia, of olfactory vesicle, 288
Cingulotomy, 82, 329
Cingulum, 75, 79
Circle of Willis, 56, 59, 359
  collateral circulation in, 359
Circuit, Papez, 334
Circulation, cerebrovascular, 358
  collateral, 359
Cistern(a)
  ambiens, 43
  cerebellomedullary, 43, 53
  chiasmatic, 43, 53, 123
  of great cerebral vein of Galen, 53
  interpeduncular, 43, 53, 123
  of lateral fossa, 43, 53
  lumbar, 44, 53
  magna, 43
  pontine, 43, 53
  subarachnoid, 53–54
  superior, 43, 53, 121
Clasp-knife phenomenon, 194
Claustrum, 7, 30, 79, 91, 113, 114
Cleft, synaptic, 137
Clonus, 194
Cochlea, 262–263
  membranous, 262
  osseous, 262
Colliculus
  facial, 104
  inferior, 65, 89, 104, 116, 228
    brachium of, 228
    development of, 18
  superior, 65, 89, 104, 116, 228, 238
    development of, 18
Coloboma, 36

Column, 4
  Clarke's, 155, 217–218
  cortical, 338–339
  dorsal, of spinal cord, 10
    lesions in, 178
    and medial lemniscus pathway,
      171–173
    subacute combined degenera-
      tion of, 178, 181–182
  of fornix, 29, 68, 112, 113
  frequency, 268
  gray
    dorsal, 10
    ventral and lateral, 10
  intermediolateral, of spinal cord,
    155
  intermediomedial, of spinal cord,
    155
  in visual cortex, 280
Coma, 235
  in uncal herniation, 45
Commissures, 6, 75–76
  anterior, 29, 68, 75, 82, 113, 114,
    116, 117, 122, 342
  habenular, 68, 76
  hippocampal, 29, 75, 87, 115
  posterior, 68, 76
Complex, olivary, superior, 266, 267,
  268, 269
Concussion, 44, 349
Cones and rods, 272
  functions of, 277–278
Confrontation method, for visual
  field defects, 282
Confusion, 235
Congenital disorders, neurologic,
  30–35
Consciousness, disorders of, 235
  in uncal herniation, 45
Contusions of brain, 44
Convergence, binocular, 279
Convolutions, 6, 69
Cord, spinal. See Spinal cord
Cornea, 272
Corona radiata, 76, 79
Corpus
  callosum, 6, 68, 75, 79, 113, 120,
    121, 122, 342
    development of, 27
    in split-brain patients, 68, 83
  cerebelli, 99
  striatum, 200
    components of, 30
    connections of amygdala, 203–
      206
    development of, 29–30
    topography of, 30
Corpuscles
  Meissner, 170
  Pacinian, 170
  Ruffini, 170

Cortex, 4
  cerebellar, 212–217
    development of, 15
    functional anatomic organiza-
      tion of, 214–217
    intrinsic circuitry of, 212–214
    layers of, 16, 212
  cerebral, 6, 86, 337–352
    agranular, 338
    association areas in, 342
      auditory, 268
      posterior parietal, 346
    auditory, 268, 346
    and autonomic function, 317
    Brodmann's map of, 338
    columns in, functional, 338–339
    commissural fibers in, 342
    connections of, 340–342
      with amygdala, 322
      with basal ganglia, 203, 204
      with thalamus, 332
    cross-control in, 342
    development of, 29
    frontal, 344–345. See also Lobe,
      frontal
    functions of, 342–350
    granular, 338
    hemisphere specialization in,
      342–344
    layers of, 338
    localization of function in, 344
    motor areas of, 69, 119, 120,
      187, 344–345
      as distribution center, 192
      supplementary, 189, 344–345
    occipital, 346. See also Lobe,
      occipital
    olfactory, 291, 346
      frontal, 291
      relation to amygdala, 322
      temporal, 291
    orbitofrontal, 293
    parastriate, 277, 346
    parietal, 345–346. See also
      Lobe, parietal
    peristriate, 277, 346
    prefrontal, 345
    premotor, 189, 344
    relation to hippocampus, 326
    somatosensory, 69, 119, 169,
      175–176, 189, 245, 345–
      346
    striate, 277
    structure of, 338–339
    temporal, 346–347. See also
      Lobe, temporal
    visual, 119, 276, 279–280, 346
      ocular dominance columns
        in, 280
      orientation columns in, 280
Coughing, 253
Craniopharyngioma, 36

Crest, neural, 10
Crura fornicis, 29, 68, 86
Cuneus, 73
Cupula, 247

Deafness, 269
   conductive, 269
   cortical, 348–349
   hereditary, 270
   sensorineural, 269
Deceleration
   linear, 247
   rotational, 247
Decussation, 6
   of medial lemniscus, 110, 173, 226–227
   pyramidal or corticospinal, 61, 108, 109, 189, 226
   sensory, 110
   of superior cerebellar peduncle, 116
   tegmental
      dorsal, 228
      ventral, 228
Defense reaction, 305
Degeneration
   anterograde or Wallerian, 143, 149
   spinocerebellar, 162
   subacute combined, of dorsal columns, 178, 181–182
Degenerative disease of spinal cord, 162
Dejerine-Roussy syndrome, 334
Dementia
   presenile, 201
   senile, 201
Dendrites, 4, 128, 132
   spines of, 132
2-Deoxyglucose methods, in neuroanatomic studies, 148
Dermatomes, 153, 154
Development of nervous system, 9–36
   brain, 11–30
   neural crest, 10
   neural tube, 10
   spinal cord, 10–11
Diabetes insipidus, 306
Diaphragma sellae, 38
Diencephalon, 7, 68
   development of, 18–21
Diplopia, 240–241
Disc
   optic, 272, 274, 283
      in papilledema, 282, 283
   spinal, prolapse of, 161–162, 163–164
Discrimination
   of odors, 293
   of pitch, 266, 268–269
   sensory, 176
   two-point, 179

Dissection of brain, 51–123
Dominance
   hemispheric, 344
   ocular, 280
Dopamine levels
   in Huntington's disease, 208
   in Parkinson's disease, 208
   in schizophrenia, 209
Dopaminergic system, 232–234
   mesolimbic, 201, 206, 233, 303
   nigrostriatal, 203, 204, 233
   tuberoinfundibular, 303
Down's syndrome, 30
Drugs, teratogenic effects of, 34
Duct
   cochlear, 262
   semicircular, 246
Dura mater
   of brain, 38–39, 53
   of spinal cord, 44
   spinal, 44
Dyskinesia, tardive, 209
Dystrophia adiposogenitalis, 306

Ear
   external, 262
   inner, 262–266
   middle, 262
Eardrum, 262
Electromyography, 185, 193
Embolism, cerebral, 362
Eminence
   lateral, 296
   medial, 104
   median, 296
Emotions
   and defense reaction, 305
   disorders in, 328
   and fainting response, 305
   and limbic system concept, 327
   and psychosomatic disorders, 306, 319
Endbrain. See Telencephalon
Endorphins, 179–180, 354–355
End-plate, motor, 185
Enkephalins, 179–180, 354–355
Enlargements
   cervical, 152
   lumbar, 152
Enophthalmos, in Horner's syndrome, 319
Envelope, nuclear, 132
Ependyma, 141
Epilepsy, 349–350
   clinical example of, 350–352
   grand mal, 350
   jacksonian seizures in, 349
   psychomotor, 329, 350
   temporal lobe, 329
Epithalamus, 18
Epithelium, olfactory, 288

Equilibrium, maintenance of, 248, 249
Extrapyramidal disorders, 206–209
   drug-induced, 209
Eye, 271–286
   autonomic innervation of, 315
   development of, 21
   disorders of, 36
   gaze centers, 238
   movements of, 238
      paralysis of, 241
      voluntary, 239–240
   visual pathway lesions, 64
Eyefield, frontal, 344

Face, pathways from
   for pain and temperature, 167
   for touch and pressure, 175
Fainting, 358
   emotional, 305
Falx
   cerebelli, 38
   cerebri, 38, 120
Fasciculations, 193
Fasciculus, 6
   arcuate, 75, 77, 340
   cuneate, 110
   dorsolateral, 173
   gracile, 110
   lenticularis, 203
   longitudinal
      dorsal, 300
      medial, 116, 227, 238, 249
      superior, 75, 77, 340
   occipitofrontal
      inferior, 75, 77, 340
      superior, 75, 340
   proprii, 159
   thalamic, 203
   uncinate, 75, 77, 340
Fastigium, 97
Fever, 306
Fibers
   afferent, 212
   aminergic, 212, 219
   arcuate, 75, 79, 340
      internal, 110, 116, 226
   association, 75, 340–342
      auditory, 268
      posterior parietal, 346
   blunt dissection of systems, 77–82
      from lateral side, 77–79
      from medial side, 79–82
   cerebelloreticular, 220
   cerebellorubral, 220
   cerebellothalamic, 220
   cerebellovestibular, 220
   classification of, 166
   climbing, 212
   collection of, 6
   commissural, 75–76, 342

corticobulbar, 77
corticofugal, 76, 82
corticopetal, 76
corticopontine, 77
corticoreticular, 77
corticospinal, 77
fusimotor, 186
hypothalamic connections, 299–302
intrafusal, 185
mossy, 212, 326
olivocerebellar, 219, 227
parallel, 212
pontocerebellar, 219
projection, 76–77, 340
reticulocerebellar, 218
trigeminocerebellar, 218
vestibulocerebellar, 218
Fibrillations, 193
Fields
  eye, frontal, 239
  of Forel, 117, 203
  visual, 64, 279
    examination of, 282
Fight or flight response, 305
Fila olfactoria, 288
Filum terminale, 11, 44
Fimbria hippocampi, 68, 87, 115
Fissures, 6, 7
  cerebellar
    horizontal, 99
    posterolateral, 99
    primary, 99
  choroid, 21, 27
  lateral, 23, 69, 119, 120, 122, 123
  transverse, 27, 29
Flexure
  cervical, 11
  midbrain, 11
  pontine, 11
Flocculus, 99, 102
Fluid, cerebrospinal, 27, 43–44, 53
  excessive. See Hydrocephalus
  lumbar puncture for, 47–48
Fluorescent substances, in neuroanatomic tract-tracing, 146
Folds
  dural, 38
  neural, 10
Folia, cerebellar, 7, 99
Foramen
  interventricular, 7, 27, 68
  of Luschka, 27, 44, 61, 65, 97
  of Magendie, 27, 44, 65, 97
  of Monro, 7, 27, 68
  stylomastoid, 243
Forel fields, 203, 204
Formation
  hippocampal. See Hippocampus

reticular, 107, 167, 228–231, 238
  ascending and descending activity in, 229–230
  connections of, 229
    with vestibular nuclei, 249
  control of spinal cord functions, 230
  intrinsic structure of, 228–229
Fornix, 27–28, 68, 86–87, 114, 115, 116, 121, 122, 300, 302
  body of, 29, 113
  columns of, 29, 112, 113
  relation to hippocampus, 326
Fossa
  interpeduncular, 61, 115
  rhomboid, 104
Fovea centralis, 272, 274
Fractures
  of skull, 44
  of spine, 163
Frequencies, tonal, organization of, 268
Froehlich syndrome, 306
Fundus oculi, 274, 282, 283
Funiculus
  dorsal, 7, 110, 159
  lateral, 6, 159
  ventral, 6, 159

Ganglia
  basal, 6, 199–209
    components of, 200–203
    connections of, 203–206
    functional aspects of, 206
    pallidosubthalamicpallidal loop in, 206
    striatonigrostriatal loop in, 203–206
    striatopallidothalamic loop in, 203
Ganglion (pl. ganglia)
  celiac, 311
  ciliary, 238, 314
  dorsal root, of spinal nerve, 13, 152
  gasserian, 241
  geniculate, 243
  mesenteric
    inferior, 311
    superior, 311
  otic, 314
  paravertebral, of sympathetic trunk, 311
  prevertebral, 311
  pterygopalatine, 314
  semilunar, 241
  spinal, 152
  submandibular, 314
  trigeminal, 241
  vestibular, 247–248
Gap, junction, 141
Genetic disorders, 30–34

Genu
  of corpus callosum, 29, 68
  of facial nerve, 228
  of internal capsule, 29–30, 95
Gland
  pineal, 18
  pituitary. See Hypophysis
Glaucoma, 280
Glial cells, 141
Globus pallidus, 31, 92, 112, 113, 117, 200
  ventral, 201
Glomerulus
  in cerebellum, 212, 213
  in olfactory bulb, 288, 290
Glomus choroideum, 86
  calcified, 120
Glutamate, 355
Glycine, 355
Gnosia, 348
Golgi apparatus, 128
Golgi cells, cerebellar, 212, 213
Golgi method, for neuroanatomic studies, 132, 143
Golgi tendon organ, 186
Granulations, arachnoid, 44
Gray matter
  of brain, 3, 4–6
  central, 18
    periaqueductal, 104, 167
  of spinal cord, 3, 152, 155–159
    intermediate, 155
Groove, neural, 10
Gyrus, 6, 23, 69
  angular, 71, 119, 346
  cingulate, 73, 327
  dentate, 68, 115, 324
  frontal
    inferior, 69, 123
    middle, 69, 120, 121, 122, 123
    superior, 69, 122
  fusiform, 73, 122
  Heschl's, 268
  lingual, 73
  long, 73
  occipitotemporal, 73
  orbital, 73
  parahippocampal, 63, 122, 123, 327
  postcentral, 69, 119, 120, 121
    lesions in, 178–179
  precentral, 69, 119, 120, 121
  rectus, 73
  short, 73
  supramarginal, 71, 119, 346
  temporal
    inferior, 71, 121, 123
    middle, 71, 120, 121, 122
    superior, 71, 119, 122
    transverse, 71, 268

Habenula, 89, 115, 116
Hair cells
  in cochlear duct, 266
  in semicircular canals, 247
Hallucinations, 349–350
Head, of caudate nucleus, 91
Head injuries, 44
Hearing, tests of, 269–270
Heart, autonomic innervation of, 315
Helicotrema, 263
Hematoma
  epidural, 45
  subdural, 44–45, 195–196
Hemianopsia
  bitemporal, 284
  homonymous
    complete, 284
    incomplete, 284
Hemiballismus, 203, 209
Hemiplegia, 193
  capsular, 95
    hypoglossal paralysis in, 254
    supranuclear facial paralysis in, 245
  spastic, 194
Hemispheres
  cerebellar, 7, 61, 99
    development of, 15
  cerebral, 6
    development of, 22–25
    dorsolateral surface of, 69–73
    medial and basal surfaces of, 73
    specialization in, 342–344
    in split-brain patients, 68, 83
Hemorrhage
  brain stem, 256
  subarachnoid, 60, 359
  subdural and extradural, 44–45
Herniation
  cingulate, 45
  of intervertebral disc, 161–162, 163–164
  tonsillar, 45, 48, 102–104
  transtentorial or uncal, 45, 46, 258–260
Herpesvirus, spread to CNS, 149
Herpes zoster, 162
  ophthalmic, 243
Hippocampus, 86, 115, 324–327
  extrinsic connections of, 326
  functional aspects of, 326–327
  histologic structure of, 324–326
  intrinsic connections of, 326
Histochemical methods, in neuroan-
    atomic studies, 146–148
Hormone
  antidiuretic, 304
  distribution in brain, 355
  hypothalamic, 303
Horn
  of Ammon, 324–327. See also
    Hippocampus

anterior, of lateral ventricle, 27, 86, 112, 120, 121, 122
  dorsal, of spinal cord, 10, 155
  lateral, of spinal cord, 10
  posterior, of lateral ventricle, 27, 86
  temporal, of lateral ventricle, 27, 86, 115
  ventral, of spinal cord, 10, 155
    motor neurons in, 157
Horner's syndrome, 319
Horseradish peroxidase, in neuroan-
    atomic tract-tracing studies, 143–145
Huntington's disease, 208–209, 354
Hydrocephalus, 36, 47, 69
Hyperesthesia, 161
Hyperthermia, 306
Hypesthesia, 161
Hypophysis, 61, 68
  adenohypophysis, 21, 304
  adenoma of, 307
  development of, 21
  disorders of, 305–306
  hypothalamohypophysial path-
    ways, 300–302
  neurohypophysis, 21, 296, 304
  portal system of, 302
  relation to hypothalamus, 300–302, 303–304
  tumors of, 68, 307
Hypothalamus, 7, 61, 68, 113, 245, 295–307
  and autonomic function, 304–305, 317
  boundaries and subdivisions of, 296
  cholinergic and monoaminergic
    pathways in, 303
  control centers in, 303
  development of, 21
  disorders of, 305–306
  fiber connections of, 299–302
  nuclei of, 296–299
  relation to amygdala, 322, 324
  relation to hypophysis, 300–302, 303–304
Hypotonus, 161

Immunohistochemical methods, in
    neuroanatomic studies, 148
Incisure, tentorial, 38
Inclusions, neuronal, 128
Incus, 262
Infarcts, lacunar, 196–197
Infections in pregnancy, affecting fe-
    tus, 34
Inferior olive, 15, 61, 108, 117, 126–127
Infundibulum of hypothalamus, 68, 296

Injuries
  of head, 44
  of spinal cord, 163
    autonomic dysfunction in, 319
Insula, 24, 69, 73, 112, 122
  development of, 23
  relation to amygdala, 322
Interneurons
  in cerebellum, 214
  in cerebral cortex, 339
  in olfactory bulb, 291
  in retina, 272
  in spinal cord, 157–158
    relationship to motor neurons, 184
Interoceptors, 166
Iris, 272
  development of, 21
Isocortex, 338
Isthmus of cingulate gyrus, 73
Itching, 166

Kinesthesia, 170
Klüver-Bucy syndrome, 323–324
Korsakoff's psychosis, 329, 349

Labyrinth, 246
  bony, 262
  membranous, 246
Lamina
  affixa, 27, 86
  medullary, internal, 90, 114
  spiral, 262
  terminalis, 21, 68
Language disorders, 350
Laryngoscopy, 254
Layers
  of cerebellar cortex, 212
  of cerebral cortex, 338
  of neural tube, 10
  of olfactory bulb, 291
Learning
  amygdala role in, 324
  and temporal lobe function, 347
Lemniscus, 6
  lateral, 108, 228, 266
  medial, 107, 108, 110, 116, 171–173, 226, 227, 228
    decussation of, 110, 173
Lens of eye, 272
  development of, 21
Lens placode, 21
Leptomeninges, 43, 53
Ligaments, denticulate, 44
Limbic system, 327, 328
Limen insulae, 73
Line of Gennari, 276–277
Lingula of cerebellum, 97, 98
Lips, rhombic, 15
Lobe(s)
  cerebellar, 99
  flocculonodular, 99, 100–102, 214

frontal, 23, 61–62, 69, 119, 120, 344–345
  lesions in, 347
  motor areas in, 344–345
  relation to amygdala, 322
occipital, 23, 69, 71, 118, 120, 121, 346
  lesions in, 348
parietal, 23, 69, 119, 120, 345–346
  lesions in, 176, 346, 348
temporal, 23, 61, 69, 71, 120, 346–347
  lesions in, 348–350
  pathology in epilepsy, 329
  relation to amygdala, 322
  tumors of, 328
Lobotomy, prefrontal, 328
Lobule
  biventer, 99
  gracile, 99
  paracentral, 73
  parietal
    inferior, 71, 346
    superior, 71, 176, 189, 346
      lesions in, 178–179
Localization of sound in space, 268, 269
Locus ceruleus, 104
  aminergic fibers from, 219
Lumbago, 161
Lumbar puncture, 47–48
Lungs, autonomic innervation of, 315
Luteinizing hormone-releasing hormone, 355

Macula lutea, 274
  sparing of, 284
Malleus, 262
Malnutrition
  and dorsal column lesions in vitamin B_{12} deficiency, 178, 181
  and Korsakoff syndrome in vitamin B_1 deficiency, 329, 349
  and neurologic maturation, 34
Mapping of central nervous system connections. See Neuroanatomic methods
Matter. See Gray matter; White matter
Meatus, auditory
  external, 253, 262
  internal, 243
Mechanoreceptors, 166
Medial forebrain bundle, 300
Medulla, adrenal, autonomic innervation of, 315
Medulla oblongata, 7, 61, 65, 108–110, 226–227
  cardiovascular centers in, 316
  development of, 11
  respiratory centers in, 316–317

Medullary syndromes
  lateral, of Wallenberg, 194, 257, 364
  medial, 364
Medulloblastoma, 104
Melanin, 201
Membrane
  basilar, 263
  otolith, 247
  postsynaptic, 137
  presynaptic, 137
  tectorial, 266
  tympanic, 262
Memory
  amygdala role in, 324
  disorders in, 349
  hippocampus role in, 316
  and temporal lobe function, 347, 349
Meniere's disease, 249
Meninges
  of brain, 53–54
  of spinal cord, 44
Meningioma, olfactory groove, 294
Meningitis, 45–47
Meningocele, 35
Mental retardation, 30–34
Mesencephalic syndrome, mediobasal, of Weber, 255, 366
Mesencephalon, 7, 61, 65, 104–107, 228
  development of, 18
Metabolic disorders, congenital, 30
Metencephalon, 7, 65
  development of, 15–16
Meyer's loop, 77, 79, 83, 276, 348
Microglia, 141
Microtubules, 128
  in axon's, 135, 136, 140
  in dendrites, 132, 140
Midbrain. See Mesencephalon
Miosis, in Horner's syndrome, 319
Mitochondria, 128
Modiolus, 262
Mongolism, 30
Monoplegia, 195
Morphine, and pain relief, 180
Motor end-plate, 185
Motor neurons. See Neurons, motor
Motor unit, 185
Movements
  basal ganglia affecting, 206
  cerebellum affecting, 222
  of eye, 238
    gaze centers for, 238
    paralysis of, 241
    voluntary, 239–240
  frontal cortex affecting, 344–345
  thalamic nuclei affecting, 333–334
Muscle(s)
  innervation of, 154
  middle ear, 262

mimetic, 243
  receptors in, 185–186
  stapedius, 262
  tensor tympani, 262
  tone of, 187
Muscle spindle, 185–186
Myasthenia gravis, 148
Myelencephalon. See Medulla oblongata
Myelin and white matter, 4
Myelin sheath, 136
Myelitis, 163
Myelomeningocele, 36
Myeloschisis, 35

Nauta-Gygax silver method, 143
Neocortex, 338
Nerve(s)
  abducens (VI), 63, 238
    lesions of, 241
  accessory (XI), 63, 254
  cochlear, 63, 245–246, 266
  cranial, 63, 237–260
  facial (VII), 63, 243–245, 314
    genu of, 228
    lesions of, 245
    parasympathetic part of, 243
    somatic motor part of, 243
    visceral sensory part of, 243–245
  glossopharyngeal (IX), 63, 243–245, 251–254, 314
    parasympathetic part of, 253
    sensory part of, 253
    somatic motor part of, 251
  hypoglossal (XII), 63, 254
  intermediate, 243
  laryngeal, recurrent, 254
  mandibular, 63, 241, 242
  maxillary, 63, 241
  oculomotor (III), 63, 238–241, 314
    lesions of, 240–241
  olfactory (I), 63, 238, 288
  ophthalmic, 63, 241
  optic (II), 21, 61, 63, 238, 276
    lesions of, 282
  pelvic, 314
  peripheral, 4, 379–387
    lesions of, 176–177
  petrosal, greater, 243
  recurrent laryngeal, 254
  regeneration of, 148–149
  sacral, 314
  of skin, 153
  spinal, 11, 152
    disorders with segmental symptoms, 161
    lesions of, 176, 177
  splanchnic, 311
  trigeminal (V), 63, 241–243
    chief sensory nucleus of, 175, 228, 241

Nerve(s) (*cont.*)
  disorders of, 242–243
    somatic motor part of, 242
    somatosensory part of, 241–242
  trochlear (IV), 63, 238
    lesions of, 241
  vagus (X), 63, 245, 251–254, 314
    parasympathetic part of, 253
    sensory part of, 253
    somatic motor part of, 251
  vestibular, 63, 247–248
  vestibulocochlear (VIII), 63, 245–249
    cochlear nerve, 245–246
    vestibular nerve, 63, 247–248
Nervi erigentes, 314
Nervous system
  autonomic, 4, 309–319
  central, 4
  peripheral, 4
    lesions of, 176–177
Neural tube, 10
  failure in closure of, 35
Neuralgia, trigeminal, 243
Neurinoma, acoustic, 249, 270
Neuroanatomic methods, 142–148, 353
  autoradiography in, 143–145, 281
  axonal transport in, 143–146
  2-deoxyglucose in, 148, 281
  fluorescent substances in, 146
  Golgi method, 132, 133, 134, 143
  histochemical methods, 146–148, 215, 353
  horseradish peroxidase in, 145
  immunocytochemical method, 148, 353
  Nissl method, 128, 129, 143
  silver in, 143
    in Nauta-Gygax method, 143
Neuroepithelial cells, 10
Neurofibril, 128
Neurofilaments, 128
Neuroglia, 141–142
Neurohypophysis, 296
  development of, 21
  relation to hypothalamus, 304
Neuroma, 149
Neuron doctrin, 140–141
Neurons, 4, 128–136
  axonal transport in, 132
  bipolar, 132
    in spiral ganglion of cochlea, 266
    in olfactory epithelium, 288
    in retina, 272
    in vestibular ganglion, 247
  cell body of, 128–132
  cell processes of, 132–136
  Golgi
    of cerebellar cortex, 212
    type I and II neurons, 132

  motor, 128, 129, 157
    alpha, 184
    alpha-gamma linkage, 187
    gamma, 184
    lower, 183–187
    somatotopic localization of, 157, 184
    upper, 187–193
    in ventral horn, 157
  multipolar, 132
  postganglionic, 310
  preganglionic, 310
  propriospinal, 157
  pseudounipolar, 132
  retrograde reaction of, 128, 129, 143
  sensory, 128, 129
  unipolar, 132
Neuropeptides, 354–355
Neuropores, anterior and posterior, 10
Neurosecretion, 303
Neurosyphilis, 163
Neurotransmitters, 353–354
Nissl method, 128, 129, 143
Nissl substance, 128
Nociceptors, 166
Nodes of Ranvier, 136
Nodule, in vermis, 99, 102
Noradrenergic pathway, 231–232
  ascending, in hypothalamus, 303
Notch
  preoccipital, 23, 69
  tentorial, 38
    in transtendorial herniation, 45
Nuclear envelope, 132
Nuclear magnetic resonance (NMR), 376
Nuclear pore, 132
Nucleolus, 132
Nucleus, 4
  abducens, 228, 238, 239
  ambiguus, 227, 239, 251
  basal, of Meynert, 201, 354
  caudate, 7, 29, 86, 87, 91, 113–117, 120–122, 200
  cerebellar, 219–220
  cervical, lateral, 155, 173
  cochlear, 239, 266
  cuneate, 110, 171, 227
  Deiters, 248
  dentate, 102, 117, 122, 220
  dorsalis, of Clarke, 155, 217
  Edinger-Westphal, 238
  emboliform, 102, 117, 220
  fastigial, 102, 192, 220
  geniculate, lateral, 276, 279
    medial, 106, 117, 286
  globose, 102, 220
  gracile, 110, 116, 171, 227
  habenular, 18

  hypoglossal, 227, 239, 254
  hypothalamic, 296–299
    dorsomedial, 298
    infundibular (arcuate), 298, 304
    paraventricular, 298, 304
    posterior, 299
    preoptic, 298
    suprachiasmatic, 298
    supraoptic, 298, 304
    ventromedial, 298, 304
  intermediolateral, 155
  intermediomedial, 155
  interstitial, of Cajal, 238
  intracerebellar, 15, 102, 219–220
  of lateral lemniscus, 268
  lentiform, 7, 29, 91–92, 200
  locus ceruleus, 231–233
  of neuron, 128
  oculomotor, 104, 228, 238–240
  olfactory, anterior, 291
  olivary, inferior, 15, 61, 108, 117, 227
  perihypoglossal, 239, 240
  pontine, 15, 65, 107, 219, 228
  posteromarginalis, 155, 167
  proprius, 155, 167
  raphe, 231, 232
  red, 18, 106, 107, 115–117, 122, 191
  salivatory
    inferior, 253, 314
    superior, 243, 314
  of solitary tract, 227, 245, 253
  of spinal trigeminal tract, 167, 227, 241
  subthalamic, 114, 117, 201
  thalamic, 332
    anterior (A), 114, 115, 332
      in Papez circuit, 334
    intralaminar, 115, 167, 334
    lateral dorsal (LD), 332, 333
    lateral posterior (LP), 332, 333
    mediodorsal (MD), 114, 116, 332
    midline, 334
    pulvinar (P), 93, 332
    reticular, 334
    ventral anterior (VA), 332
    ventral lateral (VL), 332
    ventral posterior (VP), 332
    ventral posterolateral (VPL), 167, 173, 332
    ventral posteromedial (VPM), 167, 332
  trigeminal, 227, 239
    main sensory, 175, 228, 241
    mesencephalic, 241–242
    motor, 242
    spinal, 167, 227, 241
  trochlear, 104, 228, 239, 240

tuberal, lateral, 296, 299
of vagus, dorsal motor, 227, 239, 253
vestibular, 227, 239, 248
Nutrition disorders. *See* Malnutrition
Nystagmus, 249

Obex, 104
Odors, discrimination of, 293
Olfactory system, 287–294
temporal lobe in, 346
Oligodendroglia, 141
Olive, 61
Olivocochlear bundle, 266–269
Opercula
frontal, 23
frontoparietal, 23
temporal, 23
Ophthalmoscopy, 282
Organ of Corti, 263
Orientation in space, 248, 249
and specificity of cells in visual cortex, 279, 280
Ossicles, middle ear, 262
Otoliths, 247
Otosclerosis, 270
Oxytocin, 304, 355

Pachymeninx, 38, 53
Pain
control of, 179–180
electrical stimulation in, 179
endogenous, 179–180
deep, 166
gate control hypothesis for, 169, 170, 179
pathways for, 166–169
radicular, 161
referred, 318, 319
root, 161
superficial, 166
in thalamic syndrome, 334, 367
visceral, 166, 314
Pallidum. *See* Globus pallidus
Palsy
Bell's, 245, 254–255
bulbar, chronic, 254
ocular, 241
Papez circuit, 334
Papillae
fungiform, 243
vallate, 243
Papilledema, 36, 282, 283
Paralysis, 161
agitans, 208
of eye movements, 241
facial, supranuclear, 245
flaccid, 193
lower motor neuron, 193
spastic, 194
upper motor neuron, 193–195

Paraplegia, 163, 195, 319
Paresis, 161, 193
Parkinson's disease, 148, 203, 208
Pars tuberalis, pituitary, 21
Pathway
afferent, 6
amygdalofugal, ventral, 300
amygdaloid, ventral, 322
auditory, central, 266–268
centrifugal
in auditory system, 269
to olfactory bulb, 293
in somatosensory system, 179–180, 187
cholinergic, 354
ascending, in hypothalamus, 303
descending supraspinal, 187–193
dopaminergic, 232–234
dorsal column-medial lemniscus, 171–173
efferent, 6
extrinsic, 6
hypothalamohypophysial, 300–302
intrinsic, 6
monoaminergic, 231–234
noradrenergic, 231–232
ascending, in hypothalamus, 303
olfactory, 288–292
for pain and temperature, 166–169
for position sense, 170–176
sensory, ascending, 165–182
serotonergic, 231
ascending, in hypothalamus, 303
spinocervicothalamic, 173
for taste, 243–245
for touch and pressure, 170–173
tuberoinfundibular, 233–234, 303
for vibration, 173
visual, 64, 276–277
lesions of, 282–284
Peduncle(s), 6
cerebellar, 99–100
blunt dissection of, 99–101
inferior, 61, 99, 100, 110, 116, 117, 227
middle, 61, 99, 100, 116, 123, 228
superior, 61, 99, 100, 116, 117
decussation of, 116
cerebral, 61, 65, 104
basis pedunculi, 104, 107, 115, 117, 122, 228
development of, 18
pes pedunculi, 107, 228
mammillary, 302
Peptides, and neurotransmission, 354–355
Perikaryon, 128

Perimetry, for visual defects, 282
Pes pedunculi cerebri, 107, 228
Phenylketonuria, 30
Photoreceptors, 272–274
Pia-arachnoid, 40–43, 53
Pigment cells, retinal, 272
Pineal gland, 18
Pinna, 262
Pitch discrimination, 266, 268–269
Pituitary. *See* Hypophysis
Planum temporale, 268, 346
Plasticity of CNS, 149, 347
Plate
alar, 10–11
basal, 10–11
commissural, 29
neural, 10
quadrigeminal, 89, 104
Plexus
choroid, 61, 65, 79, 86, 115, 120, 122
development of, 27
mucosal (Meissner), 315
myenteric (Auerbach), 315
Pneumoencephalography, 54, 95
Poliomyelitis, 193
Polyribosomes, in Nissl substance, 128
Pons, 7, 61, 65, 107–108, 123, 227–228
Pontine syndrome
lateral, 365–366
medial, 365
Pontocerebellum, 217, 219
Pores, nuclear, 132
Position sense, 170
pathway for, 173–175
Pouch, Rathke's, 21
Precommissural septum, 68
Precuneus, 73
Pregnancy, infections in, affecting fetus, 34
Pressure
intracranial, increased, 95, 282
pathways for, 170–173
Pretectum, 238
Projection fibers
corticofugal, 76, 340
corticopetal, 76, 340
thalamocortical and corticothalamic, 76, 175
Proprioceptors, 166
Prosopagnosia, 348
Protein deficiency, and neurologic maturation, 34
Psychosis, Korsakoff, 329, 349
Psychosomatic disorders, 306, 319
Psychosurgery, 328–329
Ptosis of eyelid, in Horner's syndrome, 319
Pulvinar, 91, 115, 332, 333
Puncture, lumbar, 47–48

Pupil, 272
Purkinje cells, 16, 132, 212
Putamen, 30, 79, 92, 112, 113, 115, 121, 122, 200
Pyramid of medulla oblongata, 15, 61, 110
Pyramis of cerebellum, 99

Quadrantanopsia, 284
Quadriplegia, *see* Tetraplegia

Rabies virus, spread to CNS, 149
Rachischisis, 35
Radiation
    auditory, 268
    optic, 77, 83, 276–277
        lesions in, 284
    thalamic, 76, 79, 332
        anterior, 117
Radiotherapy, teratogenic effects of, 34
Rage attacks, 328
Rami, 6
    communicating
        gray, 312
        white, 311
Rathke's pouch, 20
Receptors
    auditory, 263–266
    hair follicle, 170
    muscle, 185–186
    for neurotransmitters and modulators, 353
    olfactory, 288, 289
    for pain and temperature, 166
    photoreceptors, 272–274
    proprioceptive, 170
    for taste sensations, 243
    for touch and pressure, 170–171
    vestibular, 246–247
    warm-sensitive, in hypothalamus, 305
Recess
    infundibular, of third ventricle, 27, 68, 89
    lateral, of fourth ventricle, 27, 97
    optic, of third ventricle, 27, 68, 89
    pineal, of third ventricle, 27, 68, 89
Reflex(es)
    accommodation, in vision, 280
    Achilles or triceps surae, 158
    autonomic, hypothalamic control of, 304–305
    biceps, 158
    brachioradial, 158
    cardiovascular, 253
    corneal, 242–243
    coughing, 253
    crossed extensor, 158
    disynaptic, 187
    fixation, in vision, 280
    flexor withdrawal, 158

jaw, 242
light
    consensual or crossed, 280
    direct, 280
    pupillary, 241, 280
masseter, 242
middle-ear, 262
monosynaptic, 158, 187
myotatic, 158, 186
patellar, or quadriceps, 158, 159, 186–187
polysynaptic, 158
postural, 249
respiratory, 253
spinal, 158–159
stretch, 158, 186–187
swallowing, 253
triceps, 158
triceps surae, 158
vestibulo-ocular, 249
vomiting, 253
Regeneration of nerves, 148–149
Retardation, mental, 30–36
Reticular formation, 228–231
Reticulum, endoplasmic, 128
Retina, 272–276
    amacrine cells in, 272
    central artery and vein of, 21
    detachment of, 36
    development of, 21
    ganglion cells in, 272, 279
    horizontal cells in, 272
    neurons in, 272–274
        bipolar, 272
    photoreceptors in, 272, 273
    receptive fields in, 279
    topography of, 274
Retinopathy, hypertensive, 282
Retrograde cell reaction, 128, 143
Rexed's laminae, 157
Rhinencephalon, 327
Ribosomes, 128
Rinne test, 269–270
Rods and cones, 272, 277–278
Romberg's sign, 178
Roots, nerve, 6
    dorsal, of spinal nerves, 11, 152
    lumbar, compression of, 162
    sacral, compression of, 162
    ventral, of spinal nerves, 11, 152
Rostrum of corpus callosum, 29, 68, 112
Rotation, hair cell stimulation in, 247
Rubella, congenital, 34

Saccule, 246
Scala
    media, 263
    tympani, 262
    vestibuli, 262

Schizophrenia, dopamine hypothesis of, 209
Sciatica, 161–162
Sclera, 272
Sclerosis
    amyotrophic lateral, 162
    multiple, 148
Scotomas, 282
Seizures, 349–350
    uncinate, 293–294
Sensory pathways, ascending, 165–182
Sensory stimuli, responses to
    amgdala affecting, 324
    posterior parietal cortex in, 346
Septum pellucidum, 29, 68, 112, 120, 121, 122, 327
Serotonergic pathway, 231
    ascending, in hypothalamus, 303
Silver methods, in tract-tracing studies, 143
Sinus(es)
    cavernous, 38
    dural, 38–40
    petrosal
        inferior, 38–40
        superior, 38–40
    sagittal
        inferior, 38
        superior, 38
    sigmoid, 38
    straight, 38, 88, 120
    transverse, 38
Skin, innervation of, 153
Skull fractures, 44
Sleep and wakefulness, 230–231
Smell sense, 287–294
    tests of, 293
Somatostatin, 355
Somatotopic localization of motor neurons, 157, 184
Somatotopic organization
    in cerebellar cortex, 218
    in motor cortex, 189
    in somatosensory cortex, 175
    in spinothalamic tract, 167
Somnolence, 235
Sound
    intensity of, 262
        discrimination of, 269
    localization in space, 268, 279
    pitch of, 262
        discrimination of, 266, 268–269
Space
    extradural, 44
    perforated
        anterior, 62–63, 113, 291
        posterior, 61
    subarachnoid, 43, 53, 122
Spasticity, 194

Specificity
  space, 175
  stimulus, 176
Spina bifida, 35
Spinal cord
  connections with vestibular nuclei,
    248
  control by reticular formation, 230
  development of, 10–11
  disorders of, 162–163, 176, 177–
    178
    injuries of, 163
      autonomic dysfunction in, 319
  meninges of, 44
  relationship to vertebral column,
    152–154
Spines, dendritic, 132
Spinocerebellum, 215
Splenium of corpus callosum, 29, 68,
  115
Spot, blind, 274
Sprouting, collateral, in axons, 149,
  347
Stalk
  hemisphere, 27
  hypophysial, 61, 296
  optic, 21
Stapes, 262
Stereoanesthesia, 179
Steroid hormones, teratogenic effects
  of, 34
Strabismus, 240–241
Stria
  acoustic, dorsal, 266
  medullaris, 104, 114, 115, 116, 300
  terminalis, 112, 300, 322
Striatum, 29, 200
Stroke, 95, 358–359
  and transient ischemic attacks,
    362
Stupor, 235
Subiculum, 324
Substance P, 354
  and pain control, 180
Substantia
  gelatinosa, 155
    in gate control of pain, 169, 179
  innominata, 200–201
  nigra, 18, 107, 114, 116, 117, 122,
    201, 228
    pars compacta of, 201
    pars reticularis of, 201
Sulcus (Sulci), 6, 69–73
  calcarine, 71, 73, 119, 120
  central, 69
  hypothalamicus, 18, 296
  inferior frontal, 70
  inferior temporal, 70
  limitans, 10
  median, 104
  olfactory, 62
  parieto-occipital, 23, 69, 119

postcentral, 70
precentral, 70
superior frontal, 70
superior temporal, 70
Superior olivary complex, 266–269
Swallowing, 253
Synapses, 4, 137–141
  asymmetric, 138
  axoaxonic, 140
  axodendritic, 140
  axosomatic, 140
  chemical, 141
  classification of, 138–140
  dendrodendritic, in olfactory bulb,
    291
  electrical, 141
  reciprocal, in olfactory bulb, 291
  symmetric, 138
Synaptic gap, 137
Synaptic vesicle, 137–138
Syncope, 305, 358
Syringomyelia, 162–163, 177, 180–
  181
System. See also Pathway
  ascending activating, 230
  auditory, 261–270
  autonomic, 4, 309–319
  central nervous, 4
  cerebrovascular, 357–372
  hypophysial portal, 302
  limbic, 327
  olfactory, 287–294
  parasympathetic, 310, 312–314
    compared to sympathetic sys-
      tem, 310
  peripheral nervous, 4
  sympathetic, 310–312
    compared to parasympathetic
      system, 310
  vestibular, 242–249
  visual, 271–286

Tabes dorsalis, 163, 178
Tail of caudate nucleus, 91, 114, 115
Tanycytes, 141
Tardive dyskinesia, 209
Taste buds, 243
Taste pathways, 243–245
Tectum of mesencephalon, 65, 104,
  167, 228
  development of, 18
Tegmentum
  of mesencephalon, 18, 104–107
  of pons, 108
Tela choroidea, 27
  of third ventricle, 87–88
Telencephalon, 6–7, 61–63, 68
  development of, 21–30
Temperature
  pathways for, 166–169
  regulation of, 305
    disorders in, 306

Tendon organ, Golgi, 186
Tenia
  choroidea, 89
  thalami, 89
Tentorial notch, 38
Tentorium cerebelli, 38
Teratogenesis, 30–34
Terminals, axon, 4, 136
Tests
  of hearing, 269–270
  of sense of smell, 293
  of visual fields, 282
Tetanus toxin, spread to CNS, 149
Tetraplegia, 163, 195, 319
Thalamic syndrome, 334, 366–367
Thalamus, 7, 68, 86, 90–91, 113, 116,
  121, 331–334
  connections with cerebral cortex,
    332
  development of, 21
  lateral part of, 114, 115
  and motor system, 333–334
  nuclei of, 332
  in perception of pain and tempera-
    ture, 167–169
  relation to amygdala, 323
  topography of, 29–30
Thalidomide, teratogenic effect of, 34
Thermoreceptors, 166
Thiamine deficiency, and Korsakoff
  syndrome, 329, 349
Thrombosis, cerebral, 358–359
Thyrotropic-releasing hormone, 355
Tic douloureux, 243
Tinnitus, 269
Tomography
  computerized (CAT), 54, 95
  positron emission (PET), 376
Tone, muscle, 187
Tonotopic organization, in auditory
  pathway, 266, 268
Tonsil, cerebellar, 99, 123
Touch, pathways for, 170–173
Toxoplasmosis, maternal, affecting
  fetus, 34
Tracing methods. See Neuroana-
  tomic methods
Tract, 6
  bulbospinal, 192
  corticobulbar, 191, 228
  corticopontine, 108, 228
  corticospinal (pyramidal), 61, 108,
    116, 187–191, 192, 228
    cerebellar input to, 221
    course and termination of, 189–
      191
    lateral, 189, 226
    lesions of, 194
    origin of, 187–189
    ventral, 191
  cuneocerebellar, 217

Tract (cont.)
  gastrointestinal, autonomic inner-
    vation of, 315
  geniculocalcarine, 77, 276
  Lissauer, 159, 166
  mammillotegmental, 302
  mammillothalamic, 68, 114, 116,
    117, 302
  olfactory, 62, 291–292
  optic, 61, 114, 115, 117, 276
    lesions in, 284
  pontocerebellar, 108
  pontospinal, 192
  reticulospinal, 192, 193
    cerebellar input to, 221
  rubrospinal, 191, 192, 228
    cerebellar input to, 221
  solitary, nucleus of, 227, 245, 253
  spinal trigeminal, nucleus of, 167,
    227, 241
  spinocerebellar, 217–218
    dorsal, 217–218, 227
    ventral, 218, 227
  spinoreticular, 167
  spinotectal, 167
  spinothalamic, 107, 108, 166–169,
    173, 227, 228
  supraopticohypophysial, 300, 304
  tectospinal, 227
  trigeminothalamic, 175
  tuberoinfundibular, 302, 304
  vestibulospinal, 191–192, 193
    cerebellar input to, 221
    lateral, 191, 248
    medial, 192, 249
Transplantations of brain, 149
Transport, axonal, 136
Trauma
  of head, 44
  of spinal cord, 163
    autonomic dysfunction in, 319
Tremor
  cerebellar or intention, 222
  pill-rolling, in Parkinson's disease,
    208
Trigone
  hypoglossal, 104
  vagal, 104
Trunks, nerve, 6
Tube
  eustachian, 262
  neural, 10
    failure in closure of, 35
Tuber cinereum, 61, 68, 296

Tubercle
  cuneate, 110, 116
  gracile, 110, 116
  olfactory, 291
Tumors
  cerebellar, 223
  cerebellopontine angle, 64, 257–
    258
  craniopharyngioma, 36
  medulloblastoma, 104
  olfactory groove meningioma, 294
  pituitary, 68, 305, 307
  of spine, 163
  temporal lobe, 328

Uncinate seizure, 293–294
Unconsciousness, in uncal hernia-
  tion, 45
Uncus, 73
Utricle, 246
Uvula, 99

Vascular disorders
  cerebrovascular, 359–367
  of spinal cord, 163
Vasopressin, 304, 355
Vein
  central, of retina, 21
  choroid, 88
  of Galen, 38, 88, 120
  hypophysial portal, 304
  internal cerebral, 38, 88
  septal, 88
  thalamostriate, 88
Velum
  interpositum, 87
  medullary
    anterior or superior, 65, 97
    posterior or inferior, 65, 97
Ventral pallidum, 201
Ventral striatum, 113, 117, 200
Ventral tegmental area, 201
Ventricles of brain
  development of, 27
  fourth, 7, 65, 97, 123
    development of, 27
  lateral, 6, 85–86
    anterior horn of, 86, 120, 121,
      122
    central part of, 86
    development of, 27
    posterior horn of, 86
    temporal horn of, 86

third, 7, 68, 88–89, 121, 122
    anterior wall of, 89
    development of, 2, 21, 27
    floor of, 89
    lateral wall of, 89
    posterior wall of, 89
    tela choroidea of, 87–88
Vermis of cerebellum, 7, 15, 61, 97–
  99, 122, 123
Vertebral column, relationship to
  spinal cord, 152–154
Vertigo, 249
Vesicles
  brain, primary and secondary, 11
  coated, 138
  olfactory, 288
  optic, 21
  synaptic, 137–138
    agranular, 137
    granular, 137
    recycling of membrane in, 138
Vestibular system, 222–249
  cerebellum related to, 222
Vestibulocerebellum, 214–215, 218
Vibration, 170
  pathway for, 173
Villi, arachnoid, 44
Viruses, spread to CNS, 149
Visceroceptors, 166
Vision
  brain mechanisms in, 278–280
  disorders of, 280–285
  occipital lobe role in, 346
Visual system, 271–286
Vitamin B_1 deficiency, and Korsakoff syndrome, 329, 349
Vitamin B_{12} deficiency, dorsal col-
  umn lesions in, 178, 181
Vomiting, 253

Wallenberg's lateral medullary syn-
  drome, 194, 257, 364
Wallerian degeneration, 143
Walls of third ventricle, 89
Weber's mediobasal mesencephalic
  syndrome, 255, 366
Wernicke's aphasia, 350
Wernicke-Korsakoff's syndrome,
  329, 349
White matter
  of brain, 3, 4–6
    fiber systems of, 75–82
  of spinal cord, 3, 4–6, 152, 159–
    161